T0348811

Emerging and Re-Emerging Infectious Diseases

Editors

ALIMUDDIN ZUMLA
DAVID S.C. HUI

INFECTIOUS DISEASE CLINICS
OF NORTH AMERICA

www.id.theclinics.com

Consulting Editor
HELEN W. BOUCHER

December 2019 • Volume 33 • Number 4

ELSEVIER

1600 John F. Kennedy Boulevard • Suite 1800 • Philadelphia, Pennsylvania, 19103-2899.
http://www.theclinics.com

INFECTIOUS DISEASE CLINICS OF NORTH AMERICA Volume 33, Number 4
December 2019 ISSN 0891-5520, ISBN-13: 978-0-323-70845-6

Editor: Kerry Holland
Developmental Editor: Donald Mumford

Infectious Disease Clinics of North America (ISSN 0891-5520) is published in March, June, September, and December by Elsevier Inc., 360 Park Avenue South, New York, NY 10010-1710. Periodicals postage paid at New York, NY and additional mailing offices. Subscription prices are $330.00 per year for US individuals, $660.00 per year for US institutions, $100.00 per year for US students, $396.00 per year for Canadian individuals, $824.00 per year for Canadian institutions, $432.00 per year for international individuals, $824.00 per year for international institutions, and $200.00 per year for Canadian and international students. To receive student rate, orders must be accompanied by name of affiliated institution, date of term, and the *signature* of program/residency coordinator on institution letterhead. Orders will be billed at individual rate until proof of status is received. Foreign air speed delivery is included in all *Clinics* subscription prices. All prices are subject to change without notice. **POSTMASTER**: Send address changes to *Infectious Disease Clinics of North America*, Elsevier Health Sciences Division, Subcription Customer Service, 3251 Riverport Lane, Maryland Heights, MO 63043. **Customer Service: 1-800-654-2452 (US). From outside of the US and Canada, call 1-314-447-8871. Fax: 1-314-447-8029. E-mail: JournalsCustomerService-usa@elsevier.com (print support) or JournalsOnlineSupport-usa@elsevier.com (online support).**

Infectious Disease Clinics of North America is also published in Spanish by Editorial Inter-Médica, Junin 917, 1er A 1113, Buenos Aires, Argentina.

Reprints. For copies of 100 or more, of articles in this publication, please contact the Commercial Reprints Department, Elsevier Inc., 360 Park Avenue South, New York, New York 10010-1710. Tel. 212-633-3874, Fax: 212-633-3820, E-mail: reprints@elsevier.com.

Infectious Disease Clinics of North America is covered in *MEDLINE/PubMed (Index Medicus), Current Contents/Clinical Medicine, Science Citation Alert, SCISEARCH,* and *Research Alert.*

Contributors

CONSULTING EDITOR

HELEN W. BOUCHER, MD, FIDSA, FACP
Director, Infectious Diseases Fellowship Program, Division of Geographic Medicine and Infectious Diseases, Tufts Medical Center, Associate Professor of Medicine, Tufts University School of Medicine, Boston, Massachusetts, USA

EDITORS

ALIMUDDIN ZUMLA, MBChB, MSc, PhD, MD, FRCP(Lond), FRCP(Edin), FRCPath(UK), FAAS
Sir Professor, Division of Infection and Immunity, Center for Clinical Microbiology, University College London, Consultant in Infectious Diseases and Senior Investigator, NIHR Biomedical Research Center, University College London Hospitals, London, United Kingdom

DAVID S.C. HUI, MBBS, MD(UNSW), FRACP, FRCP(Lond, Edin, Glasg), FHKCP, FHKAM(Med)
Chairman & Stanley Ho Professor of Respiratory Medicine, Department of Medicine and Therapeutics, Director of Stanley Ho Center for Emerging Infectious Diseases, The Chinese University of Hong Kong, Prince of Wales Hospital, Shatin, New Territories, Hong Kong

AUTHORS

GEORGE O. AKPEDE, MBBS, FWACP, FCMPaed
Professor, Department of Paediatrics, Faculty of Clinical Sciences, College of Medicine, Ambrose Alli University, Ekpoma, Nigeria

RASHID ANSUNAMA, PhD
Mercy Hospital Research Laboratory, School of Community Health Sciences, Njala University, Bo Campus, Bo, Sierra Leone, West Africa

DANNY ASOGUN, MBBS, FWACP
Professor, Department of Public Health, College of Medicine, Ambrose Alli University, Ekpoma, Nigeria; Department of Public Health, Institute of Lassa Fever Research and Control, Irrua Specialist Teaching Hospital, Irrua, Nigeria

ESAM I. AZHAR, PhD, FRCP
Special Infectious Agents Unit, King Fahd Medical Research Centre, Faculty of Applied Medical Sciences, King Abdulaziz University, Jeddah, Saudi Arabia

ANTONINO DI CARO, MD
National Institute for Infectious Diseases, Lazzaro Spallanzani, IRCCS, Rome, Italy

CHRISTIAN DROSTEN, PhD
Institute of Virology, Campus Charité Mitte, Charité - Universitätsmedizin Berlin, Berlin Institute of Health, Berlin, Germany

DEIRDRE FITZGERALD, MBBS
Department of Respiratory Medicine, Sir Charles Gardiner Hospital, Nedlands, Perth, Australia

STEPHAN GÜNTHER, MD
Professor, Bernhard-Nocht Institute for Tropical Medicine, German Centre for Infection Research (DZIF), Hamburg, Germany

NAJMUL HAIDER, Vet PhD
The Royal Veterinary College, University of London, Hatfield, Hertfordshire, United Kingdom

RUMINA HASAN, MBBS, PhD
Department of Pathology and Laboratory Medicine, Aga Khan University, Karachi, Pakistan; Faculty of Infectious and Tropical Disease, London School of Hygiene and Tropical Medicine, London, United Kingdom

JEFFERY HO, PhD
Postdoctoral Fellow, Department of Microbiology, Faculty of Medicine, The Chinese University of Hong Kong, Shatin, Hong Kong

DAVID S.C. HUI, MBBS, MD(UNSW), FRACP, FRCP(Lond, Edin, Glasg), FHKCP, FHKAM(Med)
Chairman & Stanley Ho Professor of Respiratory Medicine, Department of Medicine and Therapeutics, Director of Stanley Ho Center for Emerging Infectious Diseases, The Chinese University of Hong Kong, Prince of Wales Hospital, Shatin, New Territories, Hong Kong

MARCO IANNETTA, MD, PhD
National Institute for Infectious Diseases, Lazzaro Spallanzani, IRCCS, Rome, Italy

CHIKWE IHEKWEAZU, MBBS, MPH, FFPH
Director-General, Nigeria Centre for Disease Control, Abuja, Nigeria

MARGARET IP, MD
Professor, Department of Microbiology, Faculty of Medicine, The Chinese University of Hong Kong, Honorary Consultant, Department of Microbiology, Prince of Wales Hospital, Shatin, Hong Kong

GIUSEPPE IPPOLITO, MD, MSc, FRCP, FRCPath
National Institute for Infectious Diseases, "Lazzaro Spallanzani" Istituto di ricovero e cura a carattere scientifico - IRCCS, Rome, Italy

MICHAEL G. ISON, MD, MS
Professor, Divisions of Infectious Diseases and Organ Transplantation, Northwestern University Feinberg School of Medicine, Chicago, Illinois, USA

ANU KANTELE, MD, PhD
Professor, Inflammation Center, Helsinki University Hospital and Helsinki University, Helsinki, Finland

GARY KOBINGER, PhD, MD
Centre de Recherche en Infectiologie, Centre Hospitalier Universitaire de Québec, Université Laval, Québec, Québec, Canada

RICHARD KOCK, MA, VetMB, Vet MD, MRCVS
The Royal Veterinary College, University of London, Hatfield, Hertfordshire, United Kingdom

MARION KOOPMANS, DVM, PhD
Professor, Viroscience Department, Erasmus Medical Centre, Rotterdam, the Netherlands

REBECCA KUMAR, MD
Division of Infectious Diseases, Northwestern University Feinberg School of Medicine, Chicago, Illinois, USA

SIMONE LANINI, MD, MSc
National Institute for Infectious Diseases, Lazzaro Spallanzani, Rome, Italy

HONORATI MASANJA, PhD
Ifakara Health Institute, Ifakara Health Research and Development Centre, Dar es Salaam, Tanzania

LEONARD E.G. MBOERA, PhD, BVM
SACIDS Foundation for One Health, Sokoine University of Agriculture, Morogoro, Tanzania

ZIAD A. MEMISH, MD, FRCP
College of Medicine, Alfaisal University, Infectious Diseases Division, Department of Medicine and Research, Prince Mohamed Bin Abdulaziz Hospital, Ministry of Health, Riyadh, Saudi Arabia

GIOVANNI BATTISTA MIGLIORI, FRCP, FERS
Istituti Clinici Scientifici Maugeri IRCCS, Tradate, Italy

ALI MIRAZIMI, MD, PhD
Division of Clinical Microbiology, Department of Laboratory Medicine, Karolinska Institutet, Stockholm, Sweden

CHIARA MONTALDO, MD
National Institute for Infectious Diseases, Lazzaro Spallanzani, IRCCS, Rome, Italy

EMANUELE NICASTRI, MD, PhD
National Institute for Infectious Diseases, Lazzaro Spallanzani, IRCCS, Rome, Italy

FRANCINE NTOUMI, PhD, FRCP
Fondation Congolaise pour la Recherche Médicale (FCRM), Faculty of Sciences and Techniques, University Marien Ngouabi, Brazzaville, Congo; Institute for Tropical Medicine, University of Tübingen, Tübingen, Germany

MALIK PEIRIS, MBBS, DPhil, FRCPath
Professor of Virology, School of Public Health, The University of Hong Kong, Pokfulam, Hong Kong

ESKILD PETERSEN, MD, DMSc, DTMH
Professor, Institute of Clinical Medicine, University of Aarhus, Aarhus N, Denmark; The Royal Hospital, Muscat, Oman; European Society for Clinical Microbiology and Infectious Diseases, Task Force for Emerging Infections, Basel, Switzerland

RAFFAELLA PISAPIA, MD
National Institute for Infectious Diseases, Lazzaro Spallanzani, Rome, Italy

JAMES A. PLATTS-MILLS, MD
Division of Infectious Diseases and International Health, University of Virginia, Charlottesville, Virginia, USA

SADIA SHAKOOR, MBBS
Pathology and Laboratory Medicine, Pediatrics and Child Health, Aga Khan University, Karachi, Pakistan

SIMON TIBERI, MD, FRCP
Department of Infection, Royal London Hospital, Blizard Institute, Barts and The London School of Medicine and Dentistry, Queen Mary, Barts Health NHS Trust, London, United Kingdom

ANDREW USTIANOWSKI, MD, PhD, FRCP
North Manchester General Hospital, Manchester, United Kingdom

TIMOTHY M. UYEKI, MD, MPH, MPP
Chief Medical Officer, Influenza Division, National Center for Immunization and Respiratory Diseases, Centers for Disease Control and Prevention, Atlanta, Georgia, USA

FRANCESCO VAIRO, MD
National Institute for Infectious Diseases, "Lazzaro Spallanzani" Istituto di ricovero e cura a carattere scientifico - IRCCS, Rome, Italy

GRANT W. WATERER, MBBS, PhD
University of Western Australia, Royal Perth Hospital, Perth, Australia

ADESOLA YINKA-OGUNLEYE, BDS, MPH
Nigeria Centre for Disease Control, Abuja, Nigeria

ALIMUDDIN ZUMLA, MBChB, MSc, PhD, MD, FRCP(Lond), FRCP(Edin), FRCPath(UK), FAAS
Sir Professor, Division of Infection and Immunity, Center for Clinical Microbiology, University College London, Consultant in Infectious Diseases and Senior Investigator, NIHR Biomedical Research Center, University College London Hospitals, London, United Kingdom

Contents

Severe acute respiratory syndrome coronavirus (SARS-CoV), emerged from China and rapidly spread worldwide. Over 8098 people fell ill and 774 died before the epidemic ended in July 2003. Bats are likely an important reservoir for SARS-CoV. SARS-like CoVs have been detected in horseshoe bats and civet cats. The main mode of transmission of SARS-CoV is through inhalation of respiratory droplets. Faeco-oral transmission has been recorded. Strict infection control procedures with respiratory and contact precautions are essential. Fever and respiratory symptoms predominate, and diarrhea is common. Treatment involves supportive care. There are no specific antiviral treatments or vaccines available.

The Middle East respiratory syndrome (MERS) is a novel lethal zoonotic disease of humans caused by the MERS coronavirus (MERS-CoV). Although MERS is endemic to the Middle East, travelers have exported MERS-CoV on return to their home countries. Clinical manifestations range from mild to severe acute respiratory disease and death. The elderly, immunocompromised, and those with chronic comorbid liver, lung, and hepatic conditions have a high mortality rate. There is no specific treatment. Person-to-person spread causes hospital and household outbreaks, and thus improved compliance with internationally recommended infection control protocols and rapid implementation of infection control measures are required.

A high index of suspicion and early diagnosis of avian influenza A virus infection is essential reduce transmission risk. Clinical suspicion relies on eliciting a history of recent exposure to poultry or to sick persons. Diagnosis requires collection of appropriate respiratory specimens. Patients with suspected infection should be isolated immediately and patients with lower respiratory tract disease should be placed on airborne precautions if possible. Antiviral treatment should be started as soon as possible based upon clinical suspicion while awaiting specific viral diagnosis. Corticosteroids and salicylates should be avoided. Clinical management focuses on supportive care of complications.

Chikungunya, a zoonotic disease caused by the Chikungunya virus (CHIKV), is transmitted by infected Aedes spp mosquitoes. CHIKV has now spread to more than 100 countries and is listed on the WHO Blueprint priority pathogens. After an incubation period of 1 to 12 days, symptoms similar to other febrile infections appear, with a sudden onset of high fever, nausea, polyarthralgia, myalgia, widespread skin rash, and conjunctivitis. Serious complications include myocarditis, uveitis, retinitis, hepatitis, acute renal disease, severe bullous lesions, meningoencephalitis, Guillain-Barré syndrome, myelitis, and cranial nerve palsies. Treatment is supportive; there is no specific antiviral treatment and no effective vaccine.

Recently, concern has been raised about the emergence of human monkeypox virus and the occasionally severe clinical presentation bearing resemblance to that of smallpox. In 2018, 3 patients in the UK were diagnosed with monkeypox, and the frequency and geographic distribution of cases across West and Central Africa have increased in recent years. In Nigeria, most monkeypox patients are aged <40 years and lack cross-protective immunity because they were born after discontinuation of the smallpox eradication campaign. This article reviews the epidemiology, clinical features, and management of monkeypox and discusses its growing public health threat in this context.

Viral hepatitis is a major global public health problem affecting hundreds of millions of people and is associated with significant morbidity and mortality. Five major biologically unrelated hepatotropic viruses cause most of the global burden of viral hepatitis. Hepatitis B and hepatitis C are associated with a significant number of chronic infections. Most deaths from viral hepatitis are due to hepatitis B and hepatitis C. An estimated 257 million people were living with HBV and 71 million people were living with HCV. Most people are asymptomatic. New diagnostics and highly effective, pangenotypic direct-acting antivirals provide opportunities to cure and eradicate chronic hepatitis C virus infection.

Multidrug-resistant tuberculosis (MDR-TB) is a growing global public health threat. MDR-TB affects more than a half-million people worldwide and is characterized by significant morbidity and mortality. New rapid diagnostic methods like GeneXpert and availability of new MDR-TB drugs and shorter treatment regimens hold promise of more patients diagnosed and put on treatment. Major challenges of lack of adequate resources, poverty, and limited access to health care continue to hamper efforts. This article reviews epidemiology, clinical features, management, and treatment, with new updates and recent changes in guidelines that offer patients better tolerated and shorter regimens for enabling therapeutic outcomes.

Antimicrobial resistance is a global concern, and prudent use of antibiotics is essential to preserve the current armamentarium of effective drugs. Acute respiratory tract infection is the most common reason for antibiotic prescription in adults. In particular, community-acquired pneumonia poses a significant health challenge and economic burden globally, especially in the current landscape of a dense and aging population. By updating the knowledge on the common antimicrobial-resistant pathogens in community-acquired respiratory tract infections, their prevalence, and resistance may pave the way to enhancing appropriate antibiotic use in the ambulatory and health care setting.

Rising rates of antimicrobial resistance (AMR) in enteric infections are now observed across the globe in low-income and middle-income as well as high-income settings owing to global travel and overlapping social drivers. Pathogen-specific risk factors for spread are now also associated with specific AMR phenotypes and profiles. Several of the drivers of AMR intersect with risk factors for enteric infections and are preventable. Concerted focus on OneHealth prevention strategies for enteric infections and AMR are likely to be of significant benefit in optimizing public health outcomes.

This review focuses on current knowledge of the epidemiology, prevention, and treatment of invasive pneumococcal (IPD) and meningococcal disease (IMD). IPD decreased significantly with the introduction of effective conjugate vaccines but is on the rise again. Effective antibiotic therapy of IPD includes the combination of a beta-lactam and a macrolide with additional considerations in meningitis. Steroids are mandatory in pneumococcal meningitis but not indicated in pneumococcal pneumonia except in the setting of refractory shock. There is increasing concern about the cardiovascular complications of IPD. IMD continues to be a significant health problem with major concerns about rising antibiotic resistance.

Rebecca Kumar and Michael G. Ison

Transplants have become common with excellent patient and graft outcomes owing to advances in surgical technique, immunosuppression, and antimicrobial prophylaxis. In 2017, 34,770 solid organ transplants were performed in the United States. For solid organ transplant recipients, infection remains a common complication owing to the regimens required to prevent rejection. Opportunistic infections, which are infections that are generally of lower virulence within a healthy host but cause more severe and frequent disease in immunosuppressed individuals, typically occur in the period 1 month to 1 year after transplantation. This article focuses on opportunistic infections in the solid organ transplant recipient.

INFECTIOUS DISEASE CLINICS OF NORTH AMERICA

THE CLINICS ARE AVAILABLE ONLINE!
Access your subscription at:
www.theclinics.com

Preface

Emerging and Reemerging Infectious Diseases: Global Overview

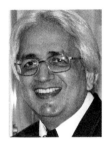

Alimuddin Zumla, MBChB,
MSc, PhD, MD, FRCP(Lond),
FRCP(Edin), FRCPath(UK),
FAAS

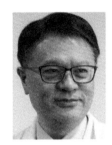

David S.C. Hui, MBBS, MD(UNSW),
FRACP, FRCP(Lond, Edin, Glasg),
FHKCP, FHKAM(Med)

Editors

BACKGROUND

New emerging and reemerging infectious disease outbreaks have continued to cause much human suffering and loss of life worldwide. During the past 2 decades, several landmark events in the field of infectious diseases with epidemic potential have occurred. The SARS (severe acute respiratory syndrome) pandemic (2002–2004), the Ebola virus disease (EVD) outbreak in West Africa (2013–2016), the cholera outbreak in Yemen (2015–2018), the Zika virus in the Americas and southeast Asia (2016–2018), Lassa fever (LF) in Nigeria (2018), diphtheria in Venezuela (2016-2017) and in Yemen (2017-2018), Yellow fever in Latin America and Africa (2016–2018), and Nipah virus in India and South Asia (2017–2018). The global media and World Health Organization (WHO) attention on Zika virus transmission at the 2016 Rio Olympic Games and the 2015 Ebola virus outbreak in West Africa had diverted the attention of global public health authorities from other lethal infectious diseases with epidemic potential. More recently, there has been growing concern of the increasing threat to global health security posed by a range of reemerging and emerging infectious diseases (**Box 1**) and the globalization of antibiotic-resistant bacterial infections.[1]

INTRODUCTION TO *INFECTIOUS DISEASE CLINICS OF NORTH AMERICA* SERIES ARTICLES
Novel Coronavirus Infections of Humans

Two new lethal zoonotic coronaviruses of humans with epidemic potential have emerged in the past 17 years. A novel β coronavirus, severe acute respiratory

Infect Dis Clin N Am 33 (2019) xiii–xix
https://doi.org/10.1016/j.idc.2019.09.001
0891-5520/19/© 2019 Published by Elsevier Inc.

id.theclinics.com

Box 1
List of priority infectious diseases that threaten global health security

Viral infections
- Middle East respiratory syndrome[a]
- Severe acute respiratory syndrome[a]
- Pandemic influenza
- Marburg[a]
- Ebola[a]
- Lassa fever[a]
- Viral hemorrhagic fevers (including Crimean-Congo hemorrhagic fever[a])
- Rift Valley fever[a]
- West Nile fever
- Dengue
- Polio (wild-type polio virus)
- Zika[a]
- Nipah and henipavirus diseases[a]
- Chikungunya[a]
- Measles
- Yellow fever
- Viral hepatitis

Bacterial infections
- Tuberculosis[a]
- Invasive meningococcal disease
- Invasive pneumococcal disease
- Drug-resistant bacterial, viral, and protozoal infections
- Cholera
- Typhoid
- Diphtheria
- Pertussis (whooping cough)

Other
- Drug-resistant malaria
- Antiretroviral-resistant human immunodeficiency virus/AIDS

  [a] WHO Blueprint priority disease.

---

syndrome coronavirus emerged in November 2002 as a lethal zoonotic human pathogen in China and rapidly spread worldwide, disappearing in 2004, never to be seen again.[2] The Middle East Respiratory Syndrome coronavirus (MERS-CoV)[3] was first identified in 2012 in a lung sample of a 60-year-old patient who had died of respiratory and multiorgan failure in Jeddah, Saudi Arabia. Since then, MERS-CoV has remained on the radar of global public health authorities because of recurrent nosocomial and community outbreaks, and its association with severe disease and high mortalities. From June 1 to July 31, 2015, MERS-CoV caused the largest outbreak outside of the Arabian Peninsula, occurring in the Republic of Korea and resulting in 186 confirmed MERS cases with 38 deaths. This occurred when a Korean traveler returning from a trip to Qatar, UAE, Saudi Arabia, and Bahrain became ill with a respiratory illness and visited several hospitals in Seoul before finally being diagnosed as having MERS-CoV infection. This outbreak clearly illustrated the epidemic potential of MERS-CoV, spreading from person to person. MERS-CoV continues to circulate in the Middle East and causes intermittent community and hospital outbreaks. As of July 2019, 2458 cases of laboratory-confirmed MERS-CoV cases (848 deaths, 34% mortality) were reported to the WHO.

Influenza Viruses

Human infections due to highly pathogenic avian influenza A(H5N1) were initially detected in Hong Kong in 1997 before spreading to other continents, with a case fatality rate close to 60%. Influenza A(H1N1)pdm09 virus emerged and led to a pandemic in 2009 and has remained a common circulating strain. Human infections with the novel avian influenza A(H7N9) virus emerged in China in March 2013, whereas sporadic human cases of avian A(H5N6), A(H10N8) and A(H6N1) have been increasingly detected since 1997.[4] An outbreak of a novel H7N9 virus caused zoonotic disease in eastern China in the early spring of 2013. Six epidemics of human cases of H7N9 virus infection with 1564 laboratory-confirmed cases and 612 deaths occurred in China through September 2017, typically during the fall, winter, and spring months, including a large fifth epidemic during 2016 to 2017. As of May 2019, 1568 laboratory-confirmed H7N9 virus infections acquired in China had occurred since 2013. At least 10 human cases of infection with avian influenza A viruses acquired in China have traveled overseas and were diagnosed elsewhere.

Zoonotic Viral Infections

EVD has focused global media attention ever since its first discovery due to its lethal nature and outbreak potential.[5] The first human case of EVD was described in 1976 near the Ebola River in the Democratic Republic of Congo (DRC), and the first outbreak of EVD affected 284 people, with a mortality of 53%. This was followed a few months later by the second outbreak of EVD in Yambuku, Zaire (now DRC). Until 2013, EVD outbreaks consisted of small numbers of cases that were contained by basic public health and containment measures. The largest EVD epidemic occurred in West Africa between 2013 and 2016, and detection of EVD cases in the United Kingdom, Sardinia, Spain, and the United States focused global attention on the epidemic. There is an ongoing EVD epidemic in the DRC. The first human case of LF was discovered in 1969 in Nigeria. Fifty years after its first discovery, LF outbreaks continue in West Africa. Annually, an estimated 300,000 to 500,000 cases of LF occur in West Africa with up to 5 to 10,000 deaths.[6] Travel-associated LF cases outside of West Africa have been recorded in the United States, Canada, United Kingdom, Netherlands, Israel, Sweden, and Germany.

Viral hemorrhagic fever can be caused by zoonotic viruses other than Ebola and LF viruses.[7] Viral hemorrhagic fevers represent a group of diseases caused by enveloped single-stranded RNA viruses belonging to 6 taxonomic families: Filoviruses (Ebola and Marburg); Arenaviruses (Lassa and other Old World arenaviruses and New World arenaviruses); Hantaviruses, Nairoviruses, and Phenuiviruses (Congo-Crimean hemorrhagic fever, Rift Valley fever, Huaiyangshan virus, and Hantavirus); and Flaviviruses (Dengue, Yellow fever, Omsk hemorrhagic fever, Kyasanur Forest disease, and Alkhumra viruses). Chikungunya (CHIK) was first described in 1952 in southern Tanzania.[8] It is a disabling and debilitating zoonotic disease of humans caused by the Chikungunya virus (CHIKV), which is transmitted by infected *Aedes* spp mosquitoes, which sustain sylvatic and human rural and urban CHIK cycles. The past 5 years has witnessed an alarming global increase and spread of CHIKV to more than 100 countries across Asia, Europe, Africa, and the Americas. The virus is maintained in a complex sylvatic and rural cycle, progressing to an urban cycle every 5 to 20 years, causing global pandemics. Recently, the Indian Ocean and Indian epidemic CHIKV strains have emerged independently from the mainland of East Africa. This Indian Ocean Lineage caused repeated outbreaks from 2005 to 2014.

Previously thought to be rare and self-limiting diseases, monkeypox has not attracted much attention since its discovery 70 years ago.[9] More recently, monkeypox is being recognized as an increasing public health threat, particularly in regions in West Africa, where there is close interaction between humans and wild animal reservoirs. Global concern has been raised about its emergence as well as the resemblance of its clinical presentation to that of smallpox, a deadly disease globally eradicated by vaccination 40 years ago. During outbreaks, it has been challenging to clinically distinguish monkeypox from chickenpox, an unrelated herpesvirus infection. Outbreaks of buffalopox have occurred with multiple human cases in India. Similarly, during outbreaks of vaccinia virus infection in cattle in Brazil, there is documented evidence of human infections.

Viral Hepatitis

Viral hepatitis affects hundreds of millions of people worldwide.[10] Five biologically unrelated hepatotropic viruses cause most of the global burden of viral hepatitis: hepatitis A virus, hepatitis B virus (HBV), hepatitis C viruses (HCV), hepatitis D (delta) virus (HDV), and hepatitis E viruses (HEV). A large proportion of deaths from viral hepatitis is due to hepatitis B and hepatitis C. Globally, an estimated 257 million people were living with HBV and 71 million people were living with HCV. In 2017, 1.4 million people died of the consequences of viral hepatitis infection, and 90% of this burden was due to cirrhosis and hepatocellular carcinoma, which are consequences of chronic hepatitis B and chronic hepatitis C. HBV, HCV, HDV, and occasionally HEV, can also produce chronic infection.

Antibiotic-Resistant Bacterial Infections

The global spread of antibiotic-resistant pathogens now threatens global health security and is a priority global public health issue. Multidrug-resistant tuberculosis (MDR-TB) affects more than half a million people worldwide, causing significant morbidity and mortality. In 2018, there were an estimated 558,000 new MDR-TB cases globally, and only a fraction of them were diagnosed. Of concern is that the number of MDR-TB cases continues to increase every year. Recent advances in rapid point-of-care diagnostics and introduction of all oral and shorter treatment regimens provide hope for improving treatment outcomes.[11]

Streptococcus pneumoniae, *Mycoplasma pneumoniae*, *Staphylococcus aureus*, *Legionella pneumophila*, and Enterobacteriaceae are common pathogens causing community-acquired pneumonia (CAP) globally. *Klebsiella pneumoniae*, *Burkholderia pseudomallei*, and *Acinetobacter baumanii* are also important causes of CAP in the Asia Pacific regions. The prevalence of antimicrobial resistance in *S pneumoniae* and *M pneumoniae* has been documented over the years, impacting the need for more prudent use of antibiotics. Antimicrobial resistance associated with the common bacterial infections causing CAP and the known mechanisms of resistance are reviewed by Margaret and Jeffery.[12]

Enteric infectious diseases cause an estimated 1.7 million deaths annually, the highest burden being borne by developing countries. Antibiotic-resistant bacterial enteric infections[13] have been reported from across the world due to travel and a convergence of multiple risk factors, including mass gathering events, conflict zones, and displaced populations.

Despite dramatic advances in the prevention of pneumococcal and meningococcal disease worldwide, case fatality rates remain static, and vaccination programs struggle to keep up with the bacterium's ability to adapt and spread.[14] Preventing further resistance by improving antimicrobial stewardship is essential. Future developments are focused on the development of universal vaccines and improved diagnostic tools rather than novel anti-infectives.

Opportunistic Infections in Transplant Recipients

Organ transplants are routinely performed worldwide. Worldwide, more than 120,000 estimated solid organ transplants are performed, with kidney, liver, heart, and lung being the top four. Despite proactive implementation of prevention and management guidelines by organ transplantation units, the threat of opportunistic known and novel infections is ever present. Advances in molecular microbiology are enabling diagnosis of an increasing number of donor and community-acquired pathogens in transplant recipients.[15]

SUMMARY

This issue of *Infectious Disease Clinics of North America* on "Emerging and Reemerging Infectious Diseases" illustrates the constant threat of a range of pathogens that can present to the physician worldwide in a variety of clinical settings. It is imperative that clinicians and other health care workers worldwide have a high degree of awareness of the possibility of an infection with pathogens with outbreak potential or antibiotic resistance. This series of up-to-date articles, written by authoritative and renowned experts in their specialist areas, is aimed at a global readership of health care practitioners, infectious disease and tropical medicine internal medicine trainees, pulmonologists, microbiologists, family physicians, and public health practitioners in both western and developing countries.

ACKNOWLEDGMENTS

Sir Prof Alimuddin Zumla is a member of the Pan-African Network for Rapid Research, Response, Relief, and Preparedness for Infectious Diseases Epidemics (PANDORA-ID-NET) Consortium funded by European and Developing Countries Clinical Trials Partnership (EDCTP) Reg/Grant RIA2016E-1609 from the EDCTP2 program, which is supported under Horizon 2020, the European Union's Framework Programme for Research and Innovation. Sir Zumla is in receipt of a National Institutes of Health Research Senior Investigator award.

We are grateful to all contributors to this excellent and comprehensive issue on emerging and reemerging infectious diseases. Our sincere thanks to Helen Boucher

(Editor-in-Chief), Kerry Holland, and Donald Mumford (Elsevier) for their due diligence and kind assistance throughout the development of this issue.

Alimuddin Zumla, MBChB, MSc, PhD, MD, FRCP(Lond), FRCP(Edin), FRCPath(UK), FAAS
Center for Clinical Microbiology
University College London
Royal Free Campus 2nd Floor, Rowland Hill Street
London NW3 2PF, United Kingdom

David S.C. Hui, MBBS, MD(UNSW), FRACP, FRCP(Lond, Edin, Glasg), FHKCP, FHKAM(Med)
Department of Medicine and Therapeutics
Clinical Science Building, Prince of Wales Hospital
30-32 Ngan Shing Street, Shatin, NT, Hong Kong

E-mail addresses:
a.zumla@ucl.ac.uk (A. Zumla)
dschui@cuhk.edu.hk (D.S.C. Hui)

REFERENCES

1. WHO. List of blueprint priority diseases. 2018 annual review. 2019. Available at: https://www.who.int/blueprint/priority-diseases/en/. Accessed August 16, 2019.
2. Hui DS, Zumla A. Severe acute respiratory syndrome (SARS)–historical, epidemiological, and clinical features. Infect Dis Clin North Am 2019;33(4):869–89.
3. Azhar EI, Hui DS, Memish ZA, et al. The Middle East respiratory syndrome (MERS). Infect Dis Clin North Am 2019;33(4):891–905.
4. Uyeki TM, Peiris M. Novel avian influenza A virus infections of humans. Infect Dis Clin North Am 2019;33(4):907–32.
5. Nicastri, Kobinger G, Mboera L, et al. Ebola virus disease (EVD): epidemiology, clinical features, management and prevention. Infect Dis Clin North Am 2019; 33(4):953–76.
6. Asogun D, Gunthner S, Akpede G, et al. Lassa fever–epidemiology, clinical features, diagnosis, management and prevention. Infect Dis Clin North Am 2019; 33(4):933–51.
7. Iannetta M, Di Caro A, Nicastri E, et al. Viral hemorrhagic fevers other than Ebola and Lassa. Infect Dis Clin North Am 2019;33(4):977–1002.
8. Vairo F, Haider N, Kock R, et al. Chikungunya–epidemiology, pathogenesis, clinical features, management and prevention. Infect Dis Clin North Am 2019;33(4): 1003–25.
9. Petersen E, Kantele A, Koopmans M, et al. Human monkeypox–epidemiological and clinical characteristics, diagnosis and prevention. Infect Dis Clin North Am 2019;33(4):1027–43.
10. Lanini S, Ustianowski A, Pisapia R, et al. Viral hepatitis: aetiology, epidemiology, transmission, diagnostics, treatment and prevention. Infect Dis Clin North Am 2019;33(4):1045–62.
11. Tiberi S, Zumla A, Migliori GB. Multi-drug/extensively drug resistant tuberculosis. Infect Dis Clin North Am 2019;33(4):1063–85.
12. Margaret IP, Jeffery HO. Antibiotic resistant community-acquired bacterial pneumonia. Infect Dis Clin North Am 2019;33(4):1087–103.

13. Shakoor S, Platts-Mills JA, Hasan R. Antibiotic resistant enteric infections. Infect Dis Clin North Am 2019;33(4):1105–23.
14. Fitzgerald D, Waterer GW. Invasive pneumococcal and meningococcal disease. Infect Dis Clin North Am 2019;33(4):1125–41.
15. Kumar R, Ison M. Opportunistic infections in transplant patient. Infect Dis Clin North Am 2019;33(4):1143–57.

Severe Acute Respiratory Syndrome
Historical, Epidemiologic, and Clinical Features

David S.C. Hui, MBBS, MD(UNSW), FRACP, FRCP(Lond, Edin, Glasg), FHKCP, FHKAM(Med)[a,*],
Alimuddin Zumla, MBChB, MSc, PhD, MD, FRCP(Lond), FRCP(Edin), FRCPath(UK), FAAS[b]

KEYWORDS

• SARS • Coronavirus • Epidemic • Epidemiology • Clinical • Prevention

KEY POINTS

- Severe acute respiratory syndrome (SARS) is highly infectious zoonotic respiratory disease of humans with significant morbidity and mortality. The specific animal host reservoir remains unknown although horseshoe bats are reservoirs of coronaviruses.
- SARS is caused by SARS-coronavirus (SARS-CoV), which first emerged in China and gained global notoriety in 2002 to 2003 causing a travel-related global outbreak with 8098 cases and 774 deaths. Nosocomial transmission of SARS-CoV was common.
- The main mode of transmission of SARS-CoV is person-to-person spread through inhalation of respiratory droplets. Feco-oral transmission via contaminated fomite on surfaces has been recorded.
- Fever and respiratory symptoms, such as influenza predominate, and diarrhea is common. About 25% of cases can rapidly progress and require intensive care.
- Treatment involves supportive care with appropriate fluid and electrolyte balance, oxygenation, and organ support. Convalescent plasma, protease inhibitors, and interferon might confer beneficial effects.
- Prevention requires strict infection control procedures, with respiratory and contact precautions for routine care, but upgrade to airborne precaution is needed for managing aerosol-generating procedures.

Disclosure: D.S. Hui and A. Zumla have an interest in global public health, emerging and re-emerging infections, particularly respiratory tract infections. Both authors have research interests in coronaviruses.
[a] Department of Medicine and Therapeutics, Stanley Ho Center for Emerging Infectious Diseases, The Chinese University of Hong Kong, Shatin, New Territories, Hong Kong; [b] Center for Clinical Microbiology, University College London, Royal Free Campus 2nd Floor, Rowland Hill Street, London NW3 2PF, United Kingdom
* Corresponding author.
E-mail address: dschui@cuhk.edu.hk

INTRODUCTION

Over the past 2 decades 2 previously unknown coronaviruses (CoVs), the severe acute respiratory syndrome CoV (SARS-CoV) and the Middle East respiratory syndrome CoV (MERS-CoV) have focused medical, scientific, and media attention because of their lethal nature and epidemic potential. In November 2002, the first case of SARS occurred in Foshan, China,[1] and in June 2012, the first case of MERS died at a hospital in Jeddah, Saudi Arabia. Both zoonotic diseases remain on the World Health Organization (WHO) list of blueprint priority diseases because they remain global threats to global public health security.[2] This review focuses on the historical, epidemiologic, and clinical features of SARS.

HISTORICAL

Before 2003, only 2 CoVs, human CoV 229E (HCoV-229E) and HCoV-OC43, were known to cause human disease. These manifest with mild symptoms like the common cold in adults and with more severe disease in infants, the elderly, and the immunosuppressed. In November 2002, unusual cases of "atypical pneumonia" of unknown cause occurred in Foshan City, Guangdong province, in China, where many health care workers became infected.[1] The infection was brought to Hong Kong on February 21, 2003, by a physician who had looked after similar cases of atypical pneumonia in mainland China, leading to subsequent outbreaks of severe pneumonia in Hong Kong and labeled by WHO as "severe acute respiratory syndrome" on March 15, 2003.[3–5] Several months elapsed and several hundred cases of SARS were observed before SARS-CoV was identified. A novel β CoV (SARS-CoV) of lineage B was confirmed as the cause of the atypical pneumonia cases on March 22, 2003.[4] The SARS-CoV epidemic spread to 29 countries and regions, and it was evident that the global public health, medical, and scientific communities were not adequately prepared for the emergence of SARS. Chains of human-to-human transmission occurred in Toronto in Canada, Hong Kong Special Administrative Region of China, Chinese Taipei, Singapore, and Hanoi, Viet Nam. The history of the SARS epidemic was short and WHO declared the end of the SARS epidemic in July 2003. There were a total of 8096 SARS cases (which included 774 deaths)[4] reported from 29 countries and regions.[5] **Fig. 1** shows the geographic map of distribution of SARS cases.

During the epidemic, SARS caused major disruptions to international air travel, and had a major impact on the health services and business in affected countries.[6] Since July 2003, there were 4 occasions when SARS has reappeared, 3 of these were attributed to breaches in laboratory biosafety in Singapore, Taipei, and Beijing, where 7 cases were associated with 1 chain of transmission and with hospital spread. The fourth incident in Guangdong province, China, resulted in 4 sporadic community-acquired cases over a 66-week period from December 2003 to January 2004. Three cases had been exposed to animals or environmental sources. There was no further community transmission.

VIROLOGY

Coronaviruses (order *Nidovirales,* family *Coronaviridae,* subfamily *Coronavirinae*) are a group of enveloped, positive-sense, single-stranded, highly diverse RNA viruses that are further divided into 4 genera: α, β, γ, and δ.[7] CoVs may cause diseases of varying severity in different systems in humans and other animal species. In March 2003, a novel group 2b β CoV was confirmed as the causative agent responsible for

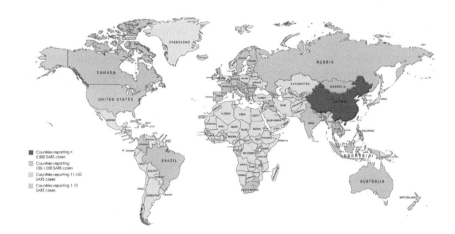

Fig. 1. Global distribution of SARS.

SARS-CoV infection.[4,8,9] The genome sequence of the SARS-CoV did not bear close relationship to any of the previously identified CoVs.[10,11]

SARS-CoV genome consists of 5′ methylated caps and 3′ polyadenylated tails. The partially overlapping 5′ terminal open reading frame 1a/b (ORF1a/b) is within the 5′ two-thirds of the CoV genome and encodes the large replicase polyprotein 1a (pp1a) and pp1ab. These polyproteins are cleaved by 3C-like serine protease and papain-like cysteine protease to produce nonstructural proteins, such as RNA polymerase and helicase, which are important enzymes involved in the transcription and replication of CoVs. The 3′ one-third of the CoV genome encodes the structural proteins (spike [S], envelope [E], membrane [M], and nucleocapsid [N]), which are important for virus-cell receptor binding and assembly of virion, and other accessory proteins and nonstructural proteins that may have immunomodulatory effects.[7]

HOST RESERVOIR

Data from a retrospective serology study done in Guangzhou in southern China, suggested that the SARS-CoV might have transmitted from animal species to humans in the wet market, because a high sero-prevalence (16.7%) was found among asymptomatic wild animal salesmen.[12] A highly similar variant of SARS-CoV was detected in palm civets at an animal market located in Shenzhen.[13] Masked palm civets were then assumed to be accountable for the transmission of SARS-CoV to humans because 30% of wild animal handlers were found to have positive serology against SARS-CoV infection compared with 1% of controls in Guangdong province.[13] In addition, up to 39% of SARS-CoV cases that arose in the early stage of the outbreak were associated with a history of exposure to animal markets.[14] This assumption was further enhanced by an epidemiology linkage in 3 of the 4 patients to indirect or direct contact with palm civets during the sporadic outbreaks of SARS-CoV infection that occurred in Guangzhou in December 2003 and January 2004.[15,16]

Subsequently, however, Chinese horseshoe bats were found to carry SARS-like CoVs in 2005,[17,18] with a high degree of nucleotide sequence similarity (88%–92%) to human or civet cat isolates, suggesting that bats could well have been the natural source of an early ancestor of SARS-CoV. It remains uncertain as to whether an intermediate mammalian host is involved before human transmission.

PATHOGENESIS

The pathogenesis of SARS is complex, and not fully defined because multiple factors govern the wide-ranging clinical manifestations from mild to severe disease.[19] Apart from the respiratory tract, SARS-CoV can infect several organs and cell types during the course of the disease, including intestinal mucosal cells, renal tubular epithelial cells, neurons, and cells of the lymphoid and reticuloendothelial system.[19]

Entry into Host Cells and Pathology

SARS-CoV invades humans through the respiratory tract as the entry site,[20] and infection occurs in 3 steps: receptor binding, conformational changes in S glycoprotein, and cathepsin L proteolysis within endosomes.[21] Entry of SARS-CoV is mediated by angiotensin-converting enzyme 2 (ACE2), a metallopeptidase that is expressed on many human organ tissues, as the host functional receptor.[22] ACE2 is present abundantly in the epithelia of human lungs and small intestine,[23] but the presence of ACE2 may not be the sole requirement for SARS-CoV tropism. One example is that, despite the abundant expression of ACE2 in vascular endothelial cells and intestinal smooth muscle cells, SARS-CoV was not detected in these cells, whereas it was found in colonic enterocytes and hepatocytes without ACE2 expression.[23,24]

Histology

Several autopsies of patients with SARS showed the predominant pathologic finding as diffuse alveolar damage (DAD). Lung histopathology in patients with SARS included DAD, loss of cilia, squamous metaplasia, denudation of bronchial epithelia, giant-cell infiltrate, with a marked increase in macrophages in the alveoli and the interstitium. ACE2 may contribute to the development of DAD. SARS-CoV infections and the S glycoprotein of the SARS-CoV could reduce ACE2 expression. In the mouse model, injection of SARS-CoV S glycoprotein worsened acute lung injury (ALI) in vivo that could be reduced by blocking the renin-angiotensin pathway.[25] In addition, overexpression of SARS-CoV proteins such as 3a and 7a, which were expressed in the lungs and intestinal tissues of patients with SARS, could induce apoptosis in vitro.[26,27]

Splenic atrophy of the white pulp, hemophagocytosis, hyaline membranes, and secondary bacterial pneumonia were observed.[28,29] Lesions resembling cryptogenic organizing pneumonia (COP) in subpleural regions were also seen.[30] Extensive expression of SARS-CoV antigen in type I pneumocytes in cynomolgus macaques experimentally infected with SARS-CoV was noted at day 4, suggesting that type I pneumocytes might be the early primary target for SARS-CoV infection.[31] Diarrhea was present in up to 70% of SARS cases.[24,32] In specimens obtained by colonoscopy or postmortem examination, active viral replication was noted within the small and large intestine with minimal architectural disruption. SARS-CoV infection was confirmed by viral culture of these specimens, while SARS-CoV RNA was detected in the stool specimens for almost 10 weeks after illness onset.[24] The presence of diarrhea and mortality were associated with a higher nasopharyngeal SARS-CoV viral load on day 10 after illness onset.[33]

Immune Responses and Immunopathology

While innate and acquired immune responses enable containment of virus and mild disease, cytokine dysregulation, viral cytopathic effects, downregulation of lung ACE 2, abnormal immune responses, and autoimmune mechanisms may lead to more severe disease and death, disease progression in SARS may be related to activation of T-helper (Th1) cell-mediated immunity and hyperinnate inflammatory response.[28,32] Marked increases in the Th1 and inflammatory cytokines (interferon-γ [IFN-γ], interleukin-1 [IL-1], IL-6, and IL-12) were noted for more than 2 weeks after illness onset in a study of 20 adults with SARS-CoV infection, together with marked increases in chemokines such as Th1 chemokine IFN-γ-inducible protein-10 (IP-10), neutrophil chemokine IL-8, and monocyte chemoattractant protein-1 (MCP-1).[34] In mice infected with SARS-CoV, T cells played an important role in SARS-CoV clearance, whereas a reduced T-cell response contributed to severe disease.[35] In another study of mice infected with SARS-CoV, robust virus replication accompanied by delayed type I IFN (IFN-I) response was observed orchestrating inflammatory responses and lung immunopathology with reduced survival, while early administration of IFN-I ameliorated immunopathology. This delayed IFN-I signaling was thought to promote the accumulation of pathogenic inflammatory monocyte-macrophages, leading to elevated lung cytokine/chemokine levels, vascular leakage, and impaired virus-specific T-cell responses, whereas genetic ablation of the IFN-$\alpha\beta$ receptor or inflammatory monocyte-macrophage depletion protected mice from fatal infection, without affecting viral load.[36]

In addition, Toll-like receptors (TLR) signaling through the TIR domain-containing adapter-inducing INF-β (TRIF) adaptor protein might play a role in protecting mice from lethal SARS-CoV disease based on a study of the innate responses in mice.[37] TLR3(−/−), TLR4(−/−), and TRIF-related adapted molecule [TRAM](−/−) mice were more prone to SARS-CoV infection than wild-type mice, although there was only transient weight loss without mortality. In contrast, mice deficient in the TLR3/TLR4 adaptor TRIF were highly susceptible to SARS-CoV infection, with marked weight loss, more pathologic conditions of the lung, higher viral titers, impaired lung function, and mortality. In TRIF(−/−) mice infected with SARS-CoV, distinct changes in inflammation occurred including excess infiltration of neutrophils and inflammatory cells that correlated with increased pathologic conditions of other known causes of acute respiratory distress syndrome (ARDS). Aberrant proinflammatory cytokines, chemokines, and INF-stimulated gene signaling programs were observed following infection of TRIF(−/−) mice that resembled those seen in human patients with poor clinical outcome following SARS-CoV infection. These findings suggest the importance of TLR adaptor signaling in generating a balanced protective innate immune response to highly pathogenic CoV infections.[37] In addition, SARS-CoV M protein may function as a cytosolic pathogen-associated molecular pattern to stimulate IFN-β production by activating a TLR-related TRAF3-independent signaling cascade.[38]

A case-control study conducted in Chinese patients with SARS-CoV infection and healthy controls has shown that genetic variants of IL-12 receptor B1 (IL12RB1) predispose to SARS-CoV infection.[39] Another case-control study has shown that mannose-binding lectin (MBL), a key molecule in innate immunity that functions as an ante-antibody before specific antibody response, contributes to the first-line host defense against SARS-CoV, and that MBL deficiency is a predisposing factor to SARS-CoV infection.[40]

In macaques infected with SARS-CoV, there is evidence that anti-spike immunoglobulin G (IgG) causes severe ALI by altering macrophage inflammation-resolving response in infected lungs. In acutely infected macaques, there was functional polarization of alveolar macrophages, demonstrating wound-healing and proinflammatory characteristics simultaneously. However, the presence of S-IgG before clearance of virus aborted wound-healing responses and promoted production of IL-8 and MCP1, with recruitment of proinflammatory monocytes/macrophages. Interestingly, the sera of patients who had succumbed to SARS-CoV infection enhanced SARS-CoV-induced MCP1 and IL-8 production by human monocyte-derived wound-healing macrophages, whereas blockade of the Fc-γ receptor reduced such effects. The findings reveal a mechanism responsible for virus-mediated ALI and define a pathologic consequence of viral-specific antibody response, in addition to providing some insight on a potential target for treatment of SARS-CoV.[41]

EPIDEMIOLOGY AND DISEASE TRANSMISSION
Discovery and Spread

In a chest hospital in Guangzhou city, a retrospective study of 55 patients hospitalized with atypical pneumonia between January 24 and February 18, 2003, showed a positive culture of SARS-CoV in the nasopharyngeal aspirates of 3 patients, and positive serology to SARS-CoV in 48 patients (87%). The genetic sequence of the virus isolated from patients in Guangdong was found subsequently to be prototypical of the SARS-CoV found in affected areas around the world.[42]

The index case for the major SARS-CoV outbreak in Hong Kong was a 64-year-old male renal physician, who traveled from the Guangdong province on February 21, 2003, to Hong Kong.[2,4] SARS-CoV was transmitted to at least 16 patrons of Hotel M where he stayed on the 9th floor. The renal physician subsequently died of severe pneumonia a few days later at a hospital near the hotel.[28] Within a few weeks, catalyzed by the speed of international air travel, the infected hotel patrons spread SARS-CoV to 29 countries/regions.[4,43] The main mode of spread of SARS-CoV seems to be through close contact with an infected person and transmitted via respiratory droplets or contact with fomite.[44]

Transmission in Hospitals

A super-spreading event at the Prince of Wales Hospital (PWH) in Hong Kong highlighted the nosocomial transmission potential of SARS-CoV infection. A 26-year-old man (and visitor who had stayed on the 9th floor of Hotel M), who was admitted to a general medical ward 8A of the hospital with fever and pneumonia on March 4, 2003,[45,46] led to 138 subjects (including previously healthy health care workers) contracting the disease within a 2-week period after exposure. An overcrowded medical ward environment, inadequate air changes in the hospital ward, and the administration of nebulized salbutamol to the index patient via a jet nebulizer, for its mucociliary clearance effects, seem to have contributed to this super-spreading event.[45,46] SARS-CoV was detected in respiratory tract secretions, urine, feces, and tears of some patients with SARS-CoV infection.[44,47] Computational fluid dynamics analysis in conjunction with investigation of the temporal-spatial pattern of spread of SARS-CoV infection among in-patients on the affected medical ward 8A, implicated airborne transmission.[48] A multiagent modeling analysis of 1744 scenarios was used to examine the contribution by different modes of transmission in the ward 8A outbreak and found that SARS-CoV most likely had spread via the combined long-range airborne and fomite routes, while fomites played a nonnegligible role in the transmission.[49]

In Toronto, SARS-CoV was found on polymerase chain reaction (PCR) testing of environmental air samples taken from a hospital room occupied by a patient with SARS-CoV infection, as well as from conventional surface swabs taken from a bed table, a patient's television remote control, and a medication refrigerator door at a nurses' station.[50] The possibility of airborne transmission as indicated by the data emphasizes that it is imperative to take appropriate respiratory protection in addition to strict surface hygiene practices. **Box 1** shows the key timeline of spread of SARS-CoV infection from China to Singapore, Taiwan, Vietnam, and Canada via

Box 1
Important timeline of spread of severe acute respiratory syndrome coronavirus infection from China to Canada, Vietnam, Taiwan, Vietnam, and Singapore via Hong Kong[51]

November 16, 2002
- First known case of atypical pneumonia in Foshan City, Guangdong province, China, but cause not identified until much later.

February 11, 2003
- WHO received reports from the Chinese Ministry of Health of an outbreak of acute respiratory syndrome with 300 cases and 5 deaths in Guangdong province.

February 21, 2003
- A 64-year-old medical doctor from Zhongshan University in Guangzhou (Guangdong province) arrived in Hong Kong to attend a wedding and was a guest on the ninth floor of Hotel M (room 911).

February 22, 2003
- The Guangdong doctor was admitted to the intensive care unit at the Kwong Wah Hospital in Hong Kong with respiratory failure (he had previously treated patients with atypical pneumonia in Guangdong). He warned medical staff that he might have contracted a "very virulent disease," with onset of symptoms on February 15, 2003.

February 26, 2003
- A 48-year-old Chinese-American businessman was admitted to the French Hospital in Hanoi with a 3-day history of fever and respiratory symptoms. He traveled to Hong Kong on February 17, departed for Hanoi on February 23, and fell ill there. Shortly before his departure from Hong Kong, he had stayed on the ninth floor of the Hotel M, in a room across the hall from the Guangdong doctor.

March 1, 2003
- A 26-year-old woman was admitted to a hospital in Singapore with respiratory symptoms. A resident of Singapore, she was a guest on the ninth floor of the Hotel M in Hong Kong from February 21 to 25.

March 4, 2003
- The Guangdong doctor died of atypical pneumonia at Kwong Wah Hospital in Hong Kong.

March 5, 2003
- In Hanoi, the Chinese-American businessman, in a stable but critical condition, was air medevaced to the Princess Margaret Hospital in Hong Kong. Seven health care workers who had cared for him in Hanoi became ill.
- A 78-year-old Toronto woman, who had checked out of the Hotel M in Hong Kong on February 23, died at Toronto's Scarborough Grace Hospital. Five members of her family were infected and admitted to the hospital. Her son, aged 43, fell ill on February 27, 2003, and was subsequently admitted to a community hospital on March 7, 2003, leading to a major nosocomial outbreak. Subsequent chains of disease transmissions resulted in numerous hospital outbreaks that involved 257 people.

March 7, 2003
- Health care workers at Hong Kong's Prince of Wales Hospital started to complain of respiratory tract infection, progressing to pneumonia. All had an identifiable link with ward 8A.

March 8, 2003
- In Taiwan, the source of SARS-CoV infection was a 54-year-old merchant who returned to Taipei via Hong Kong after visiting Guangdong on February 5, 2003. By February 25, 2003, he had developed fever, myalgia, and dry cough but was not hospitalized until March 8, 2003.

March 12, 2003
- WHO issued a global alert about cases of severe atypical pneumonia following mounting reports of spread among staff at hospitals in Hong Kong and Hanoi.

- At the French Hospital in Hanoi, 26 staff had symptoms. Of these, 25 had either pneumonia or acute respiratory syndrome, and 5 were in critical condition. The hospital was closed to new admissions.
- Hong Kong health authorities formally reported an outbreak of an unidentified flu-like illness among hospital staff at the Prince of Wales Hospital. As of midnight March 11, 50 health care workers had been screened; 23 were found to have febrile illness, and 8 showed early chest radiographic signs of pneumonia. A 26-year-old man, who had visited an acquaintance staying on the ninth floor of the Hotel M from February 15 to 23, was shown to be the source of this hospital outbreak following subsequent epidemiologic investigation.

March 13, 2003

- The Ministry of Health in Singapore reported 3 cases of atypical pneumonia in young women who had recently returned to Singapore after traveling to Hong Kong. All had stayed on the ninth floor of the Hotel M in late February.

March 15, 2003

- WHO issued a travel advisory as evidence mounted that SARS was spreading by air travel along international routes. WHO named the mysterious illness after its symptoms: severe acute respiratory syndrome (SARS) and declared it "a worldwide health threat."

March 26, 2003

- The arrival of an infected resident of the Amoy Gardens in Hong Kong to Taiwan on March 26, 2003, led to an escalation of SARS-CoV cases in Taiwan from mid-April 2003. Subsequent phylogenetic analysis of both Taiwan and Hong Kong outbreaks revealed the same strain of virus.

April 28, 2003

- In Hanoi, there was a reported total of 63 cases of SARS-CoV infection before the outbreak was declared to be over on April 28, 2003

May 5, 2003

- The SARS-CoV outbreak in Singapore was characterized by rapid nosocomial transmission involving a large number of health care workers (97 out of 238 probable SARS cases [41%]) and several super-spreading events. Transmission of SARS was finally brought to an end, with no new cases after May 5, 2003.

May 14, 2003

- Toronto was initially removed from the WHO list of areas with recent local SARS transmission and there was a province-wide scaling back of SARS control measures, such as fever surveillance and monitoring of respiratory symptoms in existing in-patients and visitors. However, 1 month after the SARS-CoV outbreak was thought to have ended, another surge of cases arose in a Toronto rehabilitation hospital involving health care workers, visitors, and patients who had been exposed to hospitalized patients with undiagnosed SARS-CoV infection.

July 2, 2003

- Toronto was finally free from local transmission.

5 July, 2003

- It was finally announced by WHO that the transmission chain of SARS-CoV in Taiwan was broken, bringing an end to the SARS-CoV epidemic.

From WHO. Update 95-SARS: Chronology of a serial killer. Accessed 10 Jan 2016. Available at: http://www.who.int/csr/don/2003_07_04/en; with permission.

Hong Kong.[51] **Box 2** summarizes the risk factors for nosocomial transmission and super-spreading events of SARS-CoV infection.[52,53]

Community Transmission

Opportunistic airborne transmission seems to have been responsible for a major community outbreak of SARS-CoV infection involving more than 300 people in Hong Kong, in a private residential complex, the Amoy Gardens.[54,55] The spread of

---

Box 2
Risk factors of nosocomial transmission of severe acute respiratory syndrome coronavirus infection

a. Independent risk factors of super-spreading nosocomial outbreaks of SARS[52]:
   - Performance of resuscitation (OR = 3.81; 95% CI, 1.04–13.87; P = .04).
   - Staff working while experiencing symptoms (OR = 10.55; 95% CI, 2.28–48.87; P = .003)
   - Patients with SARS requiring oxygen therapy at least 6 L/min (OR = 4.30; 95% CI, 1.00–18.43; P = .05)
   - Patients with SARS requiring noninvasive positive pressure ventilation (OR = 11.82; 95% CI, 1.97–70.80; P = .007)
   - Minimum distance between beds <1 m (OR = 6.98; 95% CI, 1.68–28.75; P = .008)
   - Washing or changing facilities for staff (OR = 0.12; 95% CI, 0.02–0.97; P = .05)

b. Respiratory procedures associated with increased risk of transmission to health care workers.[53]
   Procedures reported to present an increased risk of transmission included (n, pooled OR [95% CI]):
   - Tracheal intubation (n = 4 cohorts; 6.6 [2.3, 18.9], and n = 4 case-controls; 6.6 [4.1, 10.6]);
   - Noninvasive ventilation (n = 2 cohorts; OR = 3.1 [1.4, 6.8]);
   - Tracheotomy (n = 1 case-control; 4.2 [1.5, 11.5]);
   - Manual ventilation before intubation (n = 1 cohort; OR = 2.8 [1.3, 6.4]).

Adapted from Yu IT, Xie ZH, Tsoi KK, et al. Why did outbreaks of severe acute respiratory syndrome occur in some hospital wards but not in others? Clin Infect Dis 2007;44:1017–1025; and Tran K, Cimon K, Severn M, et al. Aerosol generating procedures and risk of transmission of acute respiratory infections to healthcare workers: a systematic review. PLoS One 2012;7:e35797.

SARS-CoV and creation of infectious aerosols that moved upward through the warm airshaft of the apartment building may have been because of dried up U-bend drainage on a bathroom floor and backflow of contaminated sewage (from a SARS patient with renal failure and diarrhea), in combination with negative pressure generated by the toilet exhaust fans. It was suggested via computational fluid dynamics modeling that long-range airborne transmission (>200 m) to nearby buildings was possibly caused by wind flow dispersion.[56]

Other Routes of Transmission

The main mode of SARS-CoV transmission is via respiratory droplets, although the potential of transmission by opportunistic airborne routes via aerosol-generating procedures in health care facilities,[44,50] and environmental factors, as in the case of Amoy Gardens, is known.[54–56] Other transmission routes leading to the spread of SARS-CoV included feco-oral (presence of virus in stool, and diarrhea as a symptom)[54–56] and fomite on surfaces (virus found on surfaces in hospitals treating patients with SARS-CoV).[56] The SARS-CoV that spread worldwide was due to a single virus strain.[57]

CLINICAL MANIFESTATIONS

A wide range of clinical manifestations are seen in patients with SARS from mild, moderate, to severe and rapidly progressive and fulminant disease.

Incubation Period

The estimated mean incubation period of SARS-CoV infection was 4.6 days (95% CI, 3.8–5.8 days)[58] and 95% of illness onset occurred within 10 days.[59] The mean time from symptom onset to hospitalization was between 2 and 8 days, but was shorter toward the later phase of the epidemic. The mean time from symptom onset to need for invasive mechanical ventilation (IMV) and to death was 11 and 23.7 days, respectively.[60]

Symptoms

The major clinical features of SARS are fever, rigors, chills, myalgia, dry cough, malaise, dyspnea, and headache. Sore throat, sputum production, rhinorrhea, nausea, vomiting, and dizziness are less common (**Table 1**).[3,45,61–63] Watery diarrhea was present in 40% to 70% of patients with SARS and tended to occur about 1 week after illness onset.[24,32] SARS-CoV was detected in the serum and cerebrospinal fluid of 2 patients complicated by status epilepticus.[64,65] Elderly patients with SARS-CoV infection might present with poor appetite, a decrease in general well-being, fracture as a result of fall,[66] and confusion, but some elderly subjects might not be able to mount a febrile response. In contrast, SARS-CoV infection in children aged less than 12 years was generally mild, whereas infection in teenagers resembled that in adults.[67] There was no mortality among young children and teenagers.[58,67] SARS-CoV infection acquired during pregnancy carried a case fatality rate of 25% and was associated with a high incidence of spontaneous miscarriage, preterm delivery, and intrauterine growth retardation without perinatal SARS-CoV infection among the newborn infants.[68]

Asymptomatic SARS-CoV infection was uncommon in 2003; a meta-analysis had shown overall sero-prevalence rates of 0.1% (95% CI, 0.02–0.18) for the general population and 0.23% for health care workers (95% CI, 0.02–0.45) in comparison with healthy blood donors, others from the general community, or patients without SARS-CoV infection recruited from the health care setting (0.16%, 95% CI, 0–0.37).[69]

The clinical course of patients with SARS-CoV infection seemed to manifest in different stages.[32,43,45,70] In the first week of illness of SARS-CoV infection, many patients presented with fever, dry cough, myalgia, and malaise that might improve despite the presence of lung consolidation and rising viral loads on serial samples. During the second week, many patients experienced recurrence of fever, worsening consolidation, and respiratory failure, while about 20% of patients progressed to

Table 1
Clinical features of severe acute respiratory syndrome on presentation

Symptom	% of Patients with Symptoms
Persistent fever >38°C	99–100
Nonproductive cough	57–75
Myalgia	45–61
Chills/rigor	15–73
Headache	20–56
Dyspnea	40–42
Malaise	31–45
Nausea and vomiting	20–35
Diarrhea	20–25
Sore throat	13–25
Dizziness	4.2–43
Sputum production	4.9–29
Rhinorrhea	2.1–23
Arthralgia	10.4

Data from Refs.[3,45,61–63]

ARDS requiring IMV.[32,43,45] Peaking of viral load on day 10 of illness[32] corresponded temporally to peaking of the extent of consolidation radiographically,[71] and a maximal risk of nosocomial transmission, particularly to health care workers.[72]

DIAGNOSIS AND INVESTIGATIONS
Laboratory Diagnosis

The detection rates for SARS-CoV infection in 2003 using reverse transcriptase PCR (RT-PCR) on nasopharyngeal specimens, urine, stool, and blood are shown in **Table 2**.[32,73–75] It is important to collect a combination of upper respiratory (nasal, pharyngeal, and nasopharyngeal), lower respiratory (higher yield because of higher viral levels, eg, sputum, tracheal aspirate, and bronchoalveolar lavage), blood, and fecal specimens to maximize the chance of detection. A single negative test in an upper respiratory specimen does not rule out the diagnosis. Because viral kinetics demonstrated an inverted V-shape curve peaking on day 10 of illness with progressive decrease in rates of viral shedding from nasopharynx, stool, and urine (which might persist up to day 21), clinical progression during the second week was thought to be related to immune-mediated lung injury.[32]

Specimens for viral culture require processing in biosafety level 3 facilities, but the results take too long to assist acute clinical management. Serologic diagnosis is largely retrospective and useful for epidemiologic surveillance purposes. A more robust IgG response was observed in severe SARS-CoV infections as reflected by higher IgG levels in patients who required supplemental oxygen, intensive care unit (ICU) admission, those with negative predischarge fecal RT-PCR results, and those with lymphopenia at presentation.[76] A study in Beijing has shown that, 6 years after SARS-CoV infection, specific IgG Ab to SARS-CoV eventually disappeared and peripheral memory B-cell responses became undetectable in recovered patients with SARS but specific T-cell anamnestic responses could be maintained for at least 6 years.[77]

Absolute lymphopenia (lymphocyte count <1.0 × 10^9/L) was observed in 98% of cases of SARS-CoV infection, whereas low CD4 and CD8 lymphocyte counts on hospitalization were associated with adverse clinical outcomes.[78] Liver dysfunction with abnormal alanine transaminases was noted in 29.6% of patients on presentation, but increased to 75.9% of those receiving systemic corticosteroid and ribavirin for treatment of SARS-CoV infection.[79]

Radiologic Features

The radiographic features of SARS-CoV infection were basically nonspecific. About a quarter of patients might have unremarkable chest radiographs initially,[3,45,61] with

Table 2	
Diagnostic tests for severe acute respiratory syndrome coronavirus	
RT-PCR	**Detection Rates**
Nasopharyngeal aspirate	Conventional RT-PCR: 32% day 3; 68% day 14[32] Second-generation with real-time quantitative RT-PCR assay: 80% during first 3 d[73]
Stool[32]	97% day 14 of illness
Urine[32]	42% day 15 of illness
Real-time quantitative serum SARS-CoV RNA[74,75]	80% day 1; 75% day 7; 45% day 14
Serology IgG seroconversion to SARS-CoV[32]	15% day 15; 60% day 21; >90% day 28

Data from Refs.[32,73–75]

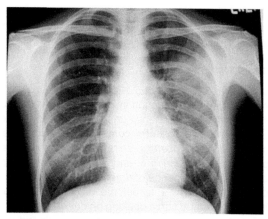

Fig. 2. Chest radiograph of a patient showing opacities at the right lower zone and left mid and lower zones.

nonspecific changes, ranging from normal to peribronchial thickening and ill-defined airspace shadowing (**Fig. 2**).

High-resolution computer tomography (HRCT) of the thorax could detect small parenchymal lesions early.[80] Common HRCT findings included interlobular septal and intralobular interstitial thickening, consolidation, and ground-glass opacification, predominantly involving peripheral lung fields and lower lobes, with features closely resembling those found in COP[45,80] (**Fig. 3**). In an ICU case series of critically ill patients, 12% of patients developed pneumo-mediastinum spontaneously, while 20% of patients developed evidence of ARDS over a period of 3 weeks.[32] Despite the use of lung protective IMV with a low tidal volume, barotrauma occurred in 26% of critically ill cases of SARS-CoV infection, possibly owing to decreased lung compliance.[81]

PROGNOSTIC MARKERS AND OUTCOME

The prognostic factors associated with a poor outcome (ICU admission or death) in SARS-CoV infection are summarized in **Box 3**.[32,45,61–63,73–75] Infants (preterm or

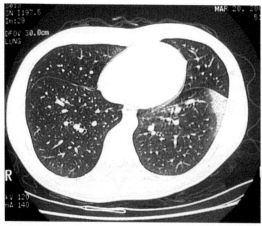

Fig. 3. Chest tomography of another patient with ground-glass opacity at the anterolateral segment of the left lower lobe.

> **Box 3**
> **Poor prognostic factors associated with intensive care unit admission and/or deaths in patients with severe acute respiratory syndrome coronavirus infection**
>
> *Factors*
>
> Advanced age[32,45,59,62,63]
>
> Viral loads: high SARS-CoV viral loads in nasopharyngeal secretions[32]; high plasma SARS-CoV concentrations[74,75]
>
> Comorbidities: chronic hepatitis B,[32] diabetes mellitus, or other co-morbid conditions[61,62]
>
> Laboratory markers: high peak lactate dehydrogenase (LDH),[45] high initial LDH level,[63] high neutrophil count on presentation,[45,63] low counts of CD4 and CD8 at presentation[78]
>
> *Data from* Refs.[32,45,61–63,74,75]

full-term) born to mothers infected with SARS-CoV infection were neither shedding SARS-CoV nor clinically infected in the postnatal period.[82] The clinical course of SARS-CoV infection in elderly patients, particularly those with comorbidities was typically fulminant and often fatal.

ANTIVIRAL THERAPY AND OTHER POTENTIAL TREATMENTS
Ribavirin

Ribavirin, a nucleoside analog, was widely prescribed for treatment of SARS-CoV infection in 2003.[32,45,61,62] Nevertheless, ribavirin monotherapy had minimal activity against SARS-CoV with concentrations that could be achieved in the clinical setting, and it led to significant hemolysis in many patients.[32,45,83]

Antiviral Therapy

The efficacy of antiviral agents including ribavirin, protease inhibitors, and INF that were used to treat patients with SARS-CoV infection in 2003 is summarized in **Table 3**.[61,83–86] Because of lack of prospective randomized, placebo-controlled clinical trial data, none of these therapies have proven benefit. Good supportive care remains the mainstay of treatment of SARS-CoV infection.

Systemic Corticosteroids

Systemic corticosteroids, in the form of intravenous pulse methylprednisolone (MP) was given to some patients with SARS-CoV infection for several reasons.[32,45,62,63,83] Firstly, there was an assumption that clinical progression of pneumonia and respiratory failure in association with peaking of SARS-CoV viral load might be mediated by the host inflammatory response.[32,71] Also, in many patients there were HRCT[3,45,80] and histologic features of COP, which was a steroid-responsive condition.[30] Systemic corticosteroids significantly reduced IL-8, MCP-1, and IP-10 concentrations from 5 to 8 days after treatment in 20 adults with SARS-CoV infection.[34] In addition, in patients with fatal SARS-CoV infection, there was evidence of hemophagocytosis in the lungs,[28] attributed to cytokine dysregulation.[87] Intervention with systemic corticosteroids was thus given to modulate these immune responses.

Although there was clinical improvement in some patients with resolution of fever and lung consolidation following treatment with intravenously pulsed MP,[3,83] a retrospective cohort analysis in Hong Kong showed that the use of pulsed MP was actually associated with an increased risk of 30-day mortality (adjusted odds ratio [OR] 26.0; 95% CI, 4.4–154.8).[88] In addition, prolonged use of systemic corticosteroid therapy

Table 3
Agents applied for treatment of humans with severe acute respiratory syndrome coronavirus infection in 2003

Agents	
Ribavirin	Ribavirin given at 1.2 g three times a day orally for 2 wk resulted in a drop in hemoglobin of >2 g/dL from baseline in 59% of patients, with evidence of hemolysis documented in 36%.[83]
	Based on a higher dosage of ribavirin for treating hemorrhagic fever virus, patients with SARS-CoV infection in Toronto developed more toxicity, including elevated transaminases and bradycardia.[61]
Protease inhibitor	Two retrospective, matched cohort studies have compared the clinical outcome of patients who received protease inhibitors (lopinavir 400 mg/ritonavir 100 mg) in addition to ribavirin, either as initial therapy within 5 d of onset of symptoms or as rescue therapy after pulsed methylprednisolone treatment for worsening respiratory symptoms; these were compared with historical controls who received ribavirin alone as initial antiviral therapy.[84,85]
	The addition of lopinavir/ritonavir as initial therapy was associated with reduced overall death rate (2.3%) and intubation rate (0%), in comparison with a matched cohort that received standard treatment (15.6% and 11%, respectively)[85]; there was also evidence of reduction in viral loads. Other beneficial effects included a reduction in methylprednisolone use and less nosocomial infections.[84]
	However, the subgroup that had received lopinavir/ritonavir as rescue therapy fared no better than the matched cohort, and received a higher mean dose of methylprednisolone.[86] The improved clinical outcome in patients who received lopinavir/ritonavir as part of the initial therapy is supported by the observations that both peak (9.6 μg/mL) and trough (5.5 μg/mL) serum concentrations of lopinavir could inhibit the virus.
Interferon	In an uncontrolled study in Toronto, interferon-alfacon-1 given within 5 d of illness resulted in improved oxygen saturation, more rapid resolution of radiographic lung opacities, and lower rates of intubation (11.1% vs 23.1%) and death (0.0% vs 7.7%); however, the sample size was small (n = 9 vs 13) and confounded by the concomitant use of systemic corticosteroid.[86]

Data from Refs.[61,83–86]

could increase the risk of nosocomial infections, such as disseminated fungal disease,[89] metabolic derangements, psychosis, and osteonecrosis.[90] A randomized controlled trial has shown that plasma SARS-CoV RNA concentrations in the second and third weeks of illness were higher in patients given initial hydrocortisone (n = 10) than those given normal saline as control (n = 7) during the early clinical course of the illness. The data suggest that systemic corticosteroids given early in the course of SARS-CoV infection might prolong viremia.[91] A systematic review concluded that systemic corticosteroid treatment was not associated with definite benefits and was potentially harmful.[92]

Convalescent Plasma/Passive Immunotherapy

Convalescent plasma, donated mostly by health care workers who had fully recovered from SARS-CoV infection, seemed to be clinically useful for treating other patients with progressive SARS-CoV infection.[93,94] In a study comparing patients with SARS-CoV infection who did and did not receive convalescent plasma, 19 patients who received such therapy had higher survival rate (100% vs 66.2%) and higher discharge rate (77.8% vs 23.0%) compared with 21 controls.[94] An exploratory post hoc meta-analysis of studies of SARS-CoV infection and severe influenza showed a significant reduction in the pooled odds of mortality following convalescent plasma versus placebo or no treatment (OR = 0.25; 95% CI, 0.14–0.45).[95] Early administration of convalescent plasma seemed to be more effective, because, among 80 patients with SARS-CoV infection who had been given convalescent plasma at PWH, the discharge rate at day 22 was 58.3% for patients (n = 48) treated within 14 days of illness onset versus 15.6% for those (n = 32) treated beyond 14 days.[93] In the absence of well-proven and effective antiviral therapy, convalescent plasma and human monoclonal antibody are worth further study for treatment of SARS-CoV if it returns.

PREVENTION
Vaccines

The S protein of SARS-CoV plays an important role in mediating viral infection via receptor binding and membrane fusion between the virion and the host cell, and is a major epitope. An adenoviral-based vaccine could induce strong SARS-CoV-specific immune responses in rhesus macaques, and hold promise for development of a protective vaccine against SARS-CoV.[96] Other investigators reported that the S gene DNA vaccine could induce the production of specific IgG antibody against SARS-CoV efficiently in mice, with a seroconversion ratio of 75% after 3 doses of immunization,[97] whereas viral replication was reduced by more than 6 orders of magnitude in the lungs of mice vaccinated with S plasmid DNA expression vectors, and protection was mediated by a humoral immune mechanism.[98] Recombinant S protein exhibited antigenicity and receptor-binding ability, whereas synthetic peptides eliciting specific antibodies against SARS-CoV S protein might provide another approach for further developing SARS vaccine.

General Preventive Measures

Prevention of transmission is crucial for managing this highly infectious disease. The primary mode of transmission of SARS-CoV infection is through direct contact and exposure to infectious respiratory droplets, or fomites, and it is therefore necessary to maintain good personal and environmental hygiene, and to implement stringent contact and droplet precautions among health care workers. To prevent community transmission, contact tracing, quarantine/isolation of close contacts, and public education are important measures.[44] Between December 16, 2003, and January 30, 2004, 4 new cases of SARS-CoV infection emerged in Guangdong, and a link was established between humans and small wild animals. The Guangdong government and Department of Public Health took public health measures and implemented strict controls over the wildlife market, including banning the rearing, transport, slaughter, sales, and food processing of small wild mammals and civet cats.[99]

Hospital Infection Control Measures

Nosocomial transmission was a hallmark of SARS-CoV infection in 2003, with 1706 out of 8096 (21%) of patients with SARS globally being health care workers.[5] A plausible reason is that viral loads reached their highest levels 10 days from disease onset, when the patient was most symptomatic and dyspneic, and close observation/treatment of these patients became necessary for the health care workers.[32] Different medical wards should be designated for patient triage (for undifferentiated fever), confirmed SARS cases, and other patients in whom SARS has been ruled out. In the event of a late detection of a nosocomial outbreak, hospital closure is required to contain onward disease transmission. However, outbreaks that are detected early and limited to few patients, may be managed by isolating the infected patients in place or, alternatively, relocating the affected patients to a designated location. Early case detection followed by isolation should ideally be performed in negative pressure isolation rooms if available. Implementing droplet precautions and contact precautions seemed adequate to reduce the risk of infection after general exposure to patients with mild SARS-CoV infection. Airborne precautions (hand hygiene, gown, gloves, N95 masks, and eye protection) should be implemented if aerosol-generating procedures are to be undertaken.[100]

SUMMARY

The SARS epidemic demonstrated that novel highly pathogenic viruses crossing the animal-human barrier remain a major threat to global health security. SARS posed a major challenge for global public health services because of its sudden appearance, rapid spread, and disappearance. The knowledge and lessons learnt from SARS-CoV epidemiology, mode of transmission, clinical course, complications, clinical management, predictors of poor outcome, and infection control have been invaluable.

Although no major outbreaks have occurred since the last reported SARS cases involving laboratory personnel in Singapore and Taiwan, and 4 residents in Guangdong, an epidemic is possible at any time. Whether SARS will reappear and cause another pandemic remains unknown. The appearance of MERS-CoV in 2012 as another highly pathogenic zoonotic CoV which continues to circulate in the Middle East is a reminder to physicians and public health authorities that the threat of CoV outbreaks is ever present.

ACKNOWLEDGMENTS

A. Zumla is in receipt of an NIH Research (NIHR) senior investigator award and acknowledges support from the PANDORA-ID-NET EDCTP Reg/Grant RIA2016E-1609, funded by the European and Developing Countries Clinical Trials Partnership (EDCTP2) programme, Horizon 2020, the European Union's Framework Programme for Research and Innovation.

REFERENCES

1. Zhao Z, Zhang F, Xu M, et al. Description and clinical treatment of an early outbreak of severe acute respiratory syndrome (SARS) in Guangzhou, PR China. J Med Microbiol 2003;52:715–20.
2. WHO. List of blue print priority diseases. Available at: https://www.who.int/blueprint/priority-diseases/en/. Accessed January7, 2019.
3. Tsang KW, Ho PL, Ooi GC, et al. A cluster of cases of severe acute respiratory syndrome in Hong Kong. N Engl J Med 2003;348:1977–85.
4. Peiris JS, Lai ST, Poon LL, et al, SARS study group. Coronavirus as a possible cause of severe acute respiratory syndrome. Lancet 2003;361(9366):1319–25.
5. WHO. Summary of probable SARS cases with onset of illness from 1 November to 31 July 2003. 2003. Available at: http://www.who.int/csr/sars/country/table2004_04_21/en/. Accessed January 10, 2016.
6. [Chapter 5] WHO. SARS: lessons from a new disease. The World Health Report; 2003. p. 71–8. Available at: http://www.who.int/whr/2003/en/whr03_en.pdf?ua=1. Accessed January 10, 2016.
7. Zumla A, Chan JF, Azhar EI, et al. Coronaviruses – drug discovery and therapeutic options. Nat Rev Drug Discov 2016;15(5):327–47.

8. Drosten C, Gunther S, Preiser W, et al. Identification of a novel coronavirus in patients with severe acute respiratory syndrome. N Engl J Med 2003;348: 1967–76.
9. Ksiazek TG, Erdman D, Goldsmith CS, et al, SARS Working Group. A novel coronavirus associated with severe acute respiratory syndrome. N Engl J Med 2003;348:1953–66.
10. Marra MA, Jones SJ, Astell CR, et al. The genome sequence of the SARS-associated coronavirus. Science 2003;300:1399–404.
11. Ruan YJ, Wei CL, Ee LA, et al. Comparative full-length genome sequence analysis of 14 SARS coronavirus isolates and common mutations associated with putative origins of infection. Lancet 2003;361:1779–85.
12. Du L, Qiu JC, Wang M, et al. Analysis on the characteristics of blood serum Ab-IgG detective result of severe acute respiratory syndrome patients in Guangzhou, China. Zhonghua Liu Xing Bing Xue Za Zhi 2004;25(11):925–8.
13. Guan Y, Zheng BJ, He YQ, et al. Isolation and characterization of viruses related to the SARS coronavirus from animals in southern China. Science 2003;302: 276–8.
14. Yu D, Li H, Xu R, et al, Centers for Disease Control and Prevention (CDC). Prevalence of IgG antibody to SARS-associated coronavirus in animal traders— Guangdong province, China, 2003. MMWR Morb Mortal Wkly Rep 2003;52: 986–7.
15. Song HD, Tu CC, Zhang GW, et al. Cross-host evolution of severe acute respiratory syndrome coronavirus in palm civet and human. Proc Natl Acad Sci U S A 2005;102:2430–5.
16. Wang M, Yan M, Xu H, et al. SARS-CoV infection in a restaurant from palm civet. Emerg Infect Dis 2005;11:1860–5.
17. Lau SK, Woo PC, Li KS, et al. Severe acute respiratory syndrome coronavirus-like virus in Chinese horseshoe bats. Proc Natl Acad Sci U S A 2005;102(39): 14040–5.
18. Li W, Shi Z, Yu M, et al. Bats are natural reservoirs of SARS-like coronaviruses. Science 2005;310:676–9.
19. Gu J, Korteweg C. Pathology and pathogenesis of severe acute respiratory syndrome. Am J Pathol 2007;170:1136–47.
20. Chan PK, To KF, Lo AW, et al. Persistent infection of SARS coronavirus in colonic cells in vitro. J Med Virol 2004;74:1–7.
21. Simmons G, Gosalia DN, Rennekamp AJ, et al. Inhibitors of cathepsin L prevent severe acute respiratory syndrome coronavirus entry. Proc Natl Acad Sci U S A 2005;102:11876–81.
22. Li W, Moore MJ, Vasilieva N, et al. Angiotensin-converting enzyme 2 is a functional receptor for the SARS coronavirus. Nature 2003;426:450–4.
23. Hamming I, Timens W, Bulthuis ML, et al. Tissue distribution of ACE2 protein, the functional receptor for SARS coronavirus. A first step in understanding SARS pathogenesis. J Pathol 2004;203:631–7.
24. Leung WK, To KF, Chan PK, et al. Enteric involvement of severe acute respiratory syndrome-associated coronavirus infection. Gastroenterology 2003;125: 1011–7.
25. Kuba K, Imai Y, Rao S, et al. A crucial role of angiotensin converting enzyme 2 (ACE2) in SARS coronavirus-induced lung injury. Nat Med 2005;11:875–9.
26. Law PT, Wong CH, Au TC, et al. The 3a protein of severe acute respiratory syndrome-associated coronavirus induces apoptosis in Vero E6 cells. J Gen Virol 2005;86(Pt 7):1921–30.

27. Tan YJ, Fielding BC, Goh PY, et al. Overexpression of 7a, a protein specifically encoded by the severe acute respiratory syndrome coronavirus, induces apoptosis via a caspase-dependent pathway. J Virol 2004;78:14043–7.
28. Nicholls JM, Poon LL, Lee KC, et al. Lung pathology of fatal severe acute respiratory syndrome. Lancet 2003;361:1773–8.
29. Franks TJ, Chong PY, Chui P, et al. Lung pathology of severe acute respiratory syndrome (SARS): a study of 8 autopsy cases from Singapore. Hum Pathol 2003;34:743–8.
30. Tse GM, To KF, Chan PK, et al. Pulmonary pathological features in coronavirus associated severe acute respiratory syndrome (SARS). J Clin Pathol 2004;57:260–5.
31. Haagmans BL, Kuiken T, Martina BE, et al. Pegulated interferon-a protects type I pneumocytes against SARS coronavirus infection in macaques. Nat Med 2004;10:290–3.
32. Peiris JS, Chu CM, Cheng VC, et al, HKU/UCH SARS Study Group. Clinical progression and viral load in a community outbreak of coronavirus-associated SARS pneumonia: a prospective study. Lancet 2003;361:1767–72.
33. Cheng VC, Hung IF, Tang BS, et al. Viral replication in the nasopharynx is associated with diarrhea in patients with severe acute respiratory syndrome. Clin Infect Dis 2004;38:467–75.
34. Wong CK, Lam CWK, Wu AK, et al. Plasma inflammatory cytokines and chemokines in severe acute respiratory syndrome. Clin Exp Immunol 2004;136:95–103.
35. Zhao J, Zhao J, Perlman S. T cell responses are required for protection from clinical disease and for virus clearance in severe acute respiratory syndrome coronavirus-infected mice. J Virol 2010;84(18):9318–25.
36. Channappanavar R, Fehr AR, Vijay R, et al. Dysregulated type I interferon and inflammatory monocyte-macrophage responses cause lethal pneumonia in SARS-CoV-infected mice. Cell Host Microbe 2016;19(2):181–93.
37. Totura AL, Whitmore A, Agnihothram S, et al. Toll-like receptor 3 signaling via TRIF contributes to a protective innate immune response to severe acute respiratory syndrome coronavirus infection. MBio 2015;6 [pii:e00638-15].
38. Wang Y, Liu L. The membrane protein of severe acute respiratory syndrome coronavirus functions as a novel cytosolic pathogen-associated molecular pattern to promote beta interferon induction via a Toll-like-receptor-related TRAF3-independent mechanism. MBio 2016;7(1) [pii:e01872-15].
39. Tang F, Liu W, Zhang F, et al. IL-12 RB1 genetic variants contribute to human susceptibility to severe acute respiratory syndrome infection among Chinese. PLoS One 2008;3(5):e2183.
40. Ip WK, Chan KH, Law HK, et al. Mannose-binding lectin in severe acute respiratory syndrome coronavirus infection. J Infect Dis 2005;191(10):1697–704.
41. Liu L, Wei Q, Lin Q, et al. Anti-spike IgG causes severe acute lung injury by skewing macrophage responses during acute SARS-CoV infection. JCI Insight 2019;4(4) [pii:123158].
42. Zhong NS, Zheng BJ, Li YM, et al. Epidemiology and cause of severe acute respiratory syndrome in Guangdong, People's Republic of China, in February 2003. Lancet 2003;362:1353–8.
43. Hui DS, Sung JJ. Severe acute respiratory syndrome. Chest 2003;124(1):12–5.
44. Peiris JS, Yuen KY, Osterhaus AD, et al. The severe acute respiratory syndrome. N Engl J Med 2003;349:2431–41.

45. Lee N, Hui DS, Wu A, et al. A major outbreak of severe acute respiratory syndrome in Hong Kong. N Engl J Med 2003;348:1986–94.
46. Wong RS, Hui DS. Index patient and SARS outbreak in Hong Kong. Emerg Infect Dis 2004;10:339–41.
47. Loon SC, Teoh SC, Oon LL, et al. The severe acute respiratory syndrome coronavirus in tears. Br J Ophthalmol 2004;88(7):861–3.
48. Yu IT, Wong TW, Chiu YL, et al. Temporal-spatial analysis of severe acute respiratory syndrome among hospital inpatients. Clin Infect Dis 2005;40:1237–43.
49. Xiao S, Li Y, Wong TW, et al. Role of fomites in SARS transmission during the largest hospital outbreak in Hong Kong. PLoS One 2017;12(7):e0181558.
50. Booth TF, Kournikakis B, Bastien N, et al. Detection of airborne severe acute respiratory syndrome (SARS) coronavirus and environmental contamination in SARS outbreak units. J Infect Dis 2005;191:1472–7.
51. WHO. Update 95-SARS: chronology of a serial killer. Available at: http://www.who.int/csr/don/2003_07_04/en. Accessed January 10, 2016.
52. Yu IT, Xie ZH, Tsoi KK, et al. Why did outbreaks of severe acute respiratory syndrome occur in some hospital wards but not in others? Clin Infect Dis 2007;44:1017–25.
53. Tran K, Cimon K, Severn M, et al. Aerosol generating procedures and risk of transmission of acute respiratory infections to healthcare workers: a systematic review. PLoS One 2012;7:e35797.
54. Chu CM, Cheng VC, Hung IF, et al. Viral load distribution in SARS outbreak. Emerg Infect Dis 2005;11:1882–6.
55. Yu IT, Li Y, Wong TW, et al. Evidence of airborne transmission of the severe acute respiratory syndrome virus. N Engl J Med 2004;350:1731–9.
56. Yu IT, Qiu H, Tse LA, et al. Severe acute respiratory syndrome beyond Amoy Gardens: completing the incomplete legacy. Clin Infect Dis 2014;58:683–6.
57. Lloyd-Smith JO, Schreiber SJ, Kopp PE, et al. Superspreading and the effect of individual variation on disease emergence. Nature 2005;438(7066):355–9.
58. Chiu WK, Cheung PCH, Ng KL, et al. Severe acute respiratory syndrome in children: experience in a regional hospital in Hong Kong. Pediatr Crit Care Med 2003;4:279–83.
59. Donnelly CA, Ghani AV, Leung GM, et al. Epidemiological determinants of spread of causal agent of severe acute respiratory syndrome in Hong Kong. Lancet 2003;361:1761–6.
60. Leung GM, Hedley AJ, Ho LM, et al. The epidemiology of severe acute respiratory syndrome in the 2003 Hong Kong epidemic: an analysis of all 1755 patients. Ann Intern Med 2004;141:662–73.
61. Booth CM, Matukas LM, Tomlinson GA, et al. Clinical features and short-term outcomes of 144 patients with SARS in the greater Toronto area. JAMA 2003;289:2801–9.
62. Chan JW, Ng CK, Chan YH, et al. Short term outcome and risk factors for adverse clinical outcomes in adults with severe acute respiratory syndrome (SARS). Thorax 2003;58:686–9.
63. Tsui PT, Kwok ML, Yuen H, et al. Severe acute respiratory syndrome: clinical outcome and prognostic correlates. Emerg Infect Dis 2003;9:1064–9.
64. Hung EC, Chim SS, Chan PK, et al. Detection of SARS coronavirus RNA in the cerebrospinal fluid of a patient with severe acute respiratory syndrome. Clin Chem 2003;49:2108–9.
65. Lau KK, Yu WC, Chu CM, et al. Possible central nervous system infection by SARS coronavirus. Emerg Infect Dis 2004;10:342–4.

66. Wong KC, Leung KS, Hui M. Severe acute respiratory syndrome (SARS) in a geriatric patient with a hip fracture. A case report. J Bone Joint Surg Am 2003;85A:1339–42.

67. Hon KL, Leung CW, Cheng WT, et al. Clinical presentations and outcome of severe acute respiratory syndrome in children. Lancet 2003;561:1701–3.

68. Wong SF, Chow KM, Leung TN, et al. Pregnancy and perinatal outcomes of women with severe acute respiratory syndrome. Am J Obstet Gynecol 2004; 191:292–7.

69. Leung GM, Lim WW, Ho LM, et al. Seroprevalence of IgG antibodies to SARS-coronavirus in asymptomatic or subclinical population groups. Epidemiol Infect 2006;134:211–21.

70. Hui DS, Wong PC, Wang C. SARS: clinical features and diagnosis. Respirology 2003;8(Suppl):S20–4.

71. Hui DS, Wong KT, Antonio GE, et al. Severe acute respiratory syndrome: correlation between clinical outcome and radiologic features. Radiology 2004;233: 579–85.

72. Pitzer VE, Leung GM, Lipstich M. Estimating variability in the transmission of severe acute respiratory syndrome to household contacts in Hong Kong, China. Am J Epidemiol 2007;166:355–63.

73. Poon LL, Chan KH, Wong OK, et al. Early diagnosis of SARS coronavirus infection by real time RT-PCR. J Clin Virol 2003;28:233–8.

74. Ng EK, Hui DS, Chan KC, et al. Quantitative analysis and prognostic implication of SARS coronavirus in the plasma and serum of patients with severe acute respiratory syndrome. Clin Chem 2003;49:1976–80.

75. Ng EK, Ng PC, Hon KL, et al. Serial analysis of the plasma concentration of SARS coronavirus RNA in pediatric patients with severe acute respiratory syndrome. Clin Chem 2003;49:2085–8.

76. Lee N, Chan PK, Ip M, et al. Anti-SARS-CoV IgG response in relation to disease severity of severe acute respiratory syndrome. J Clin Virol 2006;35:179–84.

77. Tang F, Quan Y, Xin ZT, et al. Lack of peripheral memory B cell responses in recovered patients with severe acute respiratory syndrome: a six-year follow-up study. J Immunol 2011;186:7264–8.

78. Wong RS, Wu A, To KF, et al. Haematological manifestations in patients with severe acute respiratory syndrome: retrospective analysis. Br Med J 2003;326: 1358–62.

79. Wong WM, Ho JC, Hung IF, et al. Temporal patterns of hepatic dysfunction and disease severity in patients with SARS. JAMA 2003;290:2663–5.

80. Wong KT, Antonio GE, Hui DS, et al. Thin section CT of severe acute respiratory syndrome: evaluation of 73 patients exposed to or with the disease. Radiology 2003;228:395–400.

81. Gomersall CD, Joynt GM, Lam P, et al. Short-term outcome of critically ill patients with severe acute respiratory syndrome. Intensive Care Med 2004;30: 381–7.

82. Shek CC, Ng PC, Fung GP, et al. Infants born to mothers with severe acute respiratory syndrome. Pediatrics 2003;112:e254–6.

83. Sung JJ, Wu A, Joynt GM, et al. Severe acute respiratory syndrome: report of treatment and outcome after a major outbreak. Thorax 2004;59:414–20.

84. Chu CM, Cheng VC, Hung IF, et al, HKU/UCH SARS Study Group. Role of lopinavir/ritonavir in the treatment of SARS: initial virological and clinical findings. Thorax 2004;59:252–6.

85. Chan KS, Lai ST, Chu CM, et al. Treatment of severe acute respiratory syndrome with lopinavir/ritonavir: a multicenter retrospective matched cohort study. Hong Kong Med J 2003;9:399–406.
86. Loutfy MR, Blatt LM, Siminovitch KA, et al. Interferon Alfacon-1 plus corticosteroids in severe acute respiratory syndrome. A preliminary study. JAMA 2003; 290:3222–8.
87. Fisman DN. Hemophagocytic syndrome and infection. Emerg Infect Dis 2000;6: 601–8.
88. Tsang OT, Chau TN, Choi KW, et al. Coronavirus-positive nasopharyngeal aspirate as predictor for severe acute respiratory syndrome mortality. Emerg Infect Dis 2003;9:1381–7.
89. Wang H, Ding Y, Li X, et al. Fatal aspergillosis in a patient with SARS who was treated with corticosteroids. N Engl J Med 2003;349:507–8.
90. Griffith JF, Antonio GE, Kumta SM, et al. Osteonecrosis of hip and knee in patients with severe acute respiratory syndrome treated with steroids. Radiology 2005;235:168–75.
91. Lee N, Allen Chan KC, Hui DS, et al. Effects of early corticosteroid treatment on plasma SARS-associated coronavirus RNA concentrations in adult patients. J Clin Virol 2004;31:304–9.
92. Stockman LJ, Bellamy R, Garner P. SARS: systematic review of treatment effects. PLoS Med 2006;3:e343.
93. Cheng Y, Wong R, Soo YO, et al. Use of convalescent plasma therapy in SARS patients in Hong Kong. Eur J Clin Microbiol Infect Dis 2005;24:44–6.
94. Soo Y, Cheng Y, Wong R, et al. Retrospective comparison of convalescent plasma with continuing high-dose methylprednisolone treatment in SARS patients. Clin Microbiol Infect 2004;10:676–8.
95. Mair-Jenkins J, Saavedra-Campos M, Baillie JK, et al, Convalescent Plasma Study Group. The effectiveness of convalescent plasma and hyperimmune immunoglobulin for the treatment of severe acute respiratory infections of viral etiology: a systematic review and exploratory meta-analysis. J Infect Dis 2015;211:80–90.
96. Gao W, Tamin A, Soloff A, et al. Effects of a SARS-associated coronavirus vaccine in monkeys. Lancet 2003;362:1895–6.
97. Zhao P, Ke JS, Qin ZL, et al. DNA vaccine of SARS-CoV S gene induces antibody response in mice. Acta Biochim Biophys Sin (Shanghai) 2004;36:37–41.
98. Yang ZY, Kong WP, Huang Y, et al. A DNA vaccine induces SARS coronavirus neutralization and protective immunity in mice. Nature 2004;428:561–4.
99. Zhong NS, Zeng GQ. Pandemic planning in China: applying lessons from severe acute respiratory syndrome. Respirology 2008;13(Suppl 1):S33–5.
100. Seto WH, Conly JM, Pessoa-Silva CL, et al. Infection prevention and control measures for acute respiratory infections in healthcare settings: an update. East Mediterr Health J 2013;19(Suppl 1):S39–47.

The Middle East Respiratory Syndrome (MERS)

Esam I. Azhar, PhD, FRCP[a],*,
David S.C. Hui, MBBS, MD(UNSW), FRACP, FRCP(Lond, Edin, Glasg), FHKCP, FHKAM(Med)[b],
Ziad A. Memish, MD, FRCP[c,d], Christian Drosten, PhD[e],
Alimuddin Zumla, MBChB, MSc, PhD, MD, FRCP(Lond), FRCP(Edin), FRCPath(UK), FAAS[f]

KEYWORDS

- Middle East respiratory syndrome coronavirus • MERS-CoV
- Epidemiology diagnosis • Treatment

KEY POINTS

- The Middle East respiratory syndrome (MERS) is a novel lethal zoonotic disease of humans endemic to The Middle East, caused by the MERS coronavirus (MERS-CoV).
- Humans are thought to acquire MERS-CoV though contact with camels or camel products.
- MERS carries a 35% mortality rate. There is no specific treatment for MERS. Person-to-person spread causes hospital and household outbreaks of MERS-CoV.
- Millions of visitors travel to Saudi Arabia each year from across the world, thus watchful surveillance and a high degree of clinical awareness and early diagnosis with rapid implementation of infection control measures in returning travelers is important.

Disclosures: Authors declare no conflicts of interests.
Author Declarations: All authors have an academic interest in coronaviruses.
Author Roles: All authors contributed equally to writing this article.
A. Zumla and C. Drosten are members of the PANDORA-ID-NET Consortium supported by a Grant RIA2016E-1609) funded by the European and Developing Countries Clinical Trials Partnership (EDCTP2) under Horizon 2020, the European Union's Framework Programme for Research and Innovation. A. Zumla is in receipt of a National Institutes of Health Research (NIHR) senior investigator award.
 a Special Infectious Agents Unit, King Fahd Medical Research Centre, Faculty of Applied Medical Sciences, King Abdulaziz University, Jeddah, Saudi Arabia; b Department of Medicine and Therapeutics, Stanley Ho Center for Emerging Infectious Diseases, The Chinese University of Hong Kong, Shatin, New Territories, Hong Kong; c College of Medicine, Alfaisal University, Riyadh, Saudi Arabia; d Infectious Diseases Division, Department of Medicine and Research, Prince Mohamed Bin Abdulaziz Hospital, Ministry of Health, Riyadh, Saudi Arabia; e Institute of Virology, Campus Charité Mitte, Charité - Universitätsmedizin Berlin, Berlin Institute of Health, Berlin, Germany; f Center for Clinical Microbiology, University College London, Royal Free Campus 2nd Floor, Rowland Hill Street, London NW3 2PF, United Kingdom
* Corresponding author.
E-mail address: eazhar@kau.edu.sa

Infect Dis Clin N Am 33 (2019) 891–905
https://doi.org/10.1016/j.idc.2019.08.001
0891-5520/19/© 2019 Elsevier Inc. All rights reserved.

INTRODUCTION

The Middle East respiratory syndrome coronavirus (MERS-CoV) is a new zoonotic human viral pathogen endemic to the Middle East.[1–3] It was identified in 2012 in a lung sample of a 60-year-old patient who had died of respiratory failure in Jeddah, Saudi Arabia.[4] The disease caused by MERS-CoV is named Middle East respiratory syndrome (MERS). MERS has remained on the radar of global public health authorities because of recurrent nosocomial and community outbreaks, and its association with severe disease and high mortality rates.[1–3] Intermittent sporadic cases, community clusters, and nosocomial outbreaks of MERS-CoV have continued to occur in Saudi Arabia.[1] MERS-CoV remains on the World Health Organization (WHO) Blueprint list of priority pathogens[5] because it remains a persistent threat to global health security.

EPIDEMIC POTENTIAL AND GLOBAL SPREAD

Cases of MERS from outside the Middle East have been reported from all continents, and have been linked with travel to the Middle East.[1] Nosocomial outbreaks of MERS-CoV infection accounts for approximately 40% of MERS-CoV cases globally. Large health care–associated outbreaks of MERS-CoV have occurred in Saudi Arabia, United Arab Emirates, and the Republic of Korea.[6–10] From June 1 to July 31, 2015, MERS-CoV caused the largest outbreak outside the Arabian Peninsula in the Republic of Korea, resulting in 186 confirmed MERS cases with 38 deaths.[7–9] This occurred when a Korean traveler returning from a trip to Qatar, United Arab Emirates (UAE), Saudi Arabia, and Bahrain became ill with a respiratory illness and visited several hospitals before finally being diagnosed as having MERS-CoV infection on May 20, 2015, at Samsung Medical Center.[7–9] This resulted in 186 people, including 25 health care workers (HCWs), contracting MERS-CoV infection; 181 of 186 cases were associated with hospital transmission. This outbreak clearly illustrated the epidemic potential of MERS-CoV, spreading person-to-person.

EPIDEMIOLOGY

The number of MERS-CoV cases reported to the WHO have steadily increased since the first report of MERS-CoV in September 2012.[4] MERS-CoV cases continue to be reported from the community and hospitals across the Arabian Peninsula. As of July 31st 2019, 2458 cases of laboratory-confirmed MERS cases were reported to WHO. Of these, there were 848 deaths (34% mortality)[1] (**Fig. 1**). Approximately 80% of human cases have been reported by Saudi Arabia. Twenty-seven countries have reported cases of MERS.[11] Countries in or near the Arabian Peninsula that report MERS cases are Bahrain, Iran, Jordan, Kuwait, Lebanon, Oman, Qatar, Saudi Arabia, UAE, and Yemen. Cases identified outside the Middle East are usually in travelers who were infected in the Middle East and then traveled to areas outside the Middle East. Countries outside the Arabian Peninsula that have reported travel-associated MERS cases are Algeria, Austria, China, Egypt, France, Germany, Greece, Italy, Malaysia, Netherlands, Philippines, Republic of Korea, Thailand, Tunisia, Turkey, United Kingdom, and the United States.[1]

SOURCE OF PRIMARY HUMAN MIDDLE EAST RESPIRATORY SYNDROME CORONAVIRUS INFECTIONS

The exact mode of transmission of MERS-CoV to humans is not yet accurately defined. Epidemiologic, genetic, and phenotypic studies indicate that dromedary

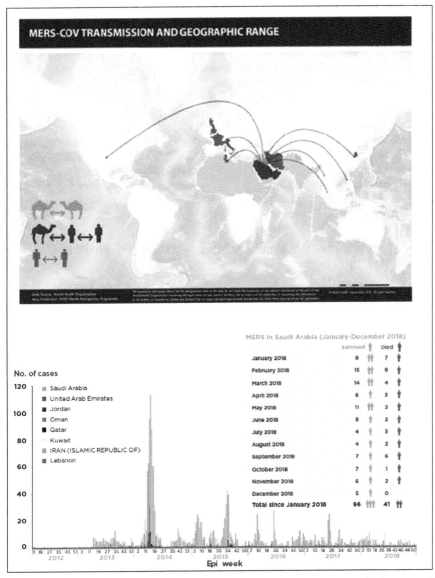

Fig. 1. Geographic distribution of MERS reported to WHO (2012–2018). (*From* WHO 2019.Middle East respiratory syndrome coronavirus (MERS-CoV. https://www.who.int/emergencies/mers-cov/en/; with permission.)

camels appear to be the main intermediary reservoirs of MERS-CoV.[12–15] Camels are assumed to be intermediary host species for the MERS-CoV, although the exact source and the mode of transmission in many primary MERS cases remain unclear. Antibodies to MERS-CoV were detected in serum and milk collected from 33 camels in Qatar in April 2014. In one study, active virus shedding in nasal secretions and in feces was observed for 7 of 12 camels.[13] MERS-CoV survives for prolonged periods in camel's milk but viable virus became undetectable after pasteurization at 63°C for

30 minutes.[16] MERS-CoV has been detected in camels from Kenya; 792 of 1163 camels studied had enzyme-linked immunosorbent assay (ELISA) seropositivity of which 11 camel nasal swabs were positive for MERS-CoV by quantitative reverse-transcription polymerase chain reaction (RT-PCR).[17] A study of humans in Kenya detected MERS-CoV neutralizing antibodies in persons living in rural areas, although no human MERS cases have been detected yet.[18]

The primary source of human MERS-CoV infections remains unknown. There are no definitive data on the epidemiologic link between human MERS-CoV infections and bats. Only one fragment of MERS-CoV with close matching to a human isolate of MERS-CoV was found in a study of more than 1000 samples from *Taphozous* bats.[19] Phylogenetic analysis of an MERS-related CoV identified from a *Neoromicia capensis* bat sampled in South Africa supports the hypothesis that bats are the evolu-tionary source of MERS-CoV but not a zoonotic reservoir.[20] To date, no sustained human-to-human transmission has been documented, although tertiary and quater-nary spread did occur in the Korean outbreak.[8,9]

RISK FACTORS FOR PRIMARY MIDDLE EAST RESPIRATORY SYNDROME CORONAVIRUS INFECTION

Several independent risk factors for increased susceptibility to acquiring primary MERS-CoV infections have been identified: direct dromedary exposure in the fortnight before illness onset, direct physical contact with dromedary camels during the previ-ous 6 months, diabetes mellitus, and heart disease. Risk factors for MERS-CoV infec-tion among camel workers include milking camels, contact with camel waste, poor hand hygiene before and after animal tasks and training activities, and workers with respiratory symptoms requiring overnight stay in hospital.[21] Viral RNA sequencing has confirmed camel to human transmission of MERS-CoV[22–24] after known exposure to the infected camels. Recent data suggest that although MERS-CoV is widespread among dromedary camels in the Middle East and Africa, zoonotic transmission of MERS-CoV from camels to humans is relatively uncommon, and human disease is not directly proportional to potential exposure. MERS-CoV does not transmit easily from person-to-person unless there is close contact, such as occurs when providing care to a patient in the household[25] or nosocomial setting when the diagnosis of MERS-CoV has not yet been recognized and there are lapses in instituting infection control measures.[2,3,6,7]

CLINICAL FEATURES

The symptoms, signs, laboratory, and imaging abnormalities associated with MERS-CoV infection are not MERS-specific and are like other respiratory tract infections (RTIs)[2,3,7,26–28] (**Box 1, Table 1**). The clinical manifestations of MERS-CoV infections range from asymptomatic infection to mild, moderate, and severe disease, often complicated by severe pneumonia, acute respiratory distress syndrome (ARDS), sep-tic shock, and multiorgan failure. The incubation period is between 2 and 14 days. Mild cases can have low-grade fever, chills, runny nose, dry cough, sore throat, and myalgia. Some patients have gastrointestinal symptoms, such as nausea, vomiting, and diarrhea. Fever may be absent in up to 15% of hospitalized cases. Laboratory ab-normalities include cytopenias and elevated transaminases (see **Table 1**). Coinfec-tions with other respiratory viruses and bacterial pathogens have been reported. Up to half of MERS cases can have acute kidney injury and one-third of very ill patients have gastrointestinal symptoms.

Box 1
Risk factors for nosocomial Middle East respiratory syndrome coronavirus (MERS-CoV) outbreaks

- Lack of awareness of the possibility of MERS in febrile patients presenting to health care facilities
- Overcrowded emergency departments where patients with MERS first present
- Exposure of health care workers and other patients to symptomatic MERS patients
- Poor compliance with infection control measures: (1) hand hygiene, (2) droplet and contact precautions, (3) inadequate environmental cleaning
- Inadequate compliance with appropriate Personal Protective Equipment
- Lack of proper isolation room facilities
- Aerosol-generating procedures on patients with MERS
- Crowded inpatient wards, including nonessential staff and visitors (family and friends)

Data from Refs.[1–3,7,8,47,51]

Severe illness can cause respiratory failure that requires mechanical ventilation and support in an intensive care unit (ICU). There is rapid progression to ARDS and multisystem disease and organ failure with a median of 2 days from hospitalization to ICU admission.[29,30] MERS-CoV infection appears to cause more severe disease in older people, people with weakened immune systems, and those with chronic diseases, such as renal disease, cancer, chronic lung disease, and diabetes.[2,3]

MORTALITY AND RISK FACTORS

A case study of 660 patients with MERS in Saudi Arabia seen between December 2, 2014, and November 12, 2016, found that 3-day, 30-day, and overall mortality were 13.8%, 28.3%, and 29.8%.[31] Patients older than 60 were more likely to die (45.2% mortality) from their infections than were younger patients (20%). Patients with preexisting medical comorbidities tend to have more severe disease and higher mortality rates.

Factors associated with poor management outcomes (severe disease or death) in patients with MERS include old age, male gender, comorbid preexisting illnesses (such as obesity, diabetes mellitus, heart and lung disease, and immunocompromised states), low serum albumin, concomitant infections, and positive plasma MERS-CoV RNA.[27–32] DPP4 receptors have been shown to be upregulated in the lungs of smokers, and this may explain why patients with comorbid lung diseases are prone to severe illness.[33]

MAKING AN EARLY DIAGNOSIS OF MIDDLE EAST RESPIRATORY SYNDROME CORONAVIRUS INFECTION

Many cases of MERS-CoV can be easily missed because the presentation is that of any community-acquired pneumonia or other respiratory illness caused by influenza A and B respiratory syncytial virus, parainfluenza viruses, rhinoviruses, adenoviruses, enteroviruses (eg, EVD68), human metapneumovirus, and endemic human coronaviruses (ie, HCoV-HKU1, -OC43, -NL63, and -229E).[2] Most nosocomial outbreaks of MERS-CoV have been associated with a delay in diagnosis.

A history of travel to the Middle East is important for patients presenting in non-Middle Eastern countries with a febrile illness.[1,2,33,34]

Table 1
Clinical and laboratory features of patients with Middle East respiratory syndrome

Clinical/Laboratory Feature(s)	
Date of first MERS case (place) (retrospective analyses)	April 2012 (Zarqa, Jordan) June 2012 (Jeddah, Kingdom of Saudi Arabia)
Incubation period	Mean: 5.2 d (95% confidence interval 1.9–14.7) Range: 2–14 d
Age group	
Adults	Adults (98%)
Children	Children (2%)
Age, y, range, median	Range:1–94; Median: 50
Gender	Male: 64.5%, Female: 35.5%
Presenting symptoms	Estimated proportion of cases, %
Fever >38°C	98
Chills/rigors	87
Cough • Dry • Productive	83 56 44
Shortness of breath	72
Myalgia	32
Malaise	38
Nausea	21
Vomiting	21
Diarrhea	26
Sore throat	14
Hemoptysis	17
Headache	11
Rhinorrhoea	6
Comorbidities (eg, obesity, diabetes, cardiac disease and lung disease), %	76
Laboratory results, %	
Chest radiograph and computed tomography abnormalities	90–100
Leukopenia (<4.0 × 10^9/L)	14
Lymphopenia (<1.5 × 10^9/L)	32
Thrombocytopenia <140 × 10^9/L)	36
Elevated lactate dehydrogenase	48
Elevated alanine transaminase	11
Elevated aspartate transaminase	14
Risk factors associated with poor outcome (severe disease or death)	Any immunocompromised state, comorbid illness, concomitant infections, low albumin, age ≥65 y
Mortality, %	
Case fatality rate (CFR), overall	34%
CFR in patients with comorbidities	60

Data from Refs.[1–3,7]

RISK FACTORS FOR NOSOCOMIAL MIDDLE EAST RESPIRATORY SYNDROME CORONAVIRUS OUTBREAKS

Early and accurate diagnosis of MERS-CoV infection is important for clinical management, and instituting infection control and epidemiologic control measures of MERS-CoV infections. Thus, a high degree of clinical awareness of the possibility of MERS-CoV infection is required in all health care settings so that an accurate diagnosis can be made and infection control measures instituted as soon as the diagnosis is entertained clinically.[33,34]

CLINICAL SAMPLES FOR LABORATORY TESTING

Upper respiratory tract samples have yielded negative results in some symptomatic close contacts of confirmed cases who later developed pneumonia and tested positive on lower respiratory specimens. For laboratory testing, WHO[35] recommends that both upper respiratory tract specimens (nasopharyngeal and oropharyngeal) and lower respiratory tract specimens (sputum, tracheal aspirate, or lavage) are collected whenever possible. Lower respiratory specimens have a higher diagnostic value than upper respiratory tract specimens for detecting MERS-CoV infection.[36] Sputum, endotracheal aspirate, or bronchoalveolar lavage should be collected for MERS-CoV testing when possible. If patients do not have signs or symptoms of lower respiratory tract disease and the collection of lower tract specimens is not possible or clinically indicated, upper respiratory tract specimens, such as a nasopharyngeal aspirate or combined nasopharyngeal and oropharyngeal swabs, should be collected.

When taking nasopharyngeal and oropharyngeal specimens, Dacron or rayon swabs specifically designed for collecting specimens for virology must be used. These swab kits should contain virus transport medium. The nasopharyngeal and oropharyngeal swabs should be placed in the same tube to increase the viral load.[35,36] A single negative test result does not exclude the diagnosis, and repeat sampling and testing is strongly recommended. To confirm clearance of the virus, respiratory samples should be collected sequentially (every 2–4 days) over ensuing days until there are 2 consecutive negative results in clinically recovered persons. Specimens for MERS-CoV detection should reach the laboratory as soon as possible after collection and be delivered promptly to the laboratory, shipped at 4°C if possible. When there is likely to be a delay of more than 72 hours in specimens reaching the laboratory, it is recommended that the specimens are frozen at −20°C or ideally −80°C and shipped on dry ice. It is important to avoid repeated freezing and thawing of specimens.[35,36]

LABORATORY TESTS FOR MIDDLE EAST RESPIRATORY SYNDROME CORONAVIRUS

Accurate laboratory molecular diagnostic tests are available using highly sensitive and specific real-time RT-PCR (rRT-PCR). Three rRT-PCR assays for routine detection of MERS-CoV have been developed targeting upstream of the E protein gene (*upE*) and the open reading frame 1b (ORF 1b), and ORF 1a.[35–37] The assay for the upE target is considered highly sensitive and is recommended for screening, with the ORF 1a assay considered of equal sensitivity. To date, these rRT-PCR assays have shown no cross-reactivity with other respiratory viruses, including human coronaviruses, and were suitable to detect all known MERS-CoV strains in humans and dromedary camels.

Laboratory confirmation of MERS-CoV infection[37] is obtained by detection of the virus by (1) MERS-CoV–specific nucleic acid amplification test with up to 2 separate targets and/or sequencing; (2) virus isolation in tissue culture; or (3) serology on serum tested in a WHO collaborating center with established testing methods.[35,36] A case confirmed by serology requires demonstration of seroconversion in 2 samples ideally taken at least 14 days apart, by a screening (ELISA, immunofluorescence assay) and a neutralization assay.

Serologic tests such as ELISAs for MERS-CoV are being developed and refined for surveillance or investigational purposes.[36,38] An indirect ELISA has been developed for sero-epidemiological testing and surveillance purposes and requires evaluation in field studies.[39]

MERS-CoV testing must be performed in appropriately equipped biosafety laboratories by staff trained in the relevant technical and safety procedures. National or WHO guidelines on laboratory biosafety should be followed in all circumstances.[40]

CLINICAL MANAGEMENT OF MIDDLE EAST RESPIRATORY SYNDROME CASES

The management of patients with MERS is largely symptomatic and supportive and aims to reduce the risk of complications, such as secondary infections, and renal and respiratory failure.[1–3] Seriously ill patients should receive intensive care.

Although a range of existing and developmental treatments may be useful[41] (**Box 2**), currently there are no specific treatments to treat MERS-CoV. A range of treatments such as lopinavir/ritonavir, pegylated interferon (IFN)-α2a, and ribavirin have been used empirically for serious cases of MERS but there is no accurate evidence base that any of them improve treatment outcomes. Treatment with either lopinavir/ritonavir or IFN-β1b in the marmoset model was associated with improved clinical, radiological, and pathologic outcomes with lower viral loads in comparison with no treatment, whereas mycophenolic acid alone increased viral loads and fatality.[42] Macrolide therapy is commonly started before the patient arrives in the ICU in Saudi Arabia. A retrospective study of 136 patients with MERS found that macrolide therapy is not associated with a reduction in mortality or improvement in MERS-CoV RNA clearance.[43]

Currently there is an ongoing randomized controlled trial in progress in the Kingdom of Saudi Arabia comparing lopinavir/ritonavir, recombinant IFN-β1b, and standard supportive care against placebo and standard supportive care in patients with laboratory-confirmed MERS requiring hospital admission.[44] Systemic corticosteroids were shown to delay viral clearance in critically ill patients with MERS-CoV infection.[30] A range of anti–MERS-CoV drugs and host-directed therapies are being considered as potential therapies for MERS-CoV.[41] Properly designed studies are needed to answer several knowledge gaps for us to understand the disease pathogenesis, viral kinetics, mode of disease transmission, and the intermediary source of MERS to guide infection control prevention measures and treatment responses in MERS-CoV infection.

INFECTION CONTROL MEASURES IN HOSPITALS WHEN MIDDLE EAST RESPIRATORY SYNDROME CORONAVIRUS INFECTION IS SUSPECTED

The main infection prevention and control measures for managing patients with MERS are well documented from the severe acute respiratory syndrome (SARS) epidemic.[45] Early identification and isolation of suspected or confirmed cases and ongoing surveillance are key to preventing nosocomial spread. Droplet precaution (wearing a surgical mask within 1 m of the patient) and contact and droplet precautions (wearing gown, gloves, mask, and eye protection on entering the room and removing them on leaving) must be used when caring for patients with suspected MERS-CoV infection.[46] HCWs should implement airborne

---

Box 2
Potential treatments for MERS-CoV infection

- Antivirals
  - Ribavirin monotherapy[a] (± interferon)
  - Human immunodeficiency virus protease inhibitors (lopinavir,[b] nelfinavir)

- Repurposed drugs:
  - Cyclophilin inhibitors (ciclosporin, alisporivir)
  - Chloroquine (active in vitro)
  - Mycophenolic acid
  - Nitazoxanide

- Interferons[b]:
  - Interferon alfa
  - Interferon beta

- Neutralizing antibodies[b]:
  - Convalescent plasma
  - Polyclonal human immunoglobulin from transgenic cows
  - Equine F(ab')2 antibody fragments
  - Camel antibodies
  - Anti-S monoclonal antibodies

- Recombinant human mannose-binding lectin

- Small interfering RNA to key MERS-CoV genes

[a] Risks likely to exceed benefits.
[b] Treatment benefits likely to exceed risks.
Adapted from Zumla A, Hui DS, Perlman S. Middle East respiratory syndrome. Lancet. 2015;386(9997):995-1007; and Zumla A, Chan JF, Azhar EI, Hui DS, Yuen KY. Coronaviruses - drug discovery and therapeutic options. Nat Rev Drug Discov. 2016 May;15(5):327-47.

---

precautions and wear a fit-tested particulate respirator (eg, The US National Institute for Occupational Safety and Health–approved N95 filtering facepiece respirator [FFR] or an European norms [EN] approved FFP2-FFR or FFP3-FFR) when performing aerosol-generating procedures for infected and potentially infected patients. Avoiding aerosolizing procedures in crowded hospital emergency or inpatient medical wards that do not have adequate infection control measures in place may decrease MERS-CoV human-to-human spread and environmental contamination. It is also prudent to use higher levels of protection for HCWs who extend close contact with patients with MERS and those who are exposed to aerosols from high-risk procedures.

Higher levels of ventilation (more air changes, higher air flow and velocity), greater effort to prevent air dispersion beyond the point of generation (enclosure, using capture ventilation), and higher levels of personal protective equipment (more coverage, more protective types of respiratory protection) are all necessary. To reduce room contamination in the hospital setting, the application of a minimum room ventilation rate of 12 air changes per hour in a single room or at least 160 L/s per patient in facilities with natural ventilation is recommended when caring for patients receiving mechanical ventilation and during aerosol-generating procedures.

DECREASING RISK OF TRANSMISSION

Instituting appropriate infection control measures as soon as the diagnosis is considered is critical to preventing spread, especially in hospitals. Because symptoms and signs of RTIs are nonspecific, it is difficult to diagnose primary cases of patients with MERS-CoV infection. Infection prevention and control measures are important to prevent the spread of MERS-CoV within households, the community, and in health care facilities.

TRANSMISSION IN HOSPITALS

Human-to-human transmission occurs within communities, households, and, more strikingly, within hospital settings. Health care–associated outbreaks have occurred in several countries, with the largest outbreaks seen in Saudi Arabia, UAE, and the Republic of Korea. Several outbreak studies have shown that MERS-CoV does not appear to transmit easily from person-to-person unless there is close contact, such as providing clinical care.[2,7,47–52] MERS-CoV has been identified in clinical specimens, such as sputum, endotracheal aspirate, bronchoalveolar lavage, nasal or nasopharyngeal swabs, urine, feces, blood, and lung tissue.[2,3] The modes of MERS-CoV transmission through direct or indirect contact, airborne, droplet, or ingestion have yet to be defined.

The upsurge in the number of human infections due to MERS-CoV over the past few years in health care facilities in the Middle East and South Korea[2,3,47,48] were related to low awareness for MERS-CoV infection resulting in nosocomial outbreaks involving existing hospitalized patients, outpatients, visitors, and HCWs within health care facilities with overcrowding, lack of isolation room facilities, environmental contamination, and inadequate infection control measures without any significant change in the transmissibility of the virus. HCWs should always undertake standard precautions consistently with all patients with fever and symptoms of RTIs. Droplet precautions should be added to the standard precautions when providing care to these patients, and contact precautions and eye protection should be included when caring for probable or confirmed cases of MERS-CoV. Airborne precautions are important when performing aerosol-generating procedures.

HOUSEHOLD TRANSMISSION

Human-to-human transmission in the community or in those living in large households and family compounds has been described.[25,50–54] An investigation of 280 household contacts of 26 index MERS-CoV–infected Saudi Arabian patients, with follow-up serologic analysis in 44 contacts performed in 2014 to determine the rate of "silent or subclinical" secondary infection after exposure to primary cases of MERS-CoV infection, found there were 12 probable cases of secondary transmission (4%; 95% confidence interval, 2–7).[51] There have been several reports of MERS-CoV carriage after exposure to patients with MERS. Apparently healthy household contacts have been found to have MERS-CoV in their upper respiratory tract. Low levels of MERS-CoV RNA have been detected in asymptomatic HCWs from nosocomial MERS-CoV outbreaks in a Jeddah hospital.[52] Of 79 relatives who were investigated after MERS-CoV infections affected an extended family in Saudi Arabia in 2014, 19 (24%) were MERS-CoV positive; 11 were hospitalized, and 2 died.

HEALTH CARE WORKER AND COMMUNITY EDUCATION

In MERS-CoV endemic countries where MERS-CoV cases can occur in the community and households, educational awareness of MERS-CoV and MERS prevention measures may reduce the risk of household transmission and prevent community clusters.[53,54] Regular hand washing before and after touching camels and avoiding contact with sick camels is advised. People should avoid drinking raw camel milk or camel urine or eating camel meat that has not been properly cooked. Persons who have diabetes, kidney disease, chronic lung disease, or cancer or are on immunosuppressive treatment are at high risk of developing severe MERS-CoV disease, thus they should avoid close contact with camels and bats.

WHO does not advise special screening for MERS-CoV at points of entry after return from the Middle East nor does it currently recommend the application of any travel or trade restrictions.[1] Persons with a history of travel from or to the Arabian Peninsula within 10 days of developing symptoms of an acute respiratory infection involving fever of 38°C or more, or cough with radiologic pulmonary changes at presentation should alert the physician to the possibility of MERS-CoV infection.[55]

MIDDLE EAST RESPIRATORY SYNDROME CORONAVIRUS VACCINES

No vaccines are yet available that can protect against MERS-CoV infection. There are several groups working on developing a vaccine using a variety of platforms and some have shown efficacy in animal models.[56]

SUMMARY

MERS-CoV remains an important public health risk and possible consequences of further international spread could be serious in view of the patterns of nosocomial transmission within health care facilities. With 10 million pilgrims visiting Saudi Arabia each year from 182 countries to perform the Hajj and Umrah pilgrimages,[57] watchful surveillance by public health systems and a high degree of clinical awareness of the possibility of MERS-CoV infection is essential.[58-61] Nosocomial transmission is often due to a delayed diagnosis of MERS-CoV infection in a patient shedding MERS-CoV in a crowded health care setting such as an inpatient ward, emergency department, or renal dialysis unit. Early recognition of cases, improved compliance with internationally recommended infection control protocols, and rapid implementation of infection control measures are required to prevent health care facility–associated outbreaks of MERS-CoV.

REFERENCES

1. WHO. Middle East respiratory syndrome coronavirus (MERS-CoV). 2019. Available at: https://www.who.int/emergencies/mers-cov/en/. Accessed June 1, 2019.
2. Zumla A, Hui DS, Perlman S. Middle East respiratory syndrome. Lancet 2015; 386(9997):995–1007.
3. Arabi YM, Balkhy HH, Hayden FG, et al. Middle East Respiratory syndrome. N Engl J Med 2017;376(6):584–94.
4. Zaki AM, van Boheemen S, Bestebroer TM, et al. Isolation of a novel coronavirus from a man with pneumonia in Saudi Arabia. N Engl J Med 2012;367:1814–20.
5. WHO. List of priority Blueprint diseases. Available at: https://www.who.int/blueprint/priority-diseases/en/. Accessed January 20, 2019.
6. Alanazi KH, Killerby ME, Biggs HM, et al. Scope and extent of healthcare-associated Middle East respiratory syndrome coronavirus transmission during two contemporaneous outbreaks in Riyadh, Saudi Arabia, 2017. Infect Control Hosp Epidemiol 2019;40(1):79–88.
7. Oh MD, Choe PG, Oh HS, et al. Middle East respiratory syndrome coronavirus superspreading event involving 81 persons, Korea 2015. J Korean Med Sci 2015;30(11):1701–5.

Azhar et al

8. Oh MD, Park WB, Choe PG, et al. Viral load kinetics of MERS coronavirus infection. N Engl J Med 2016;375(13):1303–5.

9. Kang CK, Song KH, Choe PG, et al. Clinical and epidemiologic characteristics of spreaders of Middle East respiratory syndrome coronavirus during the 2015 outbreak in Korea. J Korean Med Sci 2017;32(5):744–9.

10. Hui DS, Azhar EI, Kim YJ, et al. Middle East respiratory syndrome coronavirus: risk factors and determinants of primary, household, and nosocomial transmission. Lancet Infect Dis 2018;18(8):e217–27.

11. WHO. MERS Global summary and assessment of risk. Available at: https://www.who.int/csr/disease/coronavirus_infections/risk-assessment-august-2018.pdf. Accessed January 21, 2019.

12. Reusken CB, Haagmans BL, Müller MA, et al. Middle East respiratory syndrome coronavirus neutralising serum antibodies in dromedary camels: a comparative serological study. Lancet Infect Dis 2013;13(10):859–66.

13. Reusken CB, Farag EA, Jonges M, et al. Middle East respiratory syndrome coronavirus (MERS-CoV) RNA and neutralising antibodies in milk collected according to local customs from dromedary camels, Qatar, 2014. Euro Surveill 2014;19(23) [pii:20829].

14. Drosten C, Kellam P, Memish ZA. Evidence for camel-to-human transmission of MERS coronavirus. N Engl J Med 2014;371(14):1359–60.

15. Conzade R, Grant R, Malik MR, et al. Reported direct and indirect contact with dromedary camels among laboratory-confirmed MERS-CoV cases. Viruses 2018;10(8) [pii:E425].

16. van Doremalen N, Bushmaker T, Munster VJ. Stability of Middle East respiratory syndrome coronavirus (MERS-CoV) under different environmental conditions. Euro Surveill 2013;18(38) [pii:20590].

17. Ommeh S, Zhang W, Zohaib A, et al. Genetic evidence of Middle East respiratory syndrome coronavirus (MERS-Cov) and widespread seroprevalence among camels in Kenya. Virol Sin 2018. https://doi.org/10.1007/s12250-018-0076-4.

18. Liljander A, Meyer B, Jores J, et al. MERS-CoV Antibodies in Humans, Africa, 2013-2014. Emerg Infect Dis 2016;22(6):1086–9.

19. Memish ZA, Mishra N, Olival KJ, et al. Middle East respiratory syndrome coronavirus in bats, Saudi Arabia. Emerg Infect Dis 2013;19(11):1819–23.

20. Corman VM, Ithete NL, Richards LR, et al. Rooting the phylogenetic tree of Middle East respiratory syndrome coronavirus by characterization of a conspecific virus from an African bat. J Virol 2014;88:11297–303.

21. Sikkema RS, Farag EA, Himatt S, et al. Risk factors for primary Middle East respiratory syndrome coronavirus infection in camel workers in Qatar during 2013-2014: a case-control study. J Infect Dis 2017;215(11):1702–5.

22. Azhar EI, El-Kafrawy SA, Farraj SA, et al. Evidence for camel-to-human transmission of MERS coronavirus. N Engl J Med 2014;370(26):2499–505.

23. Memish ZA, Cotten M, Meyer B, et al. Human infection with MERS coronavirus after exposure to infected camels, Saudi Arabia, 2013. Emerg Infect Dis 2014; 20(6):1012–5.

24. Al Hammadi ZM, Chu DK, Eltahir YM, et al. Asymptomatic MERS-CoV infection in humans possibly linked to infected dromedaries imported from Oman to United Arab Emirates, May 2015. Emerg Infect Dis 2015;21(12):2197–200.

25. Arwady MA, Alraddadi B, Basler C, et al. Middle East respiratory syndrome coronavirus transmission in extended family, Saudi Arabia, 2014. Emerg Infect Dis 2016;22(8):1395–402.

26. Al-Abdallat MM, Payne DC, Alqasrawi S, et al, Jordan MERS-CoV Investigation Team. Hospital-associated outbreak of Middle East respiratory syndrome coronavirus: a serologic, epidemiologic, and clinical description. Clin Infect Dis 2014; 59(9):1225–33.

27. Garbati MA, Fagbo SF, Fang VJ, et al. Comparative study of clinical presentation and risk factors for adverse outcome in patients hospitalised with acute respiratory disease due to MERS coronavirus or other causes. PLoS One 2016;11(11): e0165978.

28. Assiri A, McGeer A, Perl TM, et al, KSA MERS-CoV Investigation Team. Hospital outbreak of Middle East respiratory syndrome coronavirus. N Engl J Med 2013; 369(5):407–16.

29. Arabi YM, Alomari A, Mandourah Y, et al. Critically ill healthcare workers with the Middle East Respiratory Syndrome (MERS). Crit Care Med 2017; 45(10):1683–95.

30. Arabi YM, Mandourah Y, Al-Hameed F, et al. Corticosteroid therapy for critically ill patients with middle east respiratory syndrome. Am J Respir Crit Care Med 2018; 197(6):757–67.

31. Ahmed AE. The predictors of 3- and 30-day mortality in 660 MERS-CoV patients. BMC Infect Dis 2017;17(1):615.

32. Yang YM, Hsu CY, Lai CC, et al. Impact of comorbidity on fatality rate of patients with middle east respiratory syndrome. Sci Rep 2017;7(1):11307.

33. Seys LJ, Widagdo W, Verhamme FM, et al. DPP4, the MERS coronavirus receptor, is upregulated in lungs of smokers and COPD patients. Clin Infect Dis 2018;66(1): 45–53.

34. Zumla A, Hui DS. Infection control and MERS-CoV in health-care workers. Lancet 2014;383(9932):1869–71.

35. WHO. Clinical management of severe acute respiratory infection when Middle East respiratory syndrome coronavirus (MERS-CoV) infection is suspected. Interim guidance January 2019. Available at: https://apps.who.int/iris/bitstream/handle/10665/178529/WHO_MERS_Clinical_15.1_eng.pdf;jsessionid=C30F54045 88BE9AA533F2B350A0FED4C?sequence=1. Accessed June 1, 2019.

36. World Health Organization. Laboratory testing for Middle East respiratory syndrome coronavirus. Interim guidance revised January 2018. Geneva (Switzerland): WHO; 2018. Available at: https://apps.who.int/iris/bitstream/handle/10665/259952/WHO-MERS-LAB-15.1-Rev1-2018-eng.pdf?sequence=1. Accessed June 1, 2019.

37. Corman VM, Muller MA, Costabel U, et al. Assays for laboratory confirmation of novel human coronavirus (hCoV-EMC) infections. Euro Surveill 2012;17:20334.

38. Corman VM, Albarrak AM, Omrani AS, et al. Viral shedding and antibody response in 37 patients with Middle East respiratory syndrome coronavirus infection. Clin Infect Dis 2016;62(4):477–83.

39. Hashem AM, Al-Amri SS, Al-Subhi TL, et al. Development and validation of different indirect ELISAs for MERS-CoV serological testing. J Immunol Methods 2019;466:41–6.

40. WHO. Laboratory biorisk management for laboratories handling human specimens suspected of confirmed to contain novel coronavirus: interim recommendations. Available at: https://www.who.int/csr/disease/coronavirus_infections/Biosafety_InterimRecommendations_NovelCoronavirus_19Feb13.pdf?ua=1. Accessed March 22, 2019.

41. Zumla A, Chan JF, Azhar EI, et al. Coronaviruses - drug discovery and therapeutic options. Nat Rev Drug Discov 2016;15(5):327–47.

42. Chan JF, Yao Y, Yeung ML, et al. Treatment with lopinavir/ritonavir or interferon-β1b improves outcome of MERS-CoV infection in a nonhuman primate model of common marmoset. J Infect Dis 2015;212(12):1904–13.

43. Arabi YM, Deeb AM, Al-Hameed F, et al. Macrolides in critically ill patients with Middle East Respiratory syndrome. Int J Infect Dis 2019;81:184–90.

44. Arabi YM, Alothman A, Balkhy HH, et al. Treatment of Middle East Respiratory Syndrome with a combination of lopinavir-ritonavir and interferon-β1b (MIRACLE trial): study protocol for a randomized controlled trial. Trials 2018;19(1):81.

45. Hui DS, Memish ZA, Zumla A. Severe acute respiratory syndrome vs. the Middle East respiratory syndrome. Curr Opin Pulm Med 2014;20(3):233–41.

46. WHO. Infection prevention and control during health care for probable or confirmed cases of Middle East respiratory syndrome coronavirus (MERS-CoV) infection -Interim guidance. Available at: https://apps.who.int/iris/bitstream/handle/10665/174652/WHO_MERS_IPC_15.1_eng.pdf;jsessionid=F6766551B38E85D0DE2FBBDEB17A0892?sequence=1. Accessed September 14, 2019.

47. Kim SW, Park JW, Jung HD, et al. Risk factors for transmission of Middle East respiratory syndrome coronavirus infection during the 2015 outbreak in South Korea. Clin Infect Dis 2017;64(5):551–7.

48. Korea Centers for Disease Control and Prevention. Middle East respiratory syndrome coronavirus outbreak in the Republic of Korea, 2015. Osong Public Health Res Perspect 2015;6:269–78.

49. Memish ZA, Zumla AI, Al-Hakeem RF, et al. Family cluster of Middle East respiratory syndrome coronavirus infections. N Engl J Med 2013;368(26):2487–94.

50. Drosten C, Meyer B, Müller MA, et al. Transmission of MERS-coronavirus in household contacts. N Engl J Med 2014;371(9):828–35.

51. Oboho IK, Tomczyk SM, Al-Asmari AM, et al. 2014 MERS-CoV outbreak in Jeddah–a link to health care facilities. N Engl J Med 2015;372(9):846–54.

52. Omrani AS, Matin MA, Haddad Q, et al. A family cluster of Middle East Respiratory Syndrome Coronavirus infections related to a likely unrecognized asymptomatic or mild case. Int J Infect Dis 2013;17(9):e668–72.

53. Siegel JD, Rhinehart E, Jackson M, et al. Health care infection control practices advisory committee. Am J Infect Control 2007;35(10 Suppl 2):S65–164.

54. MERS-CoV daily update. Saudi Arabia: Ministry of Health. Available at: https://www.moh.gov.sa/en/CCC/PressReleases/; http://www.cdc.gov/hicpac/2007IP/2007isolationPrecautions.html. Accessed July 31, 2019.

55. ISARIC and Public Health England. Treatment of MERS-CoV: Information for Clinicians. Clinical decision-making support for treatment of MERS-CoV patient. Available at: https://www.gov.uk/government/uploads/system/uploads/attachment_data/file/360424/MERS_COV_information_for_clinicians_17_July.pdf. Accessed June 21, 2019.

56. Schindewolf C, Menachery VD. Middle East respiratory syndrome vaccine candidates: cautious optimism. Viruses 2019;(1):11 [pii:E74].

57. Memish ZA, Zumla A, Alhakeem RF, et al. Hajj: infectious disease surveillance and control. Lancet 2014;383(9934):2073–82.

58. Zumla A, Mwaba P, Bates M, et al. The Hajj pilgrimage and surveillance for Middle East Respiratory syndrome coronavirus in pilgrims from African countries. Trop Med Int Health 2014;19(7):838–40.

59. Zumla A, Rustomjee R, Ntoumi F, et al. Middle East Respiratory Syndrome–need for increased vigilance and watchful surveillance for MERS-CoV in sub-Saharan Africa. Int J Infect Dis 2015;37:77–9.
60. Hui DS, Perlman S, Zumla A. Spread of MERS to South Korea and China. Lancet Respir Med 2015;3(7):509–10.
61. FAO-OIE-WHO MERS Technical Working Group. MERS: Progress on the global response, remaining challenges and the way forward. Antiviral Res 2018;159: 35–44.

Novel Avian Influenza A Virus Infections of Humans

Timothy M. Uyeki, MD, MPH, MPP[a],*, Malik Peiris, MBBS, DPhil, FRCPath[b]

KEYWORDS

- Avian influenza • H5N1 • H5N6 • H7N9

KEY POINTS

- Signs, symptoms, complications of human infection with avian influenza A viruses are nonspecific; suspicion is based on a recent history of poultry exposure or close exposure to a symptomatic person.
- Respiratory specimens for testing depend on the specific virus, time from illness onset, and the patient's symptoms and disease severity.
- Influenza tests available in clinical settings do not distinguish influenza A viruses of animal origin from seasonal influenza A viruses.
- Clinical specimens must be sent to a public health laboratory for specific testing for seasonal and avian influenza A viruses.
- Clinical management is based on prompt implementation of recommended infection prevention and control measures, antiviral treatment, and supportive care of complications.

INTRODUCTION

Influenza A viruses are RNA viruses with a segmented genome and are subtyped on the basis of the 2 virus surface glycoproteins, hemagglutinin (H) and neuraminidase (N), into 16 H and 9 N subtypes. More recently, additional virus subtypes have been discovered in bats, but these subtypes are of uncertain significance for humans. Influenza A viruses naturally circulate in a range of avian and mammalian species, including in humans. The greatest diversity of virus subtypes are found in aquatic waterfowl, which are regarded as the natural reservoir of influenza A viruses. Influenza A viruses of 3 subtypes—H1N1, H2N2, and H3N2—have been endemic in humans. Influenza A H1N1 caused the 1918 pandemic and circulated in humans

Disclaimer: The views expressed are those of the authors and do not necessarily represent the official views of the Centers for Disease Control and Prevention.
[a] Influenza Division, National Center for Immunization and Respiratory Diseases, Centers for Disease Control and Prevention, Mailstop H24-7, 1600 Clifton Road, Northeast, Atlanta, GA 30329, USA; [b] School of Public Health, The University of Hong Kong, L6-42, Laboratory Block, 21 Sassoon Road, Pokfulam, Hong Kong
* Corresponding author.
E-mail address: tmu0@cdc.gov

Infect Dis Clin N Am 33 (2019) 907–932
https://doi.org/10.1016/j.idc.2019.07.003
0891-5520/19/Published by Elsevier Inc. This is an open access article under the CC BY-NC-ND license (http://creativecommons.org/licenses/by-nc-nd/4.0/).

id.theclinics.com

until 1957 when a new pandemic H2N2 virus replaced it; which was in turn replaced by an H3N2 virus in 1968. The most recent pandemic was in 2009, caused by a 'swine-origin' H1N1 virus. Currently, influenza A subtypes H1N1 and H3N2 co-circulate in humans as seasonal influenza A viruses. Pandemics arise when novel influenza A viruses containing virus hemagglutinins from swine or birds emerge and spread efficiently and in a sustained manner among an immunologically naïve human population. In addition, avian and animal influenza A viruses may cause sporadic zoonotic human infections and disease without acquiring the ability for sustained human-to-human transmission. However, such infections cause global public health concern because they may cause significant morbidity and mortality; but the even greater concern is that they pose potential pandemic threats. Swine-origin H1 and H3 viruses have also caused zoonotic infections, but are not discussed in this article.

EPIDEMIOLOGY

Sporadic human infections with avian influenza A viruses of multiple subtypes have been increasingly detected since 1997, in part because the surveillance and laboratory capacity for molecular analyses have improved worldwide, but also because changes in poultry production marketing practices have increased the opportunity for the emergence and dissemination of potentially zoonotic viruses. The classification of avian influenza A viruses as highly pathogenic avian influenza (HPAI) or low pathogenicity avian influenza (LPAI) viruses is based on specific molecular criteria and pathogenicity in birds. Past pandemics have arisen from LPAI viruses. Although HPAI viruses have important agricultural and economic implications, both HPAI and LPAI virus infections have caused a wide range of mild to fatal human disease (**Tables 1** and **2**). Therefore, for public health impact, focus is on the virus subtype rather than virus pathogenicity in birds.

Although diverse avian influenza A virus subtypes have caused zoonotic infections (see **Tables 1** and **2**), virus subtypes H5N1 and H7N9 have caused the highest impact, both numerically and in disease severity. The first instance of a zoonotic avian influenza A virus causing severe disease was in 1997 in Hong Kong when 18 cases of H5N1 virus disease were detected leading to 6 deaths.[1] Human cases were preceded by outbreaks in poultry. The outbreak in Hong Kong was stopped by the slaughter of all poultry in markets and farms in Hong Kong in December 1997. H5N1 viruses continued to circulate and evolve among poultry in the wider region. Zoonotic disease was again observed in early 2003 with 2 deaths among 2 confirmed and 1 probable case.[2] H5N1 virus spread via the poultry trade to affect poultry in 10 countries in Asia by 2004.[3] By 2005, the virus also was established in wild migratory birds and spread via bird migration to infect poultry in Central Asia, South Asia, the Middle East, and parts of Africa. Although these poultry outbreaks were stamped out successfully and repeatedly in some countries (eg, Japan, Malaysia), they became enzootic within poultry in others, evolving into antigenically distinct and genetic diverse clades leading to zoonotic disease.[3] As of May 2019, 861 human cases of H5N1 virus infection and 455 deaths had been reported from 17 countries since November 2003, and the cumulative case fatality proportion among reported H5N1 cases has remained greater than 50%, although few cases have been reported worldwide since 2016.[4,5] Since 2013, H5N1 viruses of clade 2.3.4.4 have undergone reassortment with other avian influenza A viruses to generate H5N6, H5N8, and other related subtypes. More recently, H5N6 has become the dominant H5 lineage virus circulating in China, sometimes causing zoonotic disease.[6]

Table 1
LPAI A virus subtypes reported to cause human illness and associated clinical syndromes

Subtype	Patient Characteristics	Clinical Syndromes	Illness Severity	Countries	Years (Illness Onset)
H6N1	Young adult	Moderate lower respiratory tract disease	Moderate	Taiwan	2013
H7N2	Adults	Upper respiratory tract illness, conjunctivitis, lower respiratory tract disease	Mild to moderate	US; UK	2002, 2003, 2007, 2016[a]
H7N3	Adults	Upper respiratory tract illness, conjunctivitis	Mild	UK; Canada	2004, 2006
H7N4	Elderly adult	Pneumonia	Moderately severe	China	2017
H7N7	Adults	Conjunctivitis	Mild	US; UK	1980,[b] 1996
H7N9	All ages	Upper respiratory tract illness, lower respiratory tract disease, critical illness with multiorgan failure	Mild to severe; majority with severe to critical illness with mortality in hospitalized patients at 40%	China; exported cases identified in Hong Kong Special Administrative Region of China, Taiwan, Malaysia	2013–2018
H9N2	Young children and adults with influenza-like illness; one immunosuppressed adult with bilateral pneumonia	Upper respiratory tract illness, lower respiratory tract disease	Mild to moderately severe, fatal outcome in 1 case	China; Hong Kong Special Administrative Region of China; Bangladesh; Egypt, Oman	1998, 1999, 2003, 2007, 2008, 2009, 2011, 2013–2017, 2019
H10N7	Adults	Conjunctivitis and upper respiratory tract illness	Mild	Australia	2010
H10N8	Middle-aged and elderly adults	Severe pneumonia, critical illness with multiorgan failure	Critical illness, fatal outcome in 2 of 3 cases	China	2013, 2014

As of May 2019; excludes asymptomatic infections, infections reported by sero-epidemiology studies, or infections with illness not specified in published reports.
[a] One case of an avian-lineage H7N2 virus was transmitted from a cat to a human causing mild respiratory illness.
[b] One case of conjunctivitis occurred in a researcher through close contact with a seal that was experimentally infected with a virus that was antigenically similar to an H7N7 virus of avian origin.

Table 2
HPAI A virus subtypes reported to cause human illness and associated clinical syndromes

Subtype	Patient Characteristics	Clinical Syndromes	Illness Severity	Countries	Years
H5N1	All ages, primarily children and young adults	Upper respiratory tract illness, lower respiratory tract disease, encephalitis, respiratory failure, ARDS, multiorgan failure	Mild to critical illness; majority with severe to critical illness with mortality >50%	Hong Kong Special Administrative Region of China; China; Vietnam; Thailand; Cambodia; Indonesia; China; Turkey; Iraq; Azerbaijan; Egypt; Djibouti; Nigeria; Laos PDR; Nepal; Pakistan; Myanmar; Bangladesh; Canada (imported from China)	1997, 2003–2017, 2019
H5N6	Adults	Upper respiratory tract illness, severe pneumonia, respiratory failure, ARDS, multiorgan failure	One case with mild illness; most cases with critical illness, mortality >50%	China	2014–2018
H7N3	Adults	Conjunctivitis	Mild	Canada; UK; Mexico; Italy	2004, 2006, 2012, 2013
H7N7	All ages	Hepatitis, conjunctivitis, upper respiratory tract illness, severe pneumonia, respiratory failure, ARDS, multiorgan failure	Mild to critical illness with fatal outcome in one adult; majority with mild illness (conjunctivitis)	UK; the Netherlands, Italy	1959, 1996, 2003, 2013
H7N9		Pneumonia, respiratory failure, ARDS, multiorgan failure	Critical illness, high mortality	China	2016–2017, 2019

As of May 2019; does not include asymptomatic infections, infections reported by sero-epidemiology studies, or infections with illness not specified in published reports.

Abbreviation: ARDS, acute respiratory distress syndrome.

In 2003, an outbreak of HPAI H7N7 virus in poultry was associated with zoonotic disease affecting 89 people in the Netherlands, most of them presenting with conjunctivitis, others with influenza-like illness, and 1 fatal pneumonia in a veterinarian. There was evidence of limited human-to-human transmission to family members of persons directly exposed to infected poultry.[7]

A novel H7N9 virus caused zoonotic disease in eastern China in the early spring of 2013.[8] Six epidemics of human cases of H7N9 virus infection (1564 laboratory-confirmed cases and 612 deaths) occurred in China through September 2017, typically during the fall, winter, and spring months, including a very large fifth epidemic during 2016 to 2017.[9,10] As of May 2019, 1568 laboratory-confirmed H7N9 virus infections acquired in China had occurred since 2013. Being an LPAI virus, H7N9 caused little or no illness in poultry and spread to multiple provinces in China. The seasonal increase in human cases corresponded with a seasonal increase in virus circulation among poultry. The cumulative case fatality proportion among reported H7N9 cases has remained approximately 40% since 2013.[9] The H7N9 virus acquired properties of an HPAI virus in 2016 causing disease in poultry. This led to the introduction of a bivalent H5N1/H7N9 vaccination program in poultry in China leading to a decrease in virus activity in poultry[11] and a marked reduction of zoonotic H7N9 disease since 2017.[10] Only 2 H7N9 cases were reported in 2018, and 1 case was reported in the early spring of 2019.[12]

Most surveillance for human infections with avian influenza A viruses has been hospital based and focused on collecting respiratory specimens for virologic testing from patients with severe disease (eg, pneumonia of unknown etiology). The recognition of clinically mild infections comes from sporadic cases identified through routine influenza surveillance among outpatients with influenza-like illness,[13,14] testing of ill persons with poultry exposures during large outbreaks of avian influenza follow-up of close contacts of confirmed cases (eg, H7N9), and sero-epidemiologic studies.[7,15,16] Therefore, asymptomatic and clinically mild illness cases of infections with avian influenza A viruses are likely underestimated, the true denominator of all infections is unknown, and the case fatality proportions for hospitalized patients are likely a substantial overestimate of the overall case fatalities for different virus infections.[17,18]

Serologic studies conducted among poultry workers,[19–34] persons exposed to poultry,[35–40] close contacts of confirmed cases,[41–44] health care providers,[45–47] and the general population[20,23,39,48,49] suggest that, although the findings vary by virus subtype, except for poultry workers, human infections with avian influenza A viruses are generally infrequent. However, because some infected persons with mild illness may not mount a detectable antibody response, and limited data on the kinetics of the antibody response for HPAI H5N1 and LPAI H7N9 virus infections suggest that antibody titers decrease over time,[50] sero-surveys may underestimate some human infections with avian influenza A viruses.

Exported Cases

Several human cases of infection with avian influenza A viruses acquired in China have traveled overseas and were diagnosed elsewhere. A traveler who returned to Alberta, Canada, from a 3-week visit to Beijing, China, was hospitalized with pneumonia, progressed to respiratory failure with meningocencephalitis, and died.[51] H5N1 virus was identified in this patient's upper and lower respiratory tract and cerebrospinal fluid specimens. H7N9 virus infections acquired in China, leading to mild or critical illness, have been identified in returned travelers in Taiwan[52] and Canada,[53] and in a tourist in Malaysia.[54]

Exposure Risk Factors

Most human infections with avian influenza A viruses have been sporadic and linked to recent direct contact or close exposure with domestic poultry, including raising backyard poultry or visiting a live poultry market (**Table 3**).[55–65] Contact with dead wild swans (defeathering) was the source of infection for some cases of H5N1 virus infection in Azerbaijan.[66] However, the source of exposure is not always determined for some cases of human infection with avian influenza A viruses.[64,67] Live avian influenza A viruses have been identified in poultry carcasses sourced in endemic areas. Although cooking destroys virus infectivity, contamination from the carcass before cooking may contribute to some of the cases of zoonotic avian influenza A virus infection with no history of direct exposure to live poultry.[68] Virologically confirmed infection with avian-lineage H7N2 virus was identified in an ill veterinarian who had exposure to ill cats.[69,70] A researcher developed virologically confirmed conjunctivitis with an H7N7 virus that was antigenically related to an avian influenza A virus after close exposure to an experimentally infected seal.[71]

Infection of the human respiratory tract is likely initiated by inhalation of aerosolized avian influenza A viruses or contact transmission to mucus membranes, including conjunctivae, depending on the specific characteristics of the virus (eg, tropism for receptors with sialic acids attached to galactose by α2,6 linkages primarily in the upper respiratory tract vs sialic acids attached to galactose by α2,3 linkages primarily in the lower respiratory tract),[72] host factors (eg, age, immune function, and underlying comorbidities) and exposure (eg, virus dose, single or multiple exposures). Some avian influenza A(H7) viruses have tropism for ocular receptors and conjunctivitis has been reported in persons with H7N2, H7N3, and H7N7 virus infections.[73] In regions with enzootic poultry infections, human exposures to avian influenza A viruses such as H5N1, H5N6, and H7N9 has been extensive, but zoonotic disease is stochastic and rare. The reasons for this disconnect between exposure and disease are unclear.

Human-to-Human Transmission

Multiple clusters of epidemiologically linked human cases of H5N1 virus infection have been reported worldwide, beginning with the first outbreak described in Hong Kong

Table 3
Exposure risk factors for human infections with avian influenza A viruses

Risk Factor	Viruses
Direct contact with infected well-appearing poultry or poultry products	LPAI A viruses
Direct contact with infected sick or dead poultry or poultry products	HPAI A viruses (eg, H5N1, H5N6, H7N7, H7N9)
Close exposure to infected well-appearing poultry	LPAI A viruses
Close exposure to infected sick or dead poultry	HPAI A viruses (eg, H5N1, H5N6, H7N7, H7N9)
Visiting a live poultry market	LPAI A viruses (eg, H7N9); HPAI A viruses (eg, H5N1)
Raising backyard poultry	LPAI A viruses (eg, H7N9); HPAI A viruses (eg, H5N1, H5N6)
Close, unprotected, prolonged exposure to an ill person with avian influenza A virus infection and respiratory illness	LPAI A viruses (eg, H7N9); HPAI A viruses (eg, H5N1)

during 1997. Most cases in clusters have had recent exposure to birds, usually domestic poultry, suggesting a common exposure source.[66,67,74,75] However, some cases in clusters had close exposure to a symptomatic index case without poultry exposure. Although there is no laboratory test to confirm human-to-human transmission, epidemiologic investigations have concluded that limited, nonsustained human-to-human transmission of avian influenza A viruses likely occurred in some clusters in households or health care settings primarily among blood-related family members[67,76–79] This included 2 clusters of third-generation spread in Indonesia[80] and Pakistan.[81] Transmission has likely occurred through prolonged, unprotected close exposure to a symptomatic infected person. Similarly, at least 40 clusters of epidemiologically linked cases of H7N9 virus infection, mostly attributed to poultry exposures, were identified in China during 2013 to 2017.[82] In some of these clusters, probable limited, nonsustained human-to-human LPAI H7N9 virus transmission likely occurred in households[82–84] and in health care settings, including between blood-related family members as well as between unrelated patients.[85,86] There has been no increase identified in the transmissibility of H7N9 viruses among humans since emergence in 2013.[82,87] Probable, limited, nonsustained human-to-human transmission of HPAI H7N7 virus was also reported among family members in a few households in the Netherlands during 2004.[7]

Host Factors

The median age for reported human cases of infection with HPAI H5N1 virus is substantially younger than for infection with LPAI H7N9 virus among hospitalized patients. It has been postulated that these different age distributions are consistent with immunologic imprinting with an individual's first influenza A virus infection (belonging to either group 1 or group 2 virus hemagglutinin subtypes) and subsequent protection against future infection with influenza A viruses in the same hemagglutinin subtype grouping (group 1 or group 2).[88]

Age may also influence disease severity and thus, case detection and reporting. Older age or age 60 years or older is associated with fatal outcomes from H7N9 virus infection.[89–92] Among children with H5N1 virus infection, case fatality proportion was lowest in those aged 5 years or younger.[74] Among persons with H7N9 virus infection, mild illness was observed in young children.[64] The majority of H9N2 virus infections have occurred in children, and most cases have resulted in mild to moderate disease in patients in China, Hong Kong, Egypt, and Bangladesh.[93,94]

In contrast with H5N1 virus infection, risk factors for severe H7N9 disease include having a chronic medical condition (eg, obesity, chronic obstructive pulmonary disease, immunosuppression).[61–63,65] This finding may imply that infection in younger healthy persons occurs undetected and unreported. Epidemiologically linked clusters of H7N9 cases in China were identified in each epidemic from 2013 to 2017. Similarly, clusters of H5N1 cases have been identified in multiple countries. In zoonotic H5N1 disease, the occurrence of small clusters predominantly among blood-related family members has raised the suggestion of a genetic susceptibility.[95]

CLINICAL ISSUES
Clinical Spectrum

The clinical spectrum of infection with avian influenza A viruses is wide and depends on the specific virus and host characteristics, ranging from asymptomatic, mild focal illness (conjunctivitis), uncomplicated upper respiratory illness, to fulminant pneumonitis with multiorgan failure and sepsis leading to fatal outcomes (see **Tables 1** and **2**).

Most avian influenza A virus subtypes that have infected people have resulted in mild to moderate illness. Only a few viruses (H5N1, H5N6, H7N9) have caused a high proportion of severe illness (**Table 4**).

Asymptomatic infections have been identified by serology for several different avian influenza A viruses, although few such infections have been confirmed virologically.[16,96,97] In follow-up of household contacts of a confirmed H5N1 case, the case's adult daughter had a throat specimen collected that yielded H5N1 virus 6 days after slaughtering a chicken, and had evidence of seroconversion without experiencing any illness symptoms.[96]

Conjunctivitis has been reported for HPAI H5N1,[74,98] LPAI H7N2,[99] LPAI H7N3,[100,101] HPAI H7N3,[15,102] LPAI H7N7,[103] HPAI H7N7,[7,104] and LPAI H10N7[105] virus infections. Mild to moderate uncomplicated upper respiratory tract illness has been reported for infections with HPAI H5N1 (particularly in children),[67,74,77,106–108] HPAI H5N6,[109,110] LPAI H7N2,[69,111] LPAI H7N3,[102] HPAI H7N7,[7] LPAI H7N9,[13,14] LPAI H9N2,[93,94] and LPAI H10N7[105] viruses. Lower respiratory tract disease has been reported for HPAI H5N1,[112,113] HPAI H5N6,[114,115] LPAI H6N1,[116] LPAI H7N2,[117] LPAI H7N3, LPAI H7N4,[118] HPAI H7N7,[119] LPAI H7N9,[120] HPAI H7N9,[121] LPAI H9N2,[94] and LPAI H10N8[122] virus infections. Respiratory failure, refractory shock, acute respiratory distress syndrome, and multiorgan failure have been reported for infections with HPAI H5N1,[112,113] HPAI H5N6,[110,115] HPAI H7N7,[119] LPAI H7N9,[120] HPAI H7N9,[121,123] and LPAI H10N8[122,124] viruses. Fatal outcomes have occurred with HPAI H5N1,[60,112,113] HPAI H5N6,[110,115] HPAI H7N7,[119] LPAI H7N9,[120] HPAI H7N9,[121,123] LPAI H9N2,[125] and LPAI H10N8[109,122] virus infections.

Clinical Presentation

The clinical presentation varies by the specific virus infection, host characteristics, and time from illness onset to medical care. However, signs, symptoms, and

Table 4
Summary of clinical and clinical laboratory findings reported in patients with severe disease from avian influenza A virus infection

Admission clinical findings	History of fever and cough (productive cough, shortness of breath, dyspnea, chest pain, hypoxemia are associated with severe pneumonia), myalgia; diarrhea, malaise, headache, sore throat can occur, but are less common. Radiographic findings: bilateral patchy, interstitial, lobar, and/or diffuse infiltrates, ground glass opacities, consolidation, air bronchograms
Admission laboratory findings	White blood cell count may be low or normal; lymphopenia and moderate thrombocytopenia are common; neutropenia and elevated alanine aminotransferase associated with H5N1 mortality.
Clinical complications during hospitalization	Respiratory failure, acute respiratory distress syndrome, refractory hypoxemia, pleural effusion, cardiac failure, acute kidney injury/renal failure, multiorgan failure, septic shock, rhabdomyolysis, spontaneous miscarriage in pregnant patients, disseminated intravascular coagulation, encephalitis, bacterial co-infection, fungal co-infection, pneumothorax.
Laboratory findings during hospitalization	Elevated lactate, creatinine kinase, hepatic transaminases; hypoalbuminemia, leukopenia or leukocytosis

Associated with H5N1, H5N6, or H7N9 virus infections.

complications associated with avian influenza A virus infection are nonspecific and overlap with those caused by other respiratory pathogens, including seasonal influenza A and B viruses. Patients with avian influenza A(H7) virus infections can present with unilateral conjunctivitis only or also with fever and upper respiratory tract symptoms. The incubation period is not well-characterized for human infection with most avian influenza A viruses, but is estimated to be approximately 3 to 5 days after exposure to infected poultry for H5N1[126,127] and H7N9[127–129] virus infections, with a wider range in clusters with limited human-to-human transmission of H5N1 virus.[76,77]

In early illness with H5N1, H5N6, or H7N9 virus infections, fever or feverishness is usually present; cough, and malaise, myalgia, headache, and sore throat also may be present.[115,120,130] Gastrointestinal symptoms such as abdominal pain, vomiting, and diarrhea are variable,[60,77,120,131] but conjunctivitis is uncommon.[74,115,120] Atypical presentations have included fever and diarrhea before signs and symptoms of lower respiratory tract disease or encephalitis developed.[132,133] Dyspnea, shortness of breath, tachypnea, productive cough, and chest pain are associated with severe pneumonia. Many patients with H5N1, H5N6, or H7N9 virus infections have presented to medical care with severe pneumonia and hypoxemia approximately 5 to 7 days after illness onset.[4,64,112,113,115,123]

Routine laboratory findings are nonspecific and leukopenia, lymphopenia, and moderate thrombocytopenia are associated with more severe H5N1 disease[60,113] and lymphopenia is commonly observed at admission, but white blood cell counts may be normal initially for patients with H7N9 virus infection.[120] A high neutrophil to lymphocyte ratio 24 hours after hospital admission of H7N9 patients was independently- associated with mortality.[134] Other abnormalities reported in severely ill patients with H5N1, H5N6, or H7N9 virus infections include hypoalbuminemia[77] and elevated levels of hepatic transaminases,[60,112,113,115,120] creatinine kinase,[98,112,115,120] and lactic dehydrogenase.[112,115,120] Radiographic findings in patients with H5N1, H5N6, or H7N9 virus infections hospitalized with pneumonia include bilateral patchy, interstitial, lobar, and/or diffuse infiltrates, ground glass opacities, consolidation, pleural effusion, air bronchograms, and pneumothorax.[60,112,115,120,135]

Complications

Respiratory complications of H5N1, H5N6, or H7N9 virus infections include pneumonia, respiratory failure, and acute respiratory distress syndrome.[60,112,115,120,135] Extrapulmonary dissemination and isolation of H5N1 virus from blood, cerebrospinal fluid, brain tissues, lower respiratory tract tissues, gastrointestinal tract tissues (ileum, colon, rectum), rectal swabs, stool, ureter, and axillary lymph node have been reported.[133,136,137] Detection of H7N9 viral RNA was reported in stool.[138] Extrapulmonary complications owing to H5NI or H7N9 virus infections include cardiac failure,[60,112,120] acute kidney injury,[60,112,120] encephalitis,[51,133,139] myelitis,[140] rhabdomyolysis,[120,141] multiorgan failure and sepsis,[112,120,142] disseminated intravascular coagulation,[112,113,120,143] and spontaneous miscarriage in pregnant patients.[112] A 36-week gestational infant survived after emergency Cesarean section delivery of a critically ill pregnant woman with H5N1 virus infection who died.[144] Obstructive hydrocephalus[139] and Reye syndrome with aspirin administration[145] have been reported in pediatric cases of H5N1 virus infection. Co-infection with bacterial pathogens has been reported at hospital admission in H7N9 patients,[146] and nosocomial infection and ventilator-associated pneumonia with bacterial and fungal pathogens can occur.[8,120,147,148,149] Nosocomial bacterial infections were more common in 6 fatal cases than in 6 survivors of H7N9 virus infection.[138] H5N1 virus infection in persons with HIV has been reported.[60,150]

Neutropenia and elevated alanine aminotransferase at admission were associated with mortality for H5N1 patients in an observational study.[113] Septic shock with severe hypoxemia was an independent risk factor associated with mortality in H7N9 patients in another observational study.[151] Refractory hypoxemia is a major cause of death in H7N9 patients.[120]

Pathogenesis and pathology findings

In severe disease, the pathogenesis of H5N1, H5N6, and H7N9 virus infections is driven by high viral levels and prolonged replication in the lower respiratory tract and aggravated by innate immune dysregulation. Higher viral levels in nasal and throat swabs are associated with adverse clinical outcomes in H5N1 disease.[152] H5N1 virus infects ciliated and nonciliated tracheal epithelial cells with tropism for α2,3-linked sialic acid receptors in the lower respiratory tract,[153] and H7N9 virus has affinity for α2,6-linked sialic acid receptors in the upper respiratory tract, but preferentially binds to α2,3-linked sialic acid receptors in the lower respiratory tract.[154] Patients with severe and fatal lower respiratory tract disease have prolonged H5N1 viral replication.[153] High-dose corticosteroid treatment is associated with prolonged detection of H7N9 viral RNA.[155,156] In vitro and ex vivo studies indicate that H5N1, H5N6, and H7N9 viruses induce inflammatory mediators,[114,157–167] and data from critically ill patients indicate that virus infection of the respiratory tract triggers a dysregulated proinflammatory cytokine and chemokine response, resulting in inflammatory pulmonary damage and multiorgan injury.[2,115,168–170] H5N1 virus induces higher levels of proinflammatory cytokines and chemokines than H7N9 and seasonal influenza A viruses and infection of endothelial cells as shown in mice and ferrets may also contribute to pulmonary vascular leakage and viral pneumonia.[171,172] Limited autopsy studies have described extrapulmonary dissemination of H5N1 and H5N6 viruses,[153,173] including evidence of infection of cerebral neurons, placenta, T lymphocytes in lymph nodes, cytotrophoblasts of placental chorionic villi and fetal macrophages (transplacental transmission)[153]; pulmonary findings of diffuse alveolar damage and interstitial fibrosis for H5N1, H5N6, and H7N9 virus infections[60,138,174–179]; and other organ findings of hepatic central lobular necrosis, acute renal tubular necrosis, lymphoid depletion, and reactive hemophagocytic syndrome for H5N1 or H7N9 virus infections.[2,138,153,176,180]

CLINICAL MANAGEMENT
Infection Prevention and Control Measures

Prompt isolation and implementation of infection prevention and control measures is essential to decreasing the risk of nosocomial transmission of patients with avian influenza A virus infection associated with severe and fatal illness (eg, H5N1, H5N6, H7N9, H10N8 viruses). The Centers for Disease Control and Prevention recommend placement of patients with suspected avian influenza A virus infection associated with severe illness in a negative pressure respiratory isolation room and implementation of standard, contact (including googles), and airborne (use of fit-tested N95 respirator or higher level of respiratory protection) precautions for health care personnel[181] while providing care, including collecting respiratory specimens. The World Health Organization recommends personal protective equipment (medical mask, eye protection, gown, and gloves), performing adequate hand hygiene, and use of a separate adequately ventilated or airborne precaution room (isolation in mechanically or naturally ventilated rooms with 12 air changes per hour and controlled direction of airflow), and use of a respirator for aerosol-generating procedures.[182] Patients should wear a medical mask when outside of isolation rooms.

Diagnosis

Because the signs, symptoms, and clinical findings are nonspecific, clinical suspicion of avian influenza A virus infection (all subtypes with at least 1 human infection; see **Tables 1** and **2**) is based on eliciting a history of (1) recent poultry exposure in a virus enzootic region, in particular, visiting a market where live poultry are sold or slaughtered, or at small farms or inside/outside homes (where poultry are raised), or (2) recent close exposure to a symptomatic person with suspected or confirmed avian influenza A virus infection (eg, viruses in which limited human-to-human transmission has been reported, namely, H5N1, H7N7, and H7N9). The optimal respiratory specimens to collect depends on the time from illness onset to presentation, the presumed site of the major pathology and the patient's disease severity. For example, although a nasopharyngeal specimen might be sufficient for detecting some avian influenza A viruses associated with upper respiratory symptoms, a throat swab specimen has a higher yield for detecting H5N1 virus in patients without severe lower respiratory tract disease. For hospitalized patients, the collection of respiratory specimens from multiple respiratory sites, including sputum, can increase the likelihood of detecting avian influenza A virus infection. For critically ill patients with respiratory failure receiving invasive mechanical ventilation, an endotracheal aspirate or bronchoalveolar lavage specimen should be collected for testing.

Commercially available influenza tests available in clinical settings, including molecular assays, detect influenza A and B viruses but do not specifically distinguish between seasonal influenza A viruses circulating among people worldwide and zoonotic avian influenza A viruses. Therefore, respiratory specimens must be sent to a public health laboratory for specific testing for avian influenza A virus subtypes by reverse transcriptase polymerase chain reaction (eg, H5, H7, H9) and additional analyses, such as genetic sequencing. Antigen detection tests are less sensitive than reverse transcriptase polymerase chain reaction assays for detecting avian influenza A virus infection. Serologic testing of paired acute and convalescent sera can yield a retrospective diagnosis, but must be performed at a specialized public health or research laboratory.

Discharge Criteria

No guidelines exist on discharge criteria for hospitalized patients with avian influenza A virus infection, but key criteria are clinical recovery with demonstration of clearance of viral RNA from the respiratory tract.

Antiviral Treatment

There are no randomized controlled trials (RCTs) of antiviral treatment of patients with avian influenza A virus infection. No clinical or virologic benefit of double-dose versus standard-dose oseltamivir was found in an RCT conducted in 326 hospitalized patients with influenza, including 17 H5N1 patients.[183] Mortality was very high (88%) among the enrolled H5N1 patients.[183] Observational studies of patients with H5N1 or H7N9 virus infections have reported survival benefit of antiviral treatment with a neuraminidase inhibitor (NAI), usually oseltamivir monotherapy, particularly when treatment is initiated early in the clinical course.[74,113,184–188] One observational study reported no benefit of combination NAI treatment (oseltamivir and peramivir) compared with oseltamivir for hospitalized H7N9 patients.[189] Most severely ill H5N1, H5N6, and H7N9 patients have been admitted more than 5 days after illness onset, with late initiation of NAI treatment. One observational study reported that delayed administration of NAI treatment was an independent risk factor for prolonged H7N9 viral shedding.[156]

Currently, NAI treatment is recommended as soon as possible in patients with suspected avian influenza A virus infection, even before laboratory confirmation, because there may be a long delay until specific testing results are received. Recommended NAI dosing is the same as for the treatment of patients with seasonal influenza. Combination treatment with 2 NAIs is not recommended. The duration of antiviral treatment should continue until there is no evidence of viral shedding and be guided by testing results of respiratory tract specimens, particularly lower respiratory tract specimens, in ventilated patients. The emergence of antiviral resistance to NAIs should be considered in patients with prolonged viral replication with no decrease in viral load. Analyses of genetic markers associated with decreased antiviral susceptibility or resistance can be performed on viral RNA and phenotypic antiviral susceptibility testing on virus isolates at specialized public health reference laboratories.

The emergence of oseltamivir-resistant viruses containing an H275Y mutation in viral neuraminidase has been reported during oseltamivir treatment of H5N1 patients with sustained viral replication, clinical deterioration, and fatal outcomes,[190] and in an H5N1 patient who had received oseltamivir chemoprophylaxis followed by oseltamivir treatment and recovered.[79] Similarly, the emergence and sustained replication of H7N9 viruses with an R292 K mutation in viral neuraminidase confers resistance to NAIs.[158,191–193] This mutation confers high-level resistance to oseltamivir and moderately decreased sensitivity to peramivir and zanamivir.[194] Most H5N1, H5N6, and H7N9 viruses circulating among poultry are resistant to the adamantane antivirals (amantadine and rimantadine). Novel antivirals such as favipiravir and baloxavir marboxyl have not been used therapeutically in zoonotic avian influenza A virus infections, but may need to be considered in the event of NAI resistance.[194]

Adjunctive Therapy

Immunotherapy with convalescent plasma has been administered to a very small number of hospitalized H5N1 patients. The source of the convalescent plasma was recovered survivors of H5N1 virus infection[112,195] for 2 critically ill patients with respiratory failure receiving invasive mechanical ventilation and an H5N1 vaccine recipient for another patient[78] with pneumonia receiving noninvasive ventilation, all of whom also received antiviral treatment and survived. Convalescent plasma from a recovered survivor has also been administered to a hospitalized H7N9 patient with respiratory failure receiving invasive mechanical ventilation with no improvement from oseltamivir treatment.[196] The patient also received other medications, including methylprednisolone, and survived.[196] No conclusions can be made on the clinical benefit of convalescent plasma treatment from such limited uncontrolled data, but further studies of the clinical benefit of immunotherapy as an adjunctive treatment to antiviral therapy are warranted. IVIG has been administered to some H7N9 patients on an uncontrolled basis.[149]

No RCTs have been conducted of corticosteroid treatment for any patients with avian influenza A virus infection. Observational studies have suggested an increased mortality risk with corticosteroid treatment of H5N1[113] and H7N9[197] patients, and high-dose corticosteroids have been implicated with increased H7N9 mortality risk.[155] High-dose corticosteroids were also reported to be an independent risk factor for prolonged H7N9 viral shedding in an observational study of 478 patients with H7N9.[156] The clinical benefit or harm of low-dose or moderate-dose corticosteroid treatment for hospitalized patients with avian influenza A virus infection is unknown. However, given the observational data to date, high-dose corticosteroids should be avoided, and corticosteroids should only be administered for treatment of septic shock.

There are very limited and inconclusive observational data about the benefit of probiotic treatment of patients with H7N9 virus infection.[198–200] Salicylates should not be administered to patients with suspected or confirmed avian influenza A virus infection because of the risk of Reye syndrome.[145]

Advanced Organ Support

No RCTs are available, but advanced organ support has been administered to most critically ill hospitalized patients with H5N1, H5N6, or H7N9 virus infections, especially invasive mechanical ventilation for respiratory failure.[110,113,115,120] In H7N9 patients with acute respiratory distress syndrome, extracorporeal membrane oxygenation has been administered on an uncontrolled basis.[120,201–208] H7N9 patients with acute kidney injury have also required renal replacement therapy.[120] Plasma exchange has been used in combination with continuous venovenous hemofiltration to reduce levels of cytokines and chemokines.[209] Artificial liver therapy has been used in management of some H7N9 patients.[149]

Immune responses

During the acute illness, most H5N1 patients typically mount a robust neutralizing antibody response 14 or more days after onset.[42] In 4 H5N1 survivors of severe disease, although specific hemagglutination inhibition and neutralizing antibody titers increased from 15 days after illness onset and declined by 5 to 12 months, titers were detectable for 3 to 4 years after onset.[210] A follow-up study of 11 H5N1 patients who survived severe disease reported that 70% had a positive neutralizing antibody titer after 2 weeks and all had a neutralizing antibody titer of 1:80 or greater by 3 weeks after illness, with titers peaking at 1 to 2 months and declining by 10 to 12 months.[50]

During the acute illness, most critically ill H7N9 patients mounted a robust humoral immune response with a seroprotective titer of neutralizing antibodies ($\geq$1:40) detected significantly earlier (median, 10.5 days) in survivors than in fatal cases (median, 14 days).[211] Other studies in H7N9 survivors have reported variable kinetics and antibody titers after recovery declining, though still detectable at 1 year after illness.[212,213] T-cell (CD^8+/CD4$^+$ T-cell memory) responses are reported to play an important role in recovery from disease.[214,215]

Long-term follow-up

Few studies have assessed long-term clinical follow-up of survivors of severe or critical illness owing to avian influenza A virus infections. During follow-up of 2 adult H5N1 patients who recovered from respiratory failure and ventilator-associated bacterial pneumonia, 1 patient had bilateral patchy, as well as fibrotic reticular and linear opacities noted at 7 months that mostly had resolved by 12 months after illness onset.[216] However, the more severely ill patient had ground-glass shadows, reticular opacities, linear fibrotic opacities, interlobular thickening and intralobular lines at 12 months that persisted at 24 months after onset. Of 5 adult patients who survived H7N9 virus infection and were followed for approximately 5 to 7 months after diagnosis, only one reported mild respiratory symptoms, but all had bilateral lower lung abnormalities such as interlobular septal thickening, subpleural linear opacities, and some had cystic changes on a computed tomography scan.[217] For 3 of these 5 patients who had pulmonary function testing, 1 patient had near normal pulmonary function, but 2 patients had abnormalities in forced expiratory volume in 1 second, forced vital capacity, total lung capacity, and carbon monoxide diffusing capacity. A cohort study of 56 adult H7N9 patients followed for

---

Box 1
Gaps in the clinical management of zoonotic influenza A virus infections

- Lack of point-of-care or rapid diagnostic tests with high accuracy that can specifically identify avian influenza A viruses in respiratory specimens in a time frame relevant to inform clinical decision making.

- Lack of clinical data from randomized controlled trials on combination treatment with a neuraminidase inhibitor and an antiviral with a different mechanism of action, as well as combined with immunodulatory therapy.

- Lack of a standardized approach to clinical management of hospitalized patients with avian influenza A virus infection, such as advanced organ support of critically ill patients, and management (eg, low tidal volume lung protective strategies for acute respiratory distress syndrome).

- Lack of prospective, multiyear, multicountry, multiregional clinical influenza research networks that can serve as platforms for coordinating detailed clinical data collection, and for implementation of randomized clinical adaptive trials of interventions (pharmacologic and nonpharmacologic) for patients with seasonal influenza; sporadic patients with avian influenza A virus infections could also be enrolled.

---

2 years reported that although pulmonary function and chest computed tomography findings improved by 6 months after hospital discharge and most had returned to work, most patients had persistent abnormalities.[218] At 1 year after discharge, 42% had pulmonary fibrosis and 52% had parenchymal opacities, with bronchiectasis noted in 24% and pleural thickening reported in 22%, and 55% had evidence of ventilation dysfunction and 78% had an abnormal carbon monoxide diffusing capacity at 24 months (**Box 1**).[218]

SUMMARY

A high index of suspicion and early diagnosis of avian influenza A virus infection is essential to initiating interventions (antiviral treatment; infection prevention and control measures) as soon as possible to reduce transmission risk from symptomatic persons to close contacts, including health care personnel. Clinical suspicion relies on eliciting a history of recent exposure to poultry or to sick persons with suspected or confirmed avian influenza A virus infection. Diagnosis requires the collection of appropriate respiratory specimens, ideally from the lower respiratory tract when available, for specific testing for seasonal and avian influenza A virus subtypes at specialized public health laboratories. Patients with suspected infection should be isolated immediately and patients with lower respiratory tract disease should be placed on airborne precautions if possible, and NAI antiviral treatment should be started as soon as possible even before specific testing results are available. Corticosteroids and salicylates should be avoided and clinical management is focused on supportive care of complications, including nosocomial bacterial or fungal infections. Sporadic human infections with avian influenza A viruses resulting in mild to severe illness are expected to continue to occur in persons with close exposures to infected poultry and other birds. Options to decrease human exposure to enzootic avian influenza include interventions in live poultry markets, which serve as a major source of zoonotic infection and virus amplification.[219] Because zoonotic avian influenza A viruses pose potential pandemic threats, it is important to risk assess these viruses to prioritize countermeasure development such as vaccines.[220]

ACKNOWLEDGMENTS

M. Peiris has received research funding from the National Institute of Allergy and Infectious Diseases, National Institutes of Health, US Department of Health and Human Services, under contract number HHSN272201400006C.

REFERENCES

1. Chan PK. Outbreak of avian influenza A(H5N1) virus infection in Hong Kong in 1997. Clin Infect Dis 2002;34(Suppl 2):S58–64.
2. Peiris JS, Yu WC, Leung CW, et al. Re-emergence of fatal human influenza A subtype H5N1 disease. Lancet 2004;363(9409):617–9.
3. Webster RG, Peiris M, Chen H, et al. H5N1 outbreaks and enzootic influenza. Emerg Infect Dis 2006;12(1):3–8.
4. Lai S, Qin Y, Cowling BJ, et al. Global epidemiology of avian influenza A H5N1 virus infection in humans, 1997-2015: a systematic review of individual case data. Lancet Infect Dis 2016;16(7):e108–18.
5. Organization WH. Cumulative number of confirmed human cases of avian influenza A(H5N1) reported to WHO. 12 February 2019. 2019. Available at: https://www.who.int/influenza/human_animal_interface/2019_02_12_tableH5N1.pdf?ua=1. Accessed April 12, 2019.
6. Claes F, Morzaria SP, Donis RO. Emergence and dissemination of clade 2.3.4.4 H5Nx influenza viruses-how is the Asian HPAI H5 lineage maintained. Curr Opin Virol 2016;16:158–63.
7. Koopmans M, Wilbrink B, Conyn M, et al. Transmission of H7N7 avian influenza A virus to human beings during a large outbreak in commercial poultry farms in the Netherlands. Lancet 2004;363(9409):587–93.
8. Gao R, Cao B, Hu Y, et al. Human infection with a novel avian-origin influenza A (H7N9) virus. N Engl J Med 2013;368(20):1888–97.
9. Wang X, Jiang H, Wu P, et al. Epidemiology of avian influenza A H7N9 virus in human beings across five epidemics in mainland China, 2013-17: an epidemiological study of laboratory-confirmed case series. Lancet Infect Dis 2017; 17(8):822–32.
10. Organization WH. Influenza at the human-animal interface. Summary and assessment, 13 February to 9 April 2019 2019. Available at: https://www.who.int/influenza/human_animal_interface/Influenza_Summary_IRA_HA_interface_09_04_2019.pdf?ua=1. Accessed April 12, 2019.
11. Wu J, Ke C, Lau EHY, et al. Influenza H5/H7 virus vaccination in poultry and reduction of zoonotic infections, Guangdong Province, China, 2017-18. Emerg Infect Dis 2019;25(1):116–8.
12. Yu D, Xiang G, Zhu W, et al. The re-emergence of highly pathogenic avian influenza H7N9 viruses in humans in mainland China, 2019. Euro Surveill 2019; 24(21). pii=1900273.
13. Xu C, Havers F, Wang L, et al. Monitoring avian influenza A(H7N9) virus through national influenza-like illness surveillance, China. Emerg Infect Dis 2013;19(8): 1289–92.
14. Zeng X, Mai W, Shu B, et al. Mild influenza A/H7N9 infection among children in Guangdong Province. Pediatr Infect Dis J 2015;34(1):104–7.
15. Lopez-Martinez I, Balish A, Barrera-Badillo G, et al. Highly pathogenic avian influenza A(H7N3) virus in poultry workers, Mexico, 2012. Emerg Infect Dis 2013;19(9):1531–4.

16. Chen Z, Liu H, Lu J, et al. Asymptomatic, mild, and severe influenza A(H7N9) virus infection in humans, Guangzhou, China. Emerg Infect Dis 2014;20(9): 1535–40.

17. Yu H, Cowling BJ, Feng L, et al. Human infection with avian influenza A H7N9 virus: an assessment of clinical severity. Lancet 2013;382(9887):138–45.

18. Feng L, Wu JT, Liu X, et al. Clinical severity of human infections with avian influenza A(H7N9) virus, China, 2013/14. Euro Surveill 2014;19(49) [pii:20984].

19. Ma MJ, Zhao T, Chen SH, et al. Avian Influenza A virus infection among workers at live poultry markets, China, 2013-2016. Emerg Infect Dis 2018;24(7):1246–56.

20. Wang X, Fang S, Lu X, et al. Seroprevalence to avian influenza A(H7N9) virus among poultry workers and the general population in southern China: a longitudinal study. Clin Infect Dis 2014;59(6):e76–83.

21. Yang P, Ma C, Shi W, et al. A serological survey of antibodies to H5, H7 and H9 avian influenza viruses amongst the duck-related workers in Beijing, China. PLoS One 2012;7(11):e50770.

22. Yang P, Ma C, Cui S, et al. Avian influenza A(H7N9) and (H5N1) infections among poultry and swine workers and the general population in Beijing, China, 2013-2015. Sci Rep 2016;6:33877.

23. Yang S, Chen Y, Cui D, et al. Avian-origin influenza A(H7N9) infection in influenza A(H7N9)-affected areas of China: a serological study. J Infect Dis 2014; 209(2):265–9.

24. Huo X, Zu R, Qi X, et al. Seroprevalence of avian influenza A (H5N1) virus among poultry workers in Jiangsu Province, China: an observational study. BMC Infect Dis 2012;12:93.

25. Shimizu K, Wulandari L, Poetranto ED, et al. Seroevidence for a high prevalence of subclinical infection with avian influenza A(H5N1) virus among workers in a live-poultry market in Indonesia. J Infect Dis 2016;214(12):1929–36.

26. Nasreen S, Uddin Khan S, Azziz-Baumgartner E, et al. Seroprevalence of antibodies against highly pathogenic avian influenza A (H5N1) virus among poultry workers in Bangladesh, 2009. PLoS One 2013;8(9):e73200.

27. Nasreen S, Khan SU, Luby SP, et al. Highly pathogenic Avian Influenza A(H5N1) virus infection among workers at live bird markets, Bangladesh, 2009-2010. Emerg Infect Dis 2015;21(4):629–37.

28. Dung TC, Dinh PN, Nam VS, et al. Seroprevalence survey of avian influenza A(H5N1) among live poultry market workers in northern Viet Nam, 2011. Western Pac Surveill Response J 2014;5(4):21–6.

29. Uyeki TM, Nguyen DC, Rowe T, et al. Seroprevalence of antibodies to avian influenza A (H5) and A (H9) viruses among market poultry workers, Hanoi, Vietnam, 2001. PLoS One 2012;7(8):e43948.

30. Ortiz JR, Katz MA, Mahmoud MN, et al. Lack of evidence of avian-to-human transmission of avian influenza A (H5N1) virus among poultry workers, Kano, Nigeria, 2006. J Infect Dis 2007;196(11):1685–91.

31. Wang M, Fu CX, Zheng BJ. Antibodies against H5 and H9 avian influenza among poultry workers in China. N Engl J Med 2009;360(24):2583–4.

32. Schultsz C, Nguyen VD, Hai IT, et al. Prevalence of antibodies against avian influenza A (H5N1) virus among Cullers and poultry workers in Ho Chi Minh City, 2005. PLoS One 2009;4(11):e7948.

33. Bridges CB, Lim W, Hu-Primmer J, et al. Risk of influenza A (H5N1) infection among poultry workers, Hong Kong, 1997-1998. J Infect Dis 2002;185(8): 1005–10.

34. Wang Q, Ju L, Liu P, et al. Serological and virological surveillance of avian influenza A virus H9N2 subtype in humans and poultry in Shanghai, China, between 2008 and 2010. Zoonoses Public Health 2015;62(2):131–40.
35. Ly S, Horwood P, Chan M, et al. Seroprevalence and transmission of human influenza A(H5N1) virus before and after virus reassortment, Cambodia, 2006-2014. Emerg Infect Dis 2017;23(2):300–3.
36. Cavailler P, Chu S, Ly S, et al. Seroprevalence of anti-H5 antibody in rural Cambodia, 2007. J Clin Virol 2010;48(2):123–6.
37. Dejpichai R, Laosiritaworn Y, Phuthavathana P, et al. Seroprevalence of antibodies to avian influenza virus A (H5N1) among residents of villages with human cases, Thailand, 2005. Emerg Infect Dis 2009;15(5):756–60.
38. Wu J, Zou L, Ni H, et al. Serologic screenings for H7N9 from three sources among high-risk groups in the early stage of H7N9 circulation in Guangdong Province, China. Virol J 2014;11:184.
39. Xiang N, Bai T, Kang K, et al. Sero-epidemiologic study of influenza A(H7N9) infection among exposed populations, China 2013-2014. Influenza Other Respir Viruses 2017;11(2):170–6.
40. Khan SU, Anderson BD, Heil GL, et al. A systematic review and meta-analysis of the seroprevalence of influenza A(H9N2) infection among humans. J Infect Dis 2015;212(4):562–9.
41. Vong S, Ly S, Van Kerkhove MD, et al. Risk factors associated with subclinical human infection with avian influenza A (H5N1) virus–Cambodia, 2006. J Infect Dis 2009;199(12):1744–52.
42. Katz JM, Lim W, Bridges CB, et al. Antibody response in individuals infected with avian influenza A (H5N1) viruses and detection of anti-H5 antibody among household and social contacts. J Infect Dis 1999;180(6):1763–70.
43. Ma MJ, Ma GY, Yang XX, et al. Avian Influenza A(H7N9) virus antibodies in close contacts of infected persons, China, 2013-2014. Emerg Infect Dis 2015;21(4): 709–11.
44. Liao Q, Bai T, Zhou L, et al. Seroprevalence of antibodies to highly pathogenic avian influenza A (H5N1) virus among close contacts exposed to H5N1 cases, China, 2005-2008. PLoS One 2013;8(8):e71765.
45. Schultsz C, Dong VC, Chau NV, et al. Avian influenza H5N1 and healthcare workers. Emerg Infect Dis 2005;11(7):1158–9.
46. Buxton Bridges C, Katz JM, Seto WH, et al. Risk of influenza A (H5N1) infection among health care workers exposed to patients with influenza A (H5N1), Hong Kong. J Infect Dis 2000;181(1):344–8.
47. Uyeki TM, Chong YH, Katz JM, et al. Lack of evidence for human-to-human transmission of avian influenza A (H9N2) viruses in Hong Kong, China 1999. Emerg Infect Dis 2002;8(2):154–9.
48. Lin YP, Yang ZF, Liang Y, et al. Population seroprevalence of antibody to influenza A(H7N9) virus, Guangzhou, China. BMC Infect Dis 2016;16(1):632.
49. Ma C, Cui S, Sun Y, et al. Avian influenza A (H9N2) virus infections among poultry workers, swine workers, and the general population in Beijing, China, 2013-2016: a serological cohort study. Influenza Other Respir Viruses 2019; 13(4):415–25.
50. Buchy P, Vong S, Chu S, et al. Kinetics of neutralizing antibodies in patients naturally infected by H5N1 virus. PLoS One 2010;5(5):e10864.
51. Rajabali N, Lim T, Sokolowski C, et al. Avian influenza A (H5N1) infection with respiratory failure and meningoencephalitis in a Canadian traveller. Can J Infect Dis Med Microbiol 2015;26(4):221–3.

52. Lin PH, Chao TL, Kuo SW, et al. Virological, serological, and antiviral studies in an imported human case of avian influenza A(H7N9) virus in Taiwan. Clin Infect Dis 2014;58(2):242–6.

53. Skowronski DM, Chambers C, Gustafson R, et al. Avian Influenza A(H7N9) virus infection in 2 travelers returning from China to Canada, January 2015. Emerg Infect Dis 2016;22(1):71–4.

54. William T, Thevarajah B, Lee SF, et al. Avian influenza (H7N9) virus infection in Chinese tourist in Malaysia, 2014. Emerg Infect Dis 2015;21(1):142–5.

55. Zhou L, Liao Q, Dong L, et al. Risk factors for human illness with avian influenza A (H5N1) virus infection in China. J Infect Dis 2009;199(12):1726–34.

56. Mounts AW, Kwong H, Izurieta HS, et al. Case-control study of risk factors for avian influenza A (H5N1) disease, Hong Kong, 1997. J Infect Dis 1999;180(2):505–8.

57. Wan XF, Dong L, Lan Y, et al. Indications that live poultry markets are a major source of human H5N1 influenza virus infection in China. J Virol 2011;85(24):13432–8.

58. Yu H, Feng Z, Zhang X, et al. Human influenza A (H5N1) cases, urban areas of People's Republic of China, 2005-2006. Emerg Infect Dis 2007;13(7):1061–4.

59. Dinh PN, Long HT, Tien NT, et al. Risk factors for human infection with avian influenza A H5N1, Vietnam, 2004. Emerg Infect Dis 2006;12(12):1841–7.

60. Chotpitayasunondh T, Ungchusak K, Hanshaoworakul W, et al. Human disease from influenza A (H5N1), Thailand, 2004. Emerg Infect Dis 2005;11(2):201–9.

61. Li J, Chen J, Yang G, et al. Case-control study of risk factors for human infection with avian influenza A(H7N9) virus in Shanghai, China, 2013. Epidemiol Infect 2015;143(9):1826–32.

62. Liu B, Havers F, Chen E, et al. Risk factors for influenza A(H7N9) disease–China, 2013. Clin Infect Dis 2014;59(6):787–94.

63. Ai J, Huang Y, Xu K, et al. Case-control study of risk factors for human infection with influenza A(H7N9) virus in Jiangsu Province, China, 2013. Euro Surveill 2013;18(26):20510.

64. Li Q, Zhou L, Zhou M, et al. Epidemiology of human infections with avian influenza A(H7N9) virus in China. N Engl J Med 2014;370(6):520–32.

65. Zhou L, Ren R, Ou J, et al. Risk factors for Influenza A(H7N9) disease in China, a matched case control study, October 2014 to April 2015. Open Forum Infect Dis 2016;3(3):ofw182.

66. Gilsdorf A, Boxall N, Gasimov V, et al. Two clusters of human infection with influenza A/H5N1 virus in the Republic of Azerbaijan, February-March 2006. Euro Surveill 2006;11(5):122–6.

67. Sedyaningsih ER, Isfandari S, Setiawaty V, et al. Epidemiology of cases of H5N1 virus infection in Indonesia, July 2005-June 2006. J Infect Dis 2007;196(4):522–7.

68. Mao X, Wu J, Lau EHY, et al. Monitoring avian influenza viruses from chicken carcasses sold at markets, China, 2016. Emerg Infect Dis 2017;23(10):1714–7.

69. Lee CT, Slavinski S, Schiff C, et al. Outbreak of Influenza A(H7N2) among cats in an animal shelter with cat-to-human transmission-New York City, 2016. Clin Infect Dis 2017;65(11):1927–9.

70. Marinova-Petkova A, Laplante J, Jang Y, et al. Avian Influenza A(H7N2) virus in human exposed to sick cats, New York, USA, 2016. Emerg Infect Dis 2017;23(12).

71. Webster RG, Geraci J, Petursson G, et al. Conjunctivitis in human beings caused by influenza A virus of seals. N Engl J Med 1981;304(15):911.

72. Shinya K, Ebina M, Yamada S, et al. Avian flu: influenza virus receptors in the human airway. Nature 2006;440(7083):435–6.
73. Belser JA, Lash RR, Garg S, et al. The eyes have it: influenza virus infection beyond the respiratory tract. Lancet Infect Dis 2018;18(7):e220–7.
74. Oner AF, Dogan N, Gasimov V, et al. H5N1 avian influenza in children. Clin Infect Dis 2012;55(1):26–32.
75. Chea N, Yi SD, Rith S, et al. Two clustered cases of confirmed influenza A(H5N1) virus infection, Cambodia, 2011. Euro Surveill 2014;19(25) [pii:20839].
76. Ungchusak K, Auewarakul P, Dowell SF, et al. Probable person-to-person transmission of avian influenza A (H5N1). N Engl J Med 2005;352(4):333–40.
77. Kandun IN, Wibisono H, Sedyaningsih ER, et al. Three Indonesian clusters of H5N1 virus infection in 2005. N Engl J Med 2006;355(21):2186–94.
78. Wang H, Feng Z, Shu Y, et al. Probable limited person-to-person transmission of highly pathogenic avian influenza A (H5N1) virus in China. Lancet 2008; 371(9622):1427–34.
79. Le QM, Kiso M, Someya K, et al. Avian flu: isolation of drug-resistant H5N1 virus. Nature 2005;437(7062):1108.
80. Organization WH. H5N1 highly pathogenic avian influenza: timeline of major events 17 March 2014. 2014. 2019. Available at: https://www.who.int/influenza/human_animal_interface/H5N1_avian_influenza_update20140317.pdf. Accessed April 11, 2019.
81. Organization WH. Human cases of avian influenza A (H5N1) in North-West Frontier Province, Pakistan, October-November 2007. Wkly Epidemiol Rec 2008; 83(40):359–64.
82. Zhou L, Chen E, Bao C, et al. Clusters of human infection and human-to-human transmission of avian Influenza A(H7N9) Virus, 2013-2017. Emerg Infect Dis 2018;24(2):397–9.
83. Qi X, Qian YH, Bao CJ, et al. Probable person to person transmission of novel avian influenza A (H7N9) virus in Eastern China, 2013: epidemiological investigation. BMJ 2013;347:f4752.
84. Xiao XC, Li KB, Chen ZQ, et al. Transmission of avian influenza A(H7N9) virus from father to child: a report of limited person-to-person transmission, Guangzhou, China, January 2014. Euro Surveill 2014;19(25) [pii:20837].
85. Chen H, Liu S, Liu J, et al. Nosocomial co-transmission of avian Influenza A(H7N9) and A(H1N1)pdm09 Viruses between 2 patients with hematologic disorders. Emerg Infect Dis 2016;22(4):598–607.
86. Zhang ZH, Meng LS, Kong DH, et al. A suspected person-to-person transmission of avian Influenza A (H7N9) case in ward. Chin Med J (Engl) 2017;130(10): 1255–6.
87. Wang X, Wu P, Pei Y, et al. Assessment of human-to-human transmissibility of avian Influenza A(H7N9) virus across 5 waves by analyzing clusters of case patients in mainland China, 2013-2017. Clin Infect Dis 2019;68(4):623–31.
88. Gostic KM, Ambrose M, Worobey M, et al. Potent protection against H5N1 and H7N9 influenza via childhood hemagglutinin imprinting. Science 2016; 354(6313):722–6.
89. Cheng QL, Ding H, Sun Z, et al. Retrospective study of risk factors for mortality in human avian influenza A(H7N9) cases in Zhejiang Province, China, March 2013 to June 2014. Int J Infect Dis 2015;39:95–101.
90. Ji H, Gu Q, Chen LL, et al. Epidemiological and clinical characteristics and risk factors for death of patients with avian influenza A H7N9 virus infection from Jiangsu Province, Eastern China. PLoS One 2014;9(3):e89581.

91. Xiao YY, Cai J, Wang XY, et al. Prognosis and survival of 128 patients with severe avian influenza A(H7N9) infection in Zhejiang province, China. Epidemiol Infect 2015;143(9):1833–8.
92. Sha J, Chen X, Ren Y, et al. Differences in the epidemiology and virology of mild, severe and fatal human infections with avian influenza A (H7N9) virus. Arch Virol 2016;161(5):1239–59.
93. Peiris M, Yuen KY, Leung CW, et al. Human infection with influenza H9N2. Lancet 1999;354(9182):916–7.
94. Cheng VC, Chan JF, Wen X, et al. Infection of immunocompromised patients by avian H9N2 influenza A virus. J Infect 2011;62(5):394–9.
95. Horby P, Sudoyo H, Viprakasit V, et al. What is the evidence of a role for host genetics in susceptibility to influenza A/H5N1? Epidemiol Infect 2010;138(11):1550–8.
96. Le MQ, Horby P, Fox A, et al. Subclinical avian influenza A(H5N1) virus infection in human, Vietnam. Emerg Infect Dis 2013;19(10):1674–7.
97. Yang P, Lou X, Zheng Y, et al. Cytokines and chemokines in mild/asymptomatic cases infected with avian influenza A (H7N9) virus. J Med Microbiol 2016;65(10):1232–5.
98. Oner AF, Bay A, Arslan S, et al. Avian influenza A (H5N1) infection in eastern Turkey in 2006. N Engl J Med 2006;355(21):2179–85.
99. Editorial team C. Avian influenza A/(H7N2) outbreak in the United Kingdom. Euro Surveill 2007;12(22):3206.
100. Nguyen-Van-Tam JS, Nair P, Acheson P, et al. Outbreak of low pathogenicity H7N3 avian influenza in UK, including associated case of human conjunctivitis. Euro Surveill 2006;11(18):2952.
101. Skowronski DM, Tweed SA, Petric M, et al. Human illness and isolation of low-pathogenicity avian influenza virus of the H7N3 subtype in British Columbia, Canada. J Infect Dis 2006;193(6):899–900 [author reply 900-91].
102. Tweed SA, Skowronski DM, David ST, et al. Human illness from avian influenza H7N3, British Columbia. Emerg Infect Dis 2004;10(12):2196–9.
103. Kurtz J, Manvell RJ, Banks J. Avian influenza virus isolated from a woman with conjunctivitis. Lancet 1996;348(9031):901–2.
104. Puzelli S, Rossini G, Facchini M, et al. Human infection with highly pathogenic A(H7N7) avian influenza virus, Italy, 2013. Emerg Infect Dis 2014;20(10):1745–9.
105. Arzey GG, Kirkland PD, Arzey KE, et al. Influenza virus A (H10N7) in chickens and poultry abattoir workers, Australia. Emerg Infect Dis 2012;18(5):814–6.
106. Kandeel A, Manoncourt S, Abd el Kareem E, et al. Zoonotic transmission of avian influenza virus (H5N1), Egypt, 2006-2009. Emerg Infect Dis 2010;16(7):1101–7.
107. Brooks WA, Alamgir AS, Sultana R, et al. Avian influenza virus A (H5N1), detected through routine surveillance, in child, Bangladesh. Emerg Infect Dis 2009;15(8):1311–3.
108. Chakraborty A, Rahman M, Hossain MJ, et al. Mild respiratory illness among young children caused by highly pathogenic avian Influenza A (H5N1) virus infection in Dhaka, Bangladesh, 2011. J Infect Dis 2017;216(suppl_4):S520–8.
109. Zhang R, Chen T, Ou X, et al. Clinical, epidemiological and virological characteristics of the first detected human case of avian influenza A(H5N6) virus. Infect Genet Evol 2016;40:236–42.
110. Jiang H, Wu P, Uyeki TM, et al. Preliminary epidemiologic assessment of human infections with highly pathogenic Avian Influenza A(H5N6) Virus, China. Clin Infect Dis 2017;65(3):383–8.

111. Terebuh P, Adija A, Edwards L, et al. Human infection with avian influenza A(H7N2) virus-Virginia, 2002. Influenza Other Respir Viruses 2018;12(4): 529–32.
112. Yu H, Gao Z, Feng Z, et al. Clinical characteristics of 26 human cases of highly pathogenic avian influenza A (H5N1) virus infection in China. PLoS One 2008; 3(8):e2985.
113. Liem NT, Tung CV, Hien ND, et al. Clinical features of human influenza A (H5N1) infection in Vietnam: 2004-2006. Clin Infect Dis 2009;48(12):1639–46.
114. Li K, Liu H, Yang Z, et al. Clinical and epidemiological characteristics of a patient infected with H5N6 avian influenza A virus. J Clin Virol 2016;82:20–6.
115. Bi Y, Tan S, Yang Y, et al. Clinical and immunological characteristics of human infections with H5N6 avian influenza virus. Clin Infect Dis 2019;68(7):1100–9.
116. Wei SH, Yang JR, Wu HS, et al. Human infection with avian influenza A H6N1 virus: an epidemiological analysis. Lancet Respir Med 2013;1(10):771–8.
117. Ostrowsky B, Huang A, Terry W, et al. Low pathogenic avian influenza A (H7N2) virus infection in immunocompromised adult, New York, USA, 2003. Emerg Infect Dis 2012;18(7):1128–31.
118. Tong XC, Weng SS, Xue F, et al. First human infection by a novel avian influenza A(H7N4) virus. J Infect 2018;77(3):249–57.
119. Fouchier RA, Schneeberger PM, Rozendaal FW, et al. Avian influenza A virus (H7N7) associated with human conjunctivitis and a fatal case of acute respiratory distress syndrome. Proc Natl Acad Sci U S A 2004;101(5):1356–61.
120. Gao HN, Lu HZ, Cao B, et al. Clinical findings in 111 cases of influenza A (H7N9) virus infection. N Engl J Med 2013;368(24):2277–85.
121. Yang Y, Wong G, Yang L, et al. Comparison between human infections caused by highly and low pathogenic H7N9 avian influenza viruses in Wave Five: clinical and virological findings. J Infect 2019;78(3):241–8.
122. Chen H, Yuan H, Gao R, et al. Clinical and epidemiological characteristics of a fatal case of avian influenza A H10N8 virus infection: a descriptive study. Lancet 2014;383(9918):714–21.
123. Zhou L, Tan Y, Kang M, et al. Preliminary epidemiology of human infections with highly pathogenic Avian Influenza A(H7N9) virus, China, 2017. Emerg Infect Dis 2017;23(8):1355–9.
124. Zhang W, Wan J, Qian K, et al. Clinical characteristics of human infection with a novel avian-origin influenza A(H10N8) virus. Chin Med J (Engl) 2014;127(18): 3238–42.
125. Organization WH. Influenza at the human-animal interface. Summary and assessment 20 July to 3 October 2016. 2016. Available at: https://www.who. int/influenza/human_animal_interface/Influenza_Summary_IRA_HA_interface_10_ 03_2016.pdf?ua=1. Accessed April 11, 2019.
126. Huai Y, Xiang N, Zhou L, et al. Incubation period for human cases of avian influenza A (H5N1) infection, China. Emerg Infect Dis 2008;14(11):1819–21.
127. Cowling BJ, Jin L, Lau EH, et al. Comparative epidemiology of human infections with avian influenza A H7N9 and H5N1 viruses in China: a population-based study of laboratory-confirmed cases. Lancet 2013;382(9887):129–37.
128. Virlogeux V, Li M, Tsang TK, et al. Estimating the distribution of the incubation periods of human Avian Influenza A(H7N9) virus infections. Am J Epidemiol 2015;182(8):723–9.
129. Virlogeux V, Yang J, Fang VJ, et al. Association between the severity of Influenza A(H7N9) virus infections and length of the incubation period. PLoS One 2016; 11(2):e0148506.

130. Uyeki TM. Human infection with highly pathogenic avian influenza A (H5N1) virus: review of clinical issues. Clin Infect Dis 2009;49(2):279–90.
131. Tran TH, Nguyen TL, Nguyen TD, et al. Avian influenza A (H5N1) in 10 patients in Vietnam. N Engl J Med 2004;350(12):1179–88.
132. Apisarnthanarak A, Kitphati R, Thongphubeth K, et al. Atypical avian influenza (H5N1). Emerg Infect Dis 2004;10(7):1321–4.
133. de Jong MD, Bach VC, Phan TQ, et al. Fatal avian influenza A (H5N1) in a child presenting with diarrhea followed by coma. N Engl J Med 2005;352(7):686–91.
134. Zhang Y, Zou P, Gao H, et al. Neutrophil-lymphocyte ratio as an early new marker in AIV-H7N9-infected patients: a retrospective study. Ther Clin Risk Manag 2019;15:911–9.
135. Feng F, Jiang Y, Yuan M, et al. Association of radiologic findings with mortality in patients with avian influenza H7N9 pneumonia. PLoS One 2014;9(4):e93885.
136. Buchy P, Mardy S, Vong S, et al. Influenza A/H5N1 virus infection in humans in Cambodia. J Clin Virol 2007;39(3):164–8.
137. Gao R, Dong L, Dong J, et al. A systematic molecular pathology study of a laboratory confirmed H5N1 human case. PLoS One 2010;5(10):e13315.
138. Yu L, Wang Z, Chen Y, et al. Clinical, virological, and histopathological manifestations of fatal human infections by avian influenza A(H7N9) virus. Clin Infect Dis 2013;57(10):1449–57.
139. Mak GCK, Kwan MY, Mok CKP, et al. Influenza A(H5N1) virus infection in a child with encephalitis complicated by obstructive hydrocephalus. Clin Infect Dis 2018;66(1):136–9.
140. Xia JB, Zhu J, Hu J, et al. H7N9 influenza A-induced pneumonia associated with acute myelitis in an adult. Intern Med 2014;53(10):1093–5.
141. Shi J, Xie J, He Z, et al. A detailed epidemiological and clinical description of 6 human cases of avian-origin influenza A (H7N9) virus infection in Shanghai. PLoS One 2013;8(10):e77651.
142. Pan M, Gao R, Lv Q, et al. Human infection with a novel, highly pathogenic avian influenza A (H5N6) virus: virological and clinical findings. J Infect 2016;72(1):52–9.
143. Shu Y, Yu H, Li D. Lethal avian influenza A (H5N1) infection in a pregnant woman in Anhui Province, China. N Engl J Med 2006;354(13):1421–2.
144. Le TV, Phan LT, Ly KHK, et al. Fatal avian influenza A(H5N1) infection in a 36-week pregnant woman survived by her newborn in Sóc Trăng Province, Vietnam, 2012. Influenza Other Respir Viruses 2019;13(3):292–7.
145. Ku AS, Chan LT. The first case of H5N1 avian influenza infection in a human with complications of adult respiratory distress syndrome and Reye's syndrome. J Paediatr Child Health 1999;35(2):207–9.
146. Yang M, Gao H, Chen J, et al. Bacterial coinfection is associated with severity of avian influenza A (H7N9), and procalcitonin is a useful marker for early diagnosis. Diagn Microbiol Infect Dis 2016;84(2):165–9.
147. Luo H, Wang S, Yuan T, et al. Clinical characteristics from co-infection with avian influenza A H7N9 and Mycoplasma pneumoniae: a case report. J Med Case Rep 2018;12(1):77.
148. Liu WJ, Zou R, Hu Y, et al. Clinical, immunological and bacteriological characteristics of H7N9 patients nosocomially co-infected by Acinetobacter Baumannii: a case control study. BMC Infect Dis 2018;18(1):664.
149. Zheng S, Zou Q, Wang X, et al. Factors associated with fatality due to avian influenza A(H7N9) infection in China. Clin Infect Dis 2019. [Epub ahead of print].

150. Fox A, Horby P, Ha NH, et al. Influenza A H5N1 and HIV co-infection: case report. BMC Infect Dis 2010;10:167.
151. Yang Y, Guo F, Zhao W, et al. Novel avian-origin influenza A (H7N9) in critically ill patients in China*. Crit Care Med 2015;43(2):339–45.
152. Pawestri HA, Eggink D, Isfandari S, et al. Viral factors associated with the high mortality related to human infections with clade 2.1 influenza A/H5N1 virus in Indonesia. Clin Infect Dis 2019 [pii:ciz328].
153. Gu J, Xie Z, Gao Z, et al. H5N1 infection of the respiratory tract and beyond: a molecular pathology study. Lancet 2007;370(9593):1137–45.
154. Xiong X, Martin SR, Haire LF, et al. Receptor binding by an H7N9 influenza virus from humans. Nature 2013;499(7459):496–9.
155. Cao B, Gao H, Zhou B, et al. Adjuvant corticosteroid treatment in adults with Influenza A (H7N9) viral pneumonia. Crit Care Med 2016;44(6):e318–28.
156. Wang Y, Guo Q, Yan Z, et al. Factors associated with prolonged viral shedding in patients with Avian Influenza A(H7N9) virus infection. J Infect Dis 2018; 217(11):1708–17.
157. Guan Y, Poon LL, Cheung CY, et al. H5N1 influenza: a protean pandemic threat. Proc Natl Acad Sci U S A 2004;101(21):8156–61.
158. Hu Y, Lu S, Song Z, et al. Association between adverse clinical outcome in human disease caused by novel influenza A H7N9 virus and sustained viral shedding and emergence of antiviral resistance. Lancet 2013;381(9885):2273–9.
159. Hui KP, Chan LL, Kuok DI, et al. Tropism and innate host responses of influenza A/H5N6 virus: an analysis of ex vivo and in vitro cultures of the human respiratory tract. Eur Respir J 2017;49(3) [pii:1601710].
160. Chan MC, Chan RW, Chan LL, et al. Tropism and innate host responses of a novel avian influenza A H7N9 virus: an analysis of ex-vivo and in-vitro cultures of the human respiratory tract. Lancet Respir Med 2013;1(7):534–42.
161. Chan MC, Cheung CY, Chui WH, et al. Proinflammatory cytokine responses induced by influenza A (H5N1) viruses in primary human alveolar and bronchial epithelial cells. Respir Res 2005;6:135.
162. Yu WC, Chan RW, Wang J, et al. Viral replication and innate host responses in primary human alveolar epithelial cells and alveolar macrophages infected with influenza H5N1 and H1N1 viruses. J Virol 2011;85(14):6844–55.
163. Meliopoulos VA, Karlsson EA, Kercher L, et al. Human H7N9 and H5N1 influenza viruses differ in induction of cytokines and tissue tropism. J Virol 2014;88(22): 12982–91.
164. Zeng H, Belser JA, Goldsmith CS, et al. A(H7N9) virus results in early induction of proinflammatory cytokine responses in both human lung epithelial and endothelial cells and shows increased human adaptation compared with avian H5N1 virus. J Virol 2015;89(8):4655–67.
165. Zhou J, Wang D, Gao R, et al. Biological features of novel avian influenza A (H7N9) virus. Nature 2013;499(7459):500–3.
166. Zhao C, Qi X, Ding M, et al. Pro-inflammatory cytokine dysregulation is associated with novel avian influenza A (H7N9) virus in primary human macrophages. J Gen Virol 2016;97(2):299–305.
167. Cheung CY, Poon LL, Lau AS, et al. Induction of proinflammatory cytokines in human macrophages by influenza A (H5N1) viruses: a mechanism for the unusual severity of human disease? Lancet 2002;360(9348):1831–7.
168. de Jong MD, Simmons CP, Thanh TT, et al. Fatal outcome of human influenza A (H5N1) is associated with high viral load and hypercytokinemia. Nat Med 2006; 12(10):1203–7.

169. Wang Z, Zhang A, Wan Y, et al. Early hypercytokinemia is associated with interferon-induced transmembrane protein-3 dysfunction and predictive of fatal H7N9 infection. Proc Natl Acad Sci U S A 2014;111(2):769–74.

170. Guo J, Huang F, Liu J, et al. The serum profile of hypercytokinemia factors identified in H7N9-infected patients can predict fatal outcomes. Sci Rep 2015;5: 10942.

171. Hui KPY, Ching RHH, Chan SKH, et al. Tropism, replication competence, and innate immune responses of influenza virus: an analysis of human airway organoids and ex-vivo bronchus cultures. Lancet Respir Med 2018;6(11):846–54.

172. Tundup S, Kandasamy M, Perez JT, et al. Endothelial cell tropism is a determinant of H5N1 pathogenesis in mammalian species. PLoS Pathog 2017;13(3): e1006270.

173. Gao R, Pan M, Li X, et al. Post-mortem findings in a patient with avian influenza A (H5N6) virus infection. Clin Microbiol Infect 2016;22(6):574.e1-5.

174. Nakajima N, Van Tin N, Sato Y, et al. Pathological study of archival lung tissues from five fatal cases of avian H5N1 influenza in Vietnam. Mod Pathol 2013;26(3): 357–69.

175. Liem NT, Nakajima N, Phat IP, et al. H5N1-infected cells in lung with diffuse alveolar damage in exudative phase from a fatal case in Vietnam. Jpn J Infect Dis 2008;61(2):157–60.

176. Zhang Z, Zhang J, Huang K, et al. Systemic infection of avian influenza A virus H5N1 subtype in humans. Hum Pathol 2009;40(5):735–9.

177. Feng Y, Hu L, Lu S, et al. Molecular pathology analyses of two fatal human infections of avian influenza A(H7N9) virus. J Clin Pathol 2015;68(1):57–63.

178. Guo Q, Huang JA, Zhao D, et al. Pathological changes in a patient with acute respiratory distress syndrome and H7N9 influenza virus infection. Crit Care 2014;18(6):666.

179. Nicholls JM, Tsai PN, Chan RW, et al. Fatal H7N9 pneumonia complicated by viral infection of a prosthetic cardiac valve - an autopsy study. J Clin Virol 2014;61(3):466–9.

180. To KF, Chan PK, Chan KF, et al. Pathology of fatal human infection associated with avian influenza A H5N1 virus. J Med Virol 2001;63(3):242–6.

181. Centers for Disease Control and Prevention. Interim guidance for infection control within healthcare settings when caring for confirmed cases, probable cases, and cases under investigation for infection with novel Influenza A viruses associated with severe disease. 2019. Available at: https://www.cdc.gov/flu/avianflu/novel-flu-infection-control.htm. Accessed April 11, 2019.

182. World Health Organization. Infection prevention and control of epidemic-and pandemic prone acute respiratory infections in health care. WHO Guidelines; 2014. Available at: https://www.who.int/csr/bioriskreduction/infection_control/publication/en/. Accessed April 11, 2019.

183. South East Asia Infectious Disease Clinical Research Network. Effect of double dose oseltamivir on clinical and virological outcomes in children and adults admitted to hospital with severe influenza: double blind randomised controlled trial. BMJ 2013;346:f3039.

184. Kandun IN, Tresnaningsih E, Purba WH, et al. Factors associated with case fatality of human H5N1 virus infections in Indonesia: a case series. Lancet 2008; 372(9640):744–9.

185. Hanshaoworakul W, Simmerman JM, Narueponjirakul U, et al. Severe human influenza infections in Thailand: oseltamivir treatment and risk factors for fatal outcome. PLoS One 2009;4(6):e6051.

186. Adisasmito W, Chan PK, Lee N, et al. Effectiveness of antiviral treatment in human influenza A(H5N1) infections: analysis of a Global Patient Registry. J Infect Dis 2010;202(8):1154–60.

187. Chan PK, Lee N, Zaman M, et al. Determinants of antiviral effectiveness in influenza virus A subtype H5N1. J Infect Dis 2012;206(9):1359–66.

188. Zheng S, Tang L, Gao H, et al. Benefit of early initiation of neuraminidase inhibitor treatment to hospitalized patients with Avian Influenza A(H7N9) virus. Clin Infect Dis 2018;66(7):1054–60.

189. Zhang Y, Gao H, Liang W, et al. Efficacy of oseltamivir-peramivir combination therapy compared to oseltamivir monotherapy for Influenza A (H7N9) infection: a retrospective study. BMC Infect Dis 2016;16:76.

190. de Jong MD, Tran TT, Truong HK, et al. Oseltamivir resistance during treatment of influenza A (H5N1) infection. N Engl J Med 2005;353(25):2667–72.

191. Marjuki H, Mishin VP, Chesnokov AP, et al. Characterization of drug-resistant influenza A(H7N9) variants isolated from an oseltamivir-treated patient in Taiwan. J Infect Dis 2015;211(2):249–57.

192. Ke C, Mok CKP, Zhu W, et al. Human infection with highly pathogenic Avian Influenza A(H7N9) virus, China. Emerg Infect Dis 2017;23(8):1332–40.

193. Kile JC, Ren R, Liu L, et al. Update: increase in human infections with novel Asian lineage Avian Influenza A(H7N9) viruses during the fifth epidemic - China, October 1, 2016-August 7, 2017. MMWR Morb Mortal Wkly Rep 2017;66(35):928–32.

194. Zhang X, Song Z, He J, et al. Drug susceptibility profile and pathogenicity of H7N9 influenza virus (Anhui1 lineage) with R292K substitution. Emerg Microbes Infect 2014;3(11):e78.

195. Zhou B, Zhong N, Guan Y. Treatment with convalescent plasma for influenza A (H5N1) infection. N Engl J Med 2007;357(14):1450–1.

196. Wu XX, Gao HN, Wu HB, et al. Successful treatment of avian-origin influenza A (H7N9) infection using convalescent plasma. Int J Infect Dis 2015;41:3–5.

197. Ma W, Huang H, Chen J, et al. Predictors for fatal human infections with avian H7N9 influenza, evidence from four epidemic waves in Jiangsu Province, Eastern China, 2013-2016. Influenza Other Respir Viruses 2017;11(5):418–24.

198. Lu H, Zhang C, Qian G, et al. An analysis of microbiota-targeted therapies in patients with avian influenza virus subtype H7N9 infection. BMC Infect Dis 2014;14:359.

199. Qin N, Zheng B, Yao J, et al. Influence of H7N9 virus infection and associated treatment on human gut microbiota. Sci Rep 2015;5:14771.

200. Hu X, Zhang H, Lu H, et al. The effect of probiotic treatment on patients infected with the H7N9 influenza virus. PLoS One 2016;11(3):e0151976.

201. Liu C, Li J, Sun W, et al. Extracorporeal membrane oxygenation as rescue therapy for H7N9 influenza-associated acute respiratory distress syndrome. Chin Med J (Engl) 2014;127(9):1798.

202. Wang G, Zhou Y, Gong S, et al. A pregnant woman with avian influenza A (H7N9) virus pneumonia and ARDS managed with extracorporeal membrane oxygenation. Southeast Asian J Trop Med Public Health 2015;46(3):444–8.

203. Tang X, He H, Sun B, et al. ARDS associated with pneumonia caused by avian influenza A H7N9 virus treated with extracorporeal membrane oxygenation. Clin Respir J 2015;9(3):380–4.

204. Qian L, Zheng J, Xu H, et al. Extracorporeal membrane oxygenation treatment of a H7N9-caused respiratory failure patient with mechanical valves replacement history: a case report. Medicine (Baltimore) 2016;95(40):e5052.

205. Nie Q, Zhang DY, Wu WJ, et al. Extracorporeal membrane oxygenation for avian influenza A (H7N9) patient with acute respiratory distress syndrome: a case report and short literature review. BMC Pulm Med 2017;17(1):38.
206. Li H, Weng H, Lan C, et al. Comparison of patients with avian influenza A (H7N9) and influenza A (H1N1) complicated by acute respiratory distress syndrome. Medicine (Baltimore) 2018;97(12):e0194.
207. Huang L, Zhang W, Yang Y, et al. Application of extracorporeal membrane oxygenation in patients with severe acute respiratory distress syndrome induced by avian influenza A (H7N9) viral pneumonia: national data from the Chinese multicentre collaboration. BMC Infect Dis 2018;18(1):23.
208. Xie H, Zhou ZG, Jin W, et al. Ventilator management for acute respiratory distress syndrome associated with avian influenza A (H7N9) virus infection: a case series. World J Emerg Med 2018;9(2):118–24.
209. Liu X, Zhang Y, Xu X, et al. Evaluation of plasma exchange and continuous veno-venous hemofiltration for the treatment of severe avian influenza A (H7N9): a cohort study. Ther Apher Dial 2015;19(2):178–84.
210. Kitphati R, Pooruk P, Lerdsamran H, et al. Kinetics and longevity of antibody response to influenza A H5N1 virus infection in humans. Clin Vaccine Immunol 2009;16(7):978–81.
211. Zhang A, Huang Y, Tian D, et al. Kinetics of serological responses in influenza A(H7N9)-infected patients correlate with clinical outcome in China, 2013. Euro Surveill 2013;18(50):20657.
212. Guo L, Zhang X, Ren L, et al. Human antibody responses to avian influenza A(H7N9) virus, 2013. Emerg Infect Dis 2014;20(2):192–200.
213. Ma MJ, Liu C, Wu MN, et al. Influenza A(H7N9) virus antibody responses in survivors 1 year after infection, China, 2017. Emerg Infect Dis 2018;24(4):663–72.
214. Wang Z, Wan Y, Qiu C, et al. Recovery from severe H7N9 disease is associated with diverse response mechanisms dominated by CD8(+) T cells. Nat Commun 2015;6:6833.
215. Zhao M, Chen J, Tan S, et al. Prolonged evolution of virus-specific memory T cell immunity after severe avian Influenza A (H7N9) virus infection. J Virol 2018; 92(17) [pii:e01024-18].
216. Lu PX, Wang YX, Zhou BP, et al. Radiological features of lung changes caused by avian influenza subtype A H5N1 virus: report of two severe adult cases with regular follow-up. Chin Med J (Engl) 2010;123(1):100–4.
217. Tang XJ, Xi XH, Chen CC, et al. Long-term follow-up of 5 survivors after the first outbreak of human infections with avian Influenza A(H7N9) virus in Shanghai, China. Chin Med J (Engl) 2016;129(17):2128–30.
218. Chen J, Wu J, Hao S, et al. Long term outcomes in survivors of epidemic Influenza A (H7N9) virus infection. Sci Rep 2017;7(1):17275.
219. Peiris JS, Cowling BJ, Wu JT, et al. Interventions to reduce zoonotic and pandemic risks from avian influenza in Asia. Lancet Infect Dis 2016;16(2):252–8.
220. Cox NJ, Trock SC, Burke SA. Pandemic preparedness and the Influenza Risk Assessment Tool (IRAT). Curr Top Microbiol Immunol 2014;385:119–36.

Lassa Fever

Epidemiology, Clinical Features, Diagnosis, Management and Prevention

Danny A. Asogun, MBBS, FWACP[a,b,*], Stephan Günther, MD[c,d],
George O. Akpede, MBBS, FWACP, FCMPaed[e,1],
Chikwe Ihekweazu, MBBS, MPH, FFPH[f],
Alimuddin Zumla, MBChB, MSc, PhD, MD, FRCP(Lond), FRCP(Edin), FRCPath(UK), FAAS[g]

KEYWORDS

- Lassa fever • Epidemiology • Rodents • Clinical features • Diagnosis • Prevention
- Epidemic • Nosocomial transmission

KEY POINTS

- Lassa fever is an acute zoonotic disease of humans endemic to West Africa, caused by the Lassa virus, an enveloped, single-stranded RNA arenavirus.
- Lassa fever outbreaks continue in West Africa with up to 500,000 cases of Lassa fever annually with 10,000 deaths. Case fatality rates in hospitalized patients is up to 50%.
- Primary infection of humans occurs from contact with Lassa virus-infected rodents. Secondary person-to-person transmission occurs and can be prevented by instituting strict infection control measures.
- The incubation period ranges from 2 to 21 days. Initial presentation of Lassa fever is difficult to distinguish from other febrile illnesses.

Continued

All authors contributed equally.
Conflicts of Interest: All authors have an interest in global public health and emerging and re-emerging infections. All authors have no other conflict of interest to declare.
[a] Department of Public Health, College of Medicine, Ambrose Alli University, Ekpoma, Nigeria;
[b] Department of Public Health, Institute of Lassa Fever Research and Control, Irrua Specialist Teaching Hospital, P.M.B 008, Kilometre 87, Benin City-Auchi Road, Irrua, Nigeria; [c] Bernhard-Nocht Institute for Tropical Medicine, Strab 74, Hamburg 20359, Germany; [d] German Centre for Infection Research (DZIF), Partner Site Hamburg, Hamburg, Germany; [e] Department of Paediatrics, Faculty of Clinical Sciences, College of Medicine, Ambrose Alli University, Ekpoma, Nigeria; [f] Nigeria Centre for Disease Control, Plot 801, Ebitu Ukiwe Street, Jabi, Abuja, Nigeria; [g] Center for Clinical Microbiology, University College London, Royal Free Campus 2nd Floor, Rowland Hill Street, London NW3 2PF, United Kingdom
[1] Present address: P.M.B 008, Kilometre 87, Benin City-Auchi Road, Irrua, Nigeria.
* Corresponding author. Department of Public Health, College of Medicine, Ambrose Alli University, Ekpoma, Nigeria.
E-mail address: asogun2001@yahoo.com

Infect Dis Clin N Am 33 (2019) 933–951
https://doi.org/10.1016/j.idc.2019.08.002
0891-5520/19/© 2019 Elsevier Inc. All rights reserved.

id.theclinics.com

Continued

- Treatment involves supportive care with appropriate fluid and electrolyte balance, oxygenation, organ support and specific antiviral treatment with ribavirin or favipiravir. Vaccines are under development.

INTRODUCTION

Lassa fever, is an acute zoonotic disease of humans that is mainly endemic to West African countries of Guinea, Liberia, Nigeria, and Sierra Leone.[1–3] Other countries such as Mali, Benin, Togo, Cote d'Ivoire, Burkina Faso, and Ghana have reported sporadic Lassa fever cases.[1,4] Lassa fever is caused by the Lassa fever virus (LSAV), one of several viral causes of hemorrhagic fever, which can result in severe life-threatening systemic illness, characterized by disseminated intravascular coagulation, widespread mucosal bleeding, multiorgan failure, and shock requiring advanced life support.[5] Fifty years after its first discovery in 1969 in Nigeria, Lassa fever outbreaks have continued in West Africa and Lassa fever is now on the World Health Organization Blueprint list of priority pathogens under its research and development blue print for action.[6,7] Travel associated Lassa fever cases been recorded in several countries outside West Africa including the United States, Canada, United Kingdom, the Netherlands, Israel, Sweden, and Germany, creating much media hype.

HISTORICAL

Lassa fever first attracted global attention when missionary nurses in Nigeria developed a mysterious febrile illness in 1969.[8–11] They are thought to have acquired Lassa virus (LASV) infection while working in the mission station in the town of Lassa in the State of Borno, in northeastern Nigeria. The nurses were evacuated to the ECWA Hospital in Jos for further treatment. Two of 3 missionary nurses at ECWA Hospital died, and a doctor who performed an autopsy on 1 of the nurses[10–12] also fell ill and subsequently died. The third missionary nurse was flown to the United States, where she was diagnosed with Lassa fever and survived. The LSAV itself was first isolated from the nurse at the Yale Arbovirus Unit, Yale School of Medicine in 1970.[10,11] The chain of LASV transmission was traced back to the missionary nurses.

EPIDEMIOLOGY
Causative Agent: The Lassa Virus

LASV is an enveloped, single-stranded, bipartite RNA virus that belongs to the family Arenaviridae.[10,13] The virus is spherical with an average diameter of 110 to 130 nm, and in cross-section, they show "grainy particles" (ribosomes acquired from host cells) and thus the Latin name "arena," which means "sandy." The RNA genome encodes 4 proteins: the nucleoprotein and glycoprotein precursor on the small segment, and the RNA-dependent RNA-polymerase and matrix RING Zinc-finger protein on the large segment.[13,14] The LASV has a high level of nucleotide diversity between strains, which is correlated with clustering of strains around geographic locations. This has led to recognition of 6 major LASV clades or lineages: clades I to III in Nigeria; clade IV covering the countries of Sierra Leone, Guinea, and Liberia; and clade V in southern Mali; and a more recent clade VI, originating from Togo.[15] An important feature is the ability of these strains to evolve over time. A new lineage has recently been discovered in the recent Nigerian Lassa fever outbreak and if confirmed will make a total of 7 line-ages.[16,17] The high genetic variability of LASV is relevant for the design of diagnostic molecular assays as well as for the development of a universal Lassa fever vaccine that can be used in different geographic settings irrespective of circulating strain.[17–21] It may also have a bearing on the clinical presentation and severity of infection.[15,22–27]

Geographic Distribution

Lassa fever is endemic to West Africa (**Fig. 1**) with cases being reported from Nigeria, Benin, Liberia, Sierra Leone, Guinea, Mali, Senegal, and Ghana.[1–3,22] However, the

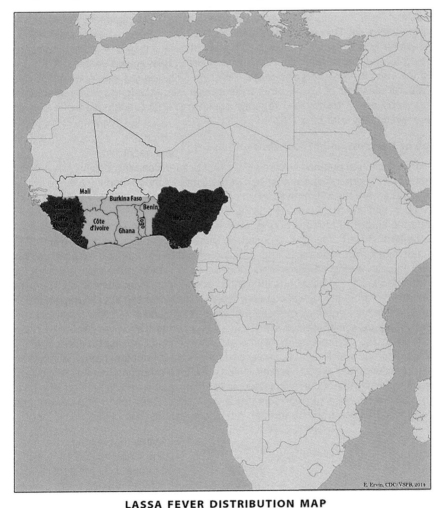

LASSA FEVER DISTRIBUTION MAP

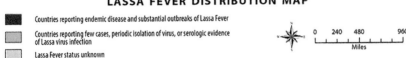

Countries reporting endemic disease and substantial outbreaks of Lassa Fever

Countries reporting few cases, periodic isolation of virus, or serologic evidence of Lassa virus infection

Lassa Fever status unknown

0   240   480   960
Miles

Fig. 1. Map of Africa – geographic distribution of Lassa fever. (*Courtesy of* the Centers for Disease Control. Lassa fever CDC. http:/www.cdc.gov/vhf/lassa/outbreaks. Accessed 6th August 2019.)

true geographic prevalence, incidence, and distribution of Lassa fever has been difficult to ascertain because a large proportion of cases are asymptomatic; the protean and nonspecific wide spectrum of clinical presentations; paucity of effective surveillance systems; lack of specific point-of-care diagnostic tests for Lassa fever, human migration, civil unrest, and deforestation, among others.[22–28] Exportation of travel associated Lassa fever cases outside West Africa to the United States, Canada, United Kingdom, the Netherlands, Israel, and Germany by aid workers, missionaries, and foreign military personnel is well-documented.[29,30]

Animal Reservoir

The animal reservoir for LASV is considered to be the "multimammate rat" *Mastomys natalensis* (**Fig. 2**). This is a rodent of the genus *Mastomys*, which is ubiquitous in West Africa and breeds prolifically.[30–35] The rats are infected in utero and remain infected for the rest of their life. Rats infected with LSAV do not become ill, but they shed the virus in their urine and feces. Although *M natalensis* was considered to be the natural reservoir of LASV, other rodent reservoirs (*Mastomys erythroleucus* and *Hylomyscus pamfi*) discovered recently could also affect distribution of LASV and Lassa fever cases over time.[34,35]

Mode of Transmission of Lassa Virus to Humans

Primary infection of humans occurs from direct or indirect contact with LASV-infected rodents.[1,35,36] Persons at greatest risk of acquiring LASV infection are those living in rural areas where the *Mastomys* rodents are usually found, especially in communities with poor sanitation or crowded living conditions.[27,37–41] The *Mastomys* rodents invade the homes of humans during the dry season in search of food. The source of LSAV infection for humans is exposure to urine, feces, blood, or meat from LSAV-infected *Mastomys* rodents. Direct contact with these materials, through touching soiled objects, eating contaminated food, or exposure to open cuts or sores, can lead to infection.[39–47] Infection is thought to occur from direct inoculation of mucous membranes or from the inhalation of aerosols produced when rodents urinate or defecate. The relative frequency of these modes of transmission remains unknown.

Secondary person-to-person spread in among humans has been recorded in people living in the community in overcrowded dwellings, families in the context of providing care to a sick person, and in communities in the context of burial practices. Health care workers are at increased risk of LASV infection.[21,22,25,48] Nosocomial transmission of LASV occurs within hospitals among and between patients and health care workers because of poor adherence to infection prevention and control practices.[46–55] LSAV can transmit through direct contact with the blood, urine, feces, or

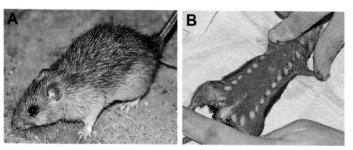

Fig. 2. (*A*) The multimammate rat *Mastomys natalensis*. (*B*) Ventral surface of *M natalensis* showing 2 rows of mammary glands. (*Courtesy of* [*A*] Danny Asogun; [*B*] Prof George Akpede.)

other bodily secretions or via accidental inoculation with sharp needles and contact with contaminated equipment.[50,51] Lassa fever outbreaks in large health care facilities are fueled by transmission where barrier nursing and infection control practices are inadequate.[52] Staff and other patients on maternity wards are at increased risk because Lassa fever is an important cause of spontaneous abortion and the virus is present in the blood and placenta of aborted fetuses.[56]

There have been reports of sexual transmission occurring months after recovery from acute disease.[51] Aerosol transmission between humans in natural settings has not been proven, but artificial production of infectious aerosols has.[36] The 1970 Lassa fever outbreak in Nigeria[9,11] was attributed to airborne transmission from a female patient with severe pulmonary disease, although definitive evidence of airborne transmission from subsequent outbreaks has not been forthcoming. Disease outbreaks seem to occur commonly through multiple independent reservoir-to-human transmissions.[16,21] The period of infectivity of patients with Lassa fever depends on the clinical state, with the highest infectivity periods being in late in the course of severe disease in the hemorrhagic phase.[48,52,57,58]

Age, Gender, and Susceptibility

Lassa fever can affect all age groups and both genders.[22,47,49] Pediatric Lassa fever is known to occur more commonly in male children for as yet unknown reasons. Presenting as an acute febrile illness, the case fatality rate may approach 30% in children with generalized edema, abdominal distension, and bleeding. Genetic and immunologic studies are ongoing in to provide better understanding of the pathogenesis and underlying protective mechanisms operating in Lassa fever.[14,57-59]

Environmental and Seasonal Factors and Risk of Transmission

Mastomys rats live in savannah and forests of west Africa, and breed frequently, producing large numbers of offspring.[32] They rapidly colonize human homes, huts, sheds, and food storage areas. Because they live in and around humans and scavenge on leftover human food items or poorly stored food, direct contact transmission is common, resulting in the relatively efficient spread from LASV-infected rats to humans. The seroprevalence of LASV antibodies among people living in houses correlates with households with large numbers of rats, owing to close contact with contaminated surfaces, utensils, and foodstuffs.[38-41,45,53,60] Human LASV infection may also occur when rodents are trapped and prepared for cooking and consumption, a common practice in some parts of West Africa.[38,45]

Factors that may affect the increase in LASV transmission and spill-over into human populations include seasonal changes, urbanization, environmental sanitation, deforestation and occurrence of disasters with involuntary migration.[37-39,60-63] This reinforces the need for a One-Human-Environmental-Animal Health (ONE HEALTH) approach for surveillance, control, early detection of spillover into human populations, and rapid emergency public response during outbreaks.[63,64]

LASSA FEVER OUTBREAKS (2016–2019)

Since 2016, there has been an increase in the number of reported Lassa fever cases from West Africa, especially in Nigeria, Benin, and Togo.[15-19,65-67] Although this increase seems unlikely to be due to the emergence of a new LASV variant, other factors may be playing a significant role: namely, increased human–rodent interactions, improved case recognition, increasing awareness and availability of diagnostics and therapy, increase in surveillance, changing demographics, and other environmental changes, or a combination of these factors.[15,16,21] Nigeria has experienced several outbreaks with large numbers of Lassa fever cases in 2018 and 2019.[9,22,67] There have been Lassa fever cases reported from Benin (54 cases and 28 deaths), Togo (2 cases), Liberia (7 cases, 3 deaths), and Sierra Leone (2 cases).[1] Cases have also been reported outside West Africa, exported by travelers to Sweden[68] and Germany.[69] The case in Germany resulted in limited secondary transmission when, 12 days after having been exposed to the corpse of a Lassa fever case imported from Togo, a symptomatic undertaker tested positive for LASV RNA.[69]

Out of the countries in West Africa that have reported Lassa fever outbreaks, Nigeria by far has had the largest Lassa fever disease burden with 23 states reporting Lassa fever cases[67] (**Fig. 3**). In Edo State, a recent spatial mapping and analysis of outbreaks supports earlier reports that some communities in the often-crowded university town of Ekpoma have geographic hotspots of Lassa fever cases.[65,66] Hotspot identification is important in planning of an effective control programs because it can reveal common environmental factor(s) causing the dense clustering of the disease in particular geographic areas.[4,23,70]

Ongoing Outbreak of Lassa Fever in Nigeria

The Nigeria Center for Disease Control reported an unusually large increase in Lassa fever cases in 2018, with a total of 3498 suspected cases from January 1 to December 31, 2018.[21,28,67] Of these, 633 cases were confirmed positive by laboratory testing. Public health officials were concerned that the Lassa fever outbreak in Nigeria in 2018 might be driven by previously unknown factors, or a new or more virulent LASV strain. From January 1 to March 24, 2019, a total of 1924 suspected cases were reported from 73 local government areas involving 21 states (see **Fig. 3**), with each state having recorded at least 1 confirmed Lassa fever case. Out of these, 495 were confirmed positive, with 117 deaths giving a case fatality rate of 22.9% for confirmed Lassa fever cases.[67] An important challenge is to define the diversity across LSAV lineages and strains and the ability of these strains to evolve over time. Global public health authorities are concerned that the 2018 to 2019 Lassa fever outbreak

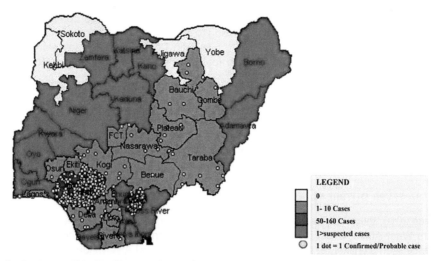

Fig. 3. Geographic distribution of Lassa fever cases in Nigeria, 2018 to 2019. (*Courtesy of* The Nigeria Center for Disease Control (2019). https:ncdc.gov.ng/diseases/sitreps. Accessed: 27th March 2019; with permission.)

in Nigeria might be driven by previously unknown factors, or a new or more virulent LSAV strain. Real-time analysis of 36 LASV genomes from the 2018 Nigeria Lassa fever outbreak[16] revealed that LSAV genomes seem to be drawn from a diverse range of viruses previously observed in Nigeria rather than from a single dominant strain. The extensive diversity and phylogenetic owing to intermingling with previous LSAV strains suggest independent zoonotic transmission events with humans becoming infected through contact with rodent feces or urine rather than human-to-human transmission.

CLINICAL FEATURES
Incubation Period, Symptoms, and Signs

The incubation period of Lassa fever ranges from 2 to 21 days.[1,2,22] Signs and symptoms of Lassa fever manifest up to 3 weeks after primary LSAV infection. The infection to disease ratio is not known. A wide spectrum of clinical manifestations occur in patients with Lassa fever, ranging from the asymptomatic, through mild, to moderate, to severe and fulminant disease (**Table 1**).[5,8,22,52] Up to 80% of LASV human infections cause mild illness and thus Lassa fever may remain undetected and undiagnosed in the community. The onset of the disease is usually gradual, starting with nonspecific symptoms of fever, general weakness, malaise, and headache. After a few days, symptoms worsen and sore throat, muscle pain, chest pain, nausea, vomiting, diarrhea, cough, arthralgia, and pain in the abdomen and back may follow. In up to one-fifth of infected individuals, the disease may progress to more serious symptoms. In severe cases, there may be facial swelling, petechiae and bruising, respiratory distress, hepatitis, renal failure, fits, tremors, gait disturbance, disorientation, loss of

Table 1
Clinical signs, symptoms, complications, and prognostic indicators

Symptoms	Signs
Fever, malaise, headache, weakness	Febrile, 1
Sore throat, muscle aches, joint pain, back pain, chest pain, cough, breathlessness	Dehydration, mouth ulcers, pharyngitis, conjunctival injection, sub-conjunctival hemorrhage, skin and mucosal petechiae/ecchymosis, jaundice, edema, ascites
Loss of appetite, nausea, vomiting, diarrhea, acute abdominal pain	
Red eyes, yellow eyes, swelling of eyes and legs, difficulty in urination	Lymphadenopathy, splenomegaly, hepatomegaly
Bruising and bleeding (skin, mouth, conjunctiva, rectal)	Lung crackles, rhonchi, bronchial breathing Pericardial effusion, pleural effusion
Tinnitus, vertigo, hearing loss	Sensorineural hearing loss (VIIIth cranial nerve)
Hand tremors, Unsteady walking, confusion, disorientation, fits, loss of consciousness	Signs of encephalitis, unsteady gait, drowsiness, coma

Complications	Poor Prognostic Indicators
Acute renal failure	High viral load and viremia
Liver failure	Grossly abnormal liver function tests (high AST levels)
Multiorgan failure	
Widespread bleeding	Renal failure (high urea and creatinine)
Disseminated intravascular coagulation	Severe bleeding
Shock (hypovolemic) and sepsis	Encephalitis
Encephalitis	Third trimester pregnancy
Fetal loss (spontaneous abortion)	Generalized edema
Deafness owing to VIIIth nerve sensorineural loss	
Death	

consciousness, and bleeding from the mucosa of the mouth, nose, vagina, or gastro-intestinal tract.[5,8,22,52] Bleeding is a feature of about 30% of patients with Lassa fever **(Fig. 4)**.[8,52,66] Lassa fever can present as an acute abdomen and should be considered as a differential diagnosis of febrile surgical acute abdomen and acute appendicitis in children in West Africa.[71,72]

Clinical Complications

Severe cases of Lassa fever manifest bleeding from mucosal surfaces (conjunctiva, mouth, and gut), disseminated intravascular coagulation, pleural or pericardial effusion, spontaneous abortion, renal failure, multiorgan failure, hypovolemic sepsis-like shock, encephalitis, encephalopathy, and bilateral or unilateral VIIIth nerve deafness.[8,22,66,73,74] The specific pathogenesis and molecular pathways that underlie these features remain poorly understood.[24,57]

A common long-term sequela of Lassa fever is deafness from sensorineural hearing loss.[74–77] Auditory nerve spiral ganglion degeneration and damage to cochlear hair cells and immune-mediated systemic vasculitis have been suggested as underlying causes.[77] Various degrees of deafness occur in approximately one-third of infections, and in many cases hearing loss is permanent. The severity of the disease does not seem to affect this complication and deafness has been reported in mild as well as in severe cases. Other long-term neurologic complications include seizures, gait disturbances, tremors, and encephalitis.

Lassa fever occurring during pregnancy can cause severe disease, high maternal death rates in the third trimester, and spontaneous abortion with an estimated 95% mortality in fetuses.[56,78,79]

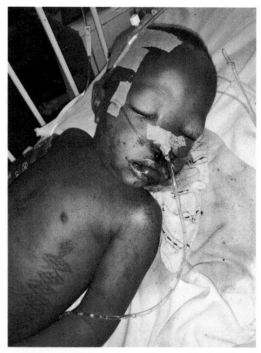

Fig. 4. Severely ill Nigerian child with Lassa fever with facial edema, spontaneously bleeding, and acute kidney injury. (*Courtesy of* George Akpede.)

Mortality, Risk, and Clinical Predictors of Management Outcomes

Although the overall mortality of Lassa fever in the community is low with only 1% of all LASV infections result in death, approximately 15% to 50% of hospitalized patients die within 14 days of the onset of disease.[79,80] Pregnant women, children under 5 years of age, and individuals with human immunodeficiency virus or other immunosuppressive conditions have an increased risk of death. Complications associated with poor management outcomes in hospitalized patients include acute kidney injury, liver failure, encephalopathy, seizures, decreased consciousness, disseminated intravascular coagulation with mucosal bleeding, septic shock progressing to multiorgan failure.[76,79,80] Studies of Lassa fever outbreaks in Nigeria show that patients with 1 or more features of severe illness such as acute kidney injury, encephalopathy, shock, disseminated intravascular coagulation, and bleeding are associated with increased case fatality rates (**Table 2**).[19,23,66,81]

LABORATORY DIAGNOSIS

The early identification of patients with Lassa fever is crucial for maximizing the benefit of available antiviral therapy, and for instituting infection control measures. Identifying the causative microbial cause of an acute febrile illness in sub-Saharan Africa can be challenging diagnostically.[70] Because the symptoms of Lassa fever are nonspecific, Lassa fever is difficult to distinguish from other common endemic microbial causes of fever such as malaria, shigellosis, typhoid fever, and other viral hemorrhagic fevers such as Ebola virus disease and yellow fever, both of which are also endemic to West Africa.

Specimen Collection

Making an accurate and specific definitive diagnosis of LSAV requires tests that are available for use only in high containment laboratories.[47] Because LSAV can spread via person-to-person virus spread via bodily fluids, laboratory staff should be aware of the risk of LSAV infection when processing potentially infectious patient specimens. Poor sample handling poses a safety hazard. The World Health Organization has issued step-by-step guidance on how to safely collect blood and other clinical samples from patients suspected to be infected with LSAV[82] and how to transport the patient samples to diagnostic reference laboratories.[83] Laboratory specimens may be hazardous and must be handled with extreme care. Ideally, every laboratory specimen for diagnosis of Lassa fever should be tested in a biosafety level 3 or 4 laboratory and should be treated as a highly infectious specimen. Lassa fever and other viral hemorrhagic fevers are category 4 pathogens. In outbreak situations, rapid deployment of mobile biosafety level 3 laboratories have been successfully used in the field.[84,85]

Lassa Virus Diagnostic Tests

A range of LASV diagnostic tests are available from cell culture, immunofluorescence assay, complement fixation tests, enzyme-linked immunosorbent assays for LASV antigens and IgM antibodies, polymerase chain reaction with several assays and targets, lateral flow assays, and other in-house rapid tests developed by research groups.[86] Definitive testing for LASV can only be done at reference laboratories, through virus isolation by cell culture. The virus itself may be cultured in 7 to 10 days, but this procedure should only be done in a high containment laboratory (biosafety level 4). Active infections can also be diagnosed by LASV-specific PCR, and LASV-specific IgG or IgM antibody response or LASV antigens shed during replication.[86–88]

Table 2
Case studies of Lassa fever at Irrua Specialist Teaching Hospital, Irrua, Nigeria

Study Reference	Adults		Children	Pregnant Women
	Asogun et al[47]	Okokhere et al[52]	Akpede et al,[66] 2019	Okogbenin et al,[81] 2010[a]
Year of study	2009–2010	2011–2015	2009–2017	2009–2018
No. of patients[a]	198	284	57	30
Deaths, n (%)	61 (30.8)	68 (24.0)	16 (28.1)	11 (36.7)
Factors associated with death (OR[c] [95% CI])				
Bleeding	Yes (6.2 [2.11–18.2])	Yes (1.9 [1.1–3.4])	Yes (17.68 [4.38–71.31])	Yes (not applicable[b])
Shock	ND	No	Yes (30.8 [3.39– 285.4])	ND
Acute kidney injury	Yes[c] (ND)	Yes 15 [8– 28])	Yes (29.57 [3.17– 275.7])	Yes (31.5 [2.98– 333.2])
Encephalopathy[d]	No (2.86 [0.78–10.58])	Yes (15 [7–34])	Yes (15.6 [4.21– 72.75])	Yes (31.5 [2.98–333.2])

Abbreviations: CI, confidence interval; ND, no data; OR, odds ratio.
[a] The same factors were associated with both maternal death and fetal loss.
[b] Nine of 11 patients with extravaginal bleeding versus none of 19 without extravaginal bleeding died.
[c] Data not available on the numbers with acute kidney injury but both the mean blood urea nitrogen (P<.001) and mean serum creatinine (P<.001) were significantly higher among those who died compared with those who survived.
[d] Defined by the presence of coma and/or seizures.

LASV RNA is detected using a nucleic acid amplification test, which can include techniques such as PCR, loop-mediated isothermal amplification, and strand displacement assays. However, reverse transcriptase PCR is the gold standard for making a definitive diagnosis of LASV infection in the early stages of the Lassa fever disease.[85,86,89,90]

Detection of LASV antibodies and antigens can be used to complement diagnosis. These can be detected by indirect immunofluorescence assay test (Immunofluorescence assay or indirect immunofluorescence test), Western blot, rapid diagnostic test formats, or by enzyme-linked immunosorbent serologic assays, which detect IgM and IgG antibodies. Many laboratories use in-house LASV assays.[87] For making a post mortem diagnosis, immunohistochemistry is performed on formalin-fixed tissue specimens.

Diagnostic Tests Under Evaluation

A rapid immunoassay for the LASV subtypes found in Sierra Leone and a similar test that is designed to detect all strains is being assessed in Nigeria.[89,90] Emerging technologies, such as CRISPR-based specific high-sensitivity enzymatic reporter unlocking, may soon provide multiplexed and portable nucleic acid detection platform for testing for new LASV strains.[91] There remains an urgent need for field-friendly, cheap, accurate, and rapid diagnostic tests for outbreak investigation and patient management.[92]

Specimen Type and Lassa Virus Detection

LASV can be present in several body fluid or tissues such as blood, urine, pleural fluid, semen, cerebrospinal fluid, throat swabs, and sputum. Acute LASV infections detected in the cerebrospinal fluid can be negative in blood[73] and LASV can persist in the central nervous system, urine, and semen long after viral clearance in the blood.[93]

MANAGEMENT OF PATIENTS
Supportive Care

Supportive care is important and appropriate fluid and electrolyte balance, oxygenation, and blood pressure control must be maintained.[1,2,22,94] To maintain renal function, dialysis is necessary (**Fig. 5**). Secondary bacterial infections should be treated with antibiotics. The treatment of patients with suspected or confirmed LSAV infections during outbreaks in dedicated Lassa fever treatment wards with facilities for enhanced supportive care including dialysis and respiratory support could decrease nosocomial case fatality and transmission rates.

Specific Antiviral Therapy

Specific antiviral therapy with the antiviral agent ribavirin can improve treatment outcome if given early in the course of illness.[94,95] However, although ribavirin has been used extensively for treatment and as postexposure prophylaxis, treatment of Lassa fever with ribavirin has been evaluated in only a single nonrandomized clinical[96] and in retrospective analyses of field studies.[80] Animal and/or human studies of the efficacy of ribavirin against the multiple LASV lineages and at various stages of Lassa fever disease progression are needed, as well as an assessment of the different administration routes and dosing regimens.[6]

Newer Therapies

Favipiravir is another broad-spectrum RNA inhibitor that has broad-spectrum activity against RNA viruses and has been shown to decrease LASV viremia in animal

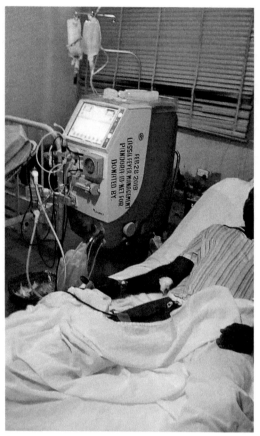

Fig. 5. A patient with Lassa fever undergoing renal dialysis in a Lassa isolation ward at Irrua Lassa Fever Hospital, Irrua, Nigeria. (*Courtesy of* Danny Asogun.)

models.[97] Monoclonal antibodies specific for LASV neutralization cloned from West African Lassa fever survivors[98] seem to bind to individual or combined Lassa GP protein subunits, which can potently neutralize all 4 LASV lineages—an early start to immunotherapeutic development. Human monoclonal antibody therapy seems to protect nonhuman primates against advanced Lassa fever.[99]

PREVENTION
Avoiding or Reducing Contact with Rats

Avoiding contact with *Mastomys* rodents can reduce the risk of primary transmission of LASV to humans.[37] Placing food away in rodent-proof containers and keeping the home and surroundings clean, as well as trapping in and around homes, can help to decrease rodent populations and contact with their droppings or urine. Further, educating people in high-risk areas about ways to decrease rodent populations in their homes will reduce risk of LASV infection.

Preventing Nosocomial Spread

Strict adherence to standard infection prevention and control precautions is mandatory for prevention of human LSAV infection spread in health care settings, especially when caring for patients with fever of undetermined origin and suspected viral hemorrhagic fevers. These measures include basic hand hygiene, respiratory hygiene, use of personal protective equipment (to block splashes or other contact with infected materials), safe injection practices, and safe burial practices. Health care workers caring for patients with suspected or confirmed Lassa fever should take measures to prevent contact with the patient's blood and body fluids and contaminated surfaces or materials, such as clothing and bedding. Laboratory workers should be trained to handle and process biological samples and process these in suitably equipped laboratories under maximum biological containment conditions.

When caring for patients with confirmed or suspected Lassa fever, transmission of LSAV in health care facilities through person-to-person contact or nosocomial routes can be avoided by following strict infection control procedures and using viral hemorrhagic fever isolation precautions and barrier nursing methods.[100] All health care facilities caring for suspected or confirmed Lassa fever cases should use generic precautions include wearing protective clothing, such as masks, gloves, gowns, and goggles; using infection control measures, such as complete equipment sterilization; and isolating infected patients from contact with unprotected persons until the disease has run its course.

Vaccines

The recurrent and increasing epidemic of Lassa fever has had major socioeconomic consequences on West Africa countries making the development of effective medical countermeasures urgent. One of these measures is the development of effective vaccines against Lassa fever.[101] Currently there are no effective Lassa fever vaccines. In 2017, the World Health Organization released a Target Product Profile for LASV vaccine development, and in 2018, the US Food and Drug Administration added Lassa fever to its priority list of infections for development of preventive measures. Several vaccines are under development, including LASSARAB and an inactivated recombinant LASV. The recombinant vesicular stomatitis virus (VSV) vaccine expressing LASV glycoprotein (VSV-LASV-GPC) is among one of the leading candidates developed thus far and is targeted for accelerated development by The Coalition for Epidemic Preparedness Innovations,[102,103] who are supporting the development of Lassa vaccine candidates.

SUMMARY

Although malaria, typhoid fever, and many other tropical infections are much more common, the diagnosis of Lassa fever should be considered in febrile patients returning from West Africa, especially if they have had exposures in rural areas or hospitals in countries where Lassa fever is known to be endemic. Health care workers should have a high index of clinical suspicion of the possibility of Lassa in returning travelers to Europe or the United States with Lassa fever. When a patient suspected to have Lassa fever is seen, the health care worker or attending physician should immediately contact local and national public health authorities for advice and to arrange for laboratory testing. There is a great need for point-of-care diagnostics for detecting Lassa fever cases to enable timely isolation and treatment and for defining outbreaks more accurately.

ACKNOWLEDGMENTS

All authors are members of the PANDORA-ID-NET consortium and acknowledge support from the European and Developing Countries Clinical Trials Partnership (EDCTP2) programme (Grant Agreement RIA2016E-1609) which is supported under

Horizon 2020, the European Union's Framework Programme for Research and Innovation. Sir A. Zumla is in receipt of a UK NIHR Senior Investigator Award.

REFERENCES

1. WHO 2019. Lassa fever. Available at: https://www.who.int/emergencies/diseases/lassa-fever/en/. Accessed March 18, 2019.
2. CDC 2019. Lassa fever. Available at: https://www.cdc.gov/vhf/lassa/index.html. Accessed March 18, 2019.
3. Owolabi JB, Mamah CM, Okoro CC, et al. Re-emerging human viral hemorrhagic fevers: a review. Am J Infect Dis Microbiol 2016;4(4):79–90.
4. Mylne AQ, Pigott DM, Longbottom J. Mapping the zoonotic niche of Lassa fever in Africa. Trans R Soc Trop Med Hyg 2015;109(8):483–92.
5. Ippolito G, Feldmann H, Lanini S, et al. Viral hemorrhagic fevers: advancing the level of treatment. BMC Med 2012;10:31.
6. WHO. Blueprint for action to prevent epidemics. May 2016 WHO, 2017. R&D Blueprint for action to prevent epidemics. 2016. Available at: http://www.who.int/blueprint/en/. Accessed October 26, 2018.
7. WHO. List of Blueprint priority diseases. 2018 annual review. 2018. Available at: https://www.who.int/blueprint/priority-diseases/en/. Accessed March 18, 2019.
8. Frame JD, Baldwin JM Jr, Gocke DJ, et al. Lassa fever, a new virus disease of man from West Africa. I. Clinical description and pathological findings. Am J Trop Med Hyg 1970;19(4):670–6.
9. Troup JM, White HA, Fom AL, et al. An outbreak of Lassa fever on the Jos plateau, Nigeria, in January-February 1970. A preliminary report. Am J Trop Med Hyg 1970;19(4):695–6.
10. Buckley SM, Casals J. Lassa fever, a new virus disease of man from West Africa. III. Isolation and Characterization of the virus. Am J Trop Med Hyg 1970;19:670–6.
11. Carey DE, Kemp GE, White HA, et al. Lassa fever. Epidemiological aspects of the 1970 epidemic, Jos, Nigeria. Trans R Soc Trop Med Hyg 1972;66(3):402–8.
12. Bond N, Schieffelin JS, Moses LM, et al. A historical look at the first reported cases of Lassa fever: IgG antibodies 40 years after acute infection. Am J Trop Med Hyg 2013;88(2):241–4.
13. Radoshitzky SR, Bào Y, Buchmeier MJ, et al. Past, present, and future of arenavirus taxonomy. Arch Virol 2015;160(7):1851–74.
14. Andersen KG, Shapiro J, Matranga CB, et al. Clinical sequence uncovers origins and evolution of Lassa virus. Cell 2015;162:736–50.
15. Whitmer SLM, Strecker T, Cadar D, et al. New Lineage of Lassa Virus, Togo, 2016. Emerg Infect Dis 2018;24(3):599–602.
16. Kafetzopoulou LE, Pullan ST, Lemey P, et al. Metagenomic sequencing at the epicenter of the Nigeria 2018 Lassa fever outbreak. Science 2019;363(6422):74–7.
17. Lukashevich IS. The search for animal models for Lassa fever vaccine development. Expert Rev Vaccines 2013;12(1):71–86.
18. Bowen MD, Rollin PE, Ksiazek TG, et al. Genetic diversity among Lassa virus strains. J Virol 2000;74(15):6992–7004.
19. Ehichioya DU, Hass M, Becker-Ziaja B, et al. Current molecular epidemiology of Lassa virus in Nigeria. J Clin Microbiol 2011;49(3):1157–61.
20. Hallam HJ, Hallam S, Rodriguez SE, et al. Baseline mapping of Lassa fever virology, epidemiology and vaccine research and development. NPJ Vaccin 2018;3:11. 1–8.

21. Siddle KJ, Eromon P, Barnes KG, et al. Genomic Analysis of Lassa Virus during an Increase in Cases in Nigeria in 2018. N Engl J Med 2018;379(18):1745–53.
22. Akpede GO, Asogun DA, Okogbenin SA, et al. Lassa fever outbreaks in Nigeria. Expert Rev Anti Infect Ther 2018;16(9):663–6.
23. Gibb R, Moses LM, Redding DW, et al. Understanding the cryptic nature of Lassa fever in West Africa. Pathog Glob Health 2017. https://doi.org/10.1080/20477724.2017.1369643.
24. Yun NE, Walker DH. Pathogenesis of Lassa fever. Viruses 2012;4(10):2031–48.
25. Safronetz D, Sogoba N, Lopez JE, et al. Geographic distribution and genetic characterization of Lassa virus in sub-Saharan Mali. PLoS Negl Trop Dis 2013; 7(12):e2582.
26. Sogoba N, Feldmann H, Safronetz D. Lassa fever in West Africa: evidence for an expanded region of endemicity. Zoonoses Public Health 2012. https://doi.org/10.1111/j.1863-2378.2012.01469.x.
27. Adebayo D, Nwobi EA, Vincent T, et al. Response preparedness to viral hemorrhagic fever in Nigeria: risk perception, attitude towards lassa fever. Epidemiology (Sunnyvale) 2015;5(199):1161–5.
28. Roberts L. Nigeria hit by unprecedented Lassa fever outbreak. Science 2018; 359(6381):1201–2.
29. Kofman A, Choi MJ, Rollin PE. Lassa Fever in Travelers from West Africa, 1969-2016. Emerg Infect Dis 2019;25(2):245–8.
30. Nikisins S, Rieger T, Patel P, et al. International external quality assessment study for molecular detection of Lassa virus. PLoS Negl Trop Dis 2015;9(5): e0003793.
31. Lecompte E, Fichet-Calvet E, Daffis S, et al. Mastomys natalensis and Lassa fever, West Africa. Emerg Infect Dis 2006. https://doi.org/10.3201/eid1212.060812.
32. Monath TP, Newhouse VF, Kemp GE, et al. Lassa virus isolation from *Mastomys natalensis* rodents during an epidemic in Sierra Leone. Science 1974; 185(4147):263–5.
33. Olayemi A, Obadare A, Oyeyiola A, et al. Arenavirus diversity and phylogeography of mastomys natalensis rodents, Nigeria. Emerg Infect Dis 2016;22(4): 694–7.
34. Coulibaly-N'Golo D, Allali B, Kouassi SK, et al. Novel arenavirus sequences in hylomyscus sp. and Mus (Nannomys) setulosus from Co ˆte d'Ivoire: implications for evolution of arenaviruses in Africa. PLoS One 2011;6(6):e20893.
35. Olayemi A, Cadar D, Magassouba N, et al. New hosts of the Lassa virus. Sci Rep 2016;6:25280.
36. CDC. Transmission: Lassa fever. 2014. Available at: https://www.cdc.gov. Accessed March 17, 2019.
37. Bonwitt J, Kandeh M, Dawson M, et al. Participation of women and children in hunting activities in Sierra Leone and implications for control of zoonotic infections. PLoS Negl Trop Dis 2017;11(7):e0005699.
38. Bonwitt J, Kelly AH, Ansumana R, et al. Rat-atouille: a mixed method study to characterize rodent hunting and consumption in the context of Lassa fever. Ecohealth 2016;13(2):234–47.
39. Bonwitt J, Sáez AM, Lamin J, et al. At home with mastomys and rattus: human-rodent interactions and potential for primary transmission of lassa virus in domestic spaces. Am J Trop Med Hyg 2017;96(4):935–43.
40. McCormick JB. Epidemiology and control of Lassa fever. Curr Top Microbiol Immunol 1987;134:69–78.

41. McCormick JB, Webb PA, Krebs JW, et al. A prospective study of the epidemiology and ecology of Lassa fever. J Infect Dis 1987;155:437–44.

42. Akhuemokhan OC, Ewah-Odiase RO, Akpede N, et al. Prevalence of Lassa Virus Disease (LVD) in Nigerian children with fever or fever and convulsions in an endemic area. PLoS Negl Trop Dis 2017;11(7):e0005711.

43. Bello OO, Akinajo OR, Odubamowo KH, et al. Lassa fever in pregnancy: report of 2 cases seen at the University College Hospital, Ibadan. Case Rep Obstet Gynecol 2016;2016:9673683.

44. Dan-Nwafor CC, Ipadeola O, Smout E, et al. A cluster of nosocomial Lassa fever cases in a tertiary health facility in Nigeria: description and lessons learned, 2018. Int J Infect Dis 2019;83:88–94.

45. Ter Meulen J, Lukashevich I, Sidibe K, et al. Hunting of peridomestic rodents and consumption of their meat as possible risk factors for rodent-to-human transmission of Lassa virus in the Republic of Guinea. Am J Trop Med Hyg 1996;55:661–6.

46. Brosh-Nissimov T. Lassa fever: another threat from West Africa. Disaster Mil Med 2016;2(1):8.

47. Asogun DA, Adomeh DI, Ehimuna J, et al. Molecular diagnostics for Lassa fever at Irrua specialist teaching hospital, Nigeria: lessons learnt from two years of laboratory operation. PLoS Negl Trop Dis 2012;6(9):e1839.

48. Bajani MD, Tomori O, Rollin PE, et al. A survey for antibodies to Lassa virus among health workers in Nigeria. Trans R Soc Trop Med Hyg 1997;91(4): 379–81.

49. Woyessa AB, Maximore L, Keller D, et al. Lesson learned from the investigation and response of Lassa fever outbreak, Margibi County, Liberia, 2018: case report. BMC Infect Dis 2019 Jul 11;19(1):610.

50. Simonsen L, Kane A, Lloyd J, et al. Unsafe injections in the developing world and transmission of bloodborne pathogens: a review. Bull World Health Organ 1999;77(10):789–800.

51. Arias A, Watson SJ, Asogun D, et al. Rapid outbreak sequencing of Ebola virus in Sierra Leone identifies transmission chains linked to sporadic cases. Virus Evol 2016;2(1):vew016.

52. Okokhere P, Colubri A, Azubike C, et al. Clinical and laboratory predictors of Lassa fever outcome in a dedicated treatment facility in Nigeria: a retrospective, observational cohort study. Lancet Infect Dis 2018;18(6):684–95.

53. Isere EE, Fatiregun AA, Ilesanmi O, et al. Lessons Learnt from Epidemiological Investigation of Lassa Fever Outbreak in a Southwest State of Nigeria December 2015 to April 2016. PLoS Curr 2018;10 [pii: ecurrents.outbreaks.bc4396a6650d0ed1985d731583bf5ded].

54. Garnett LE, Strong JE. Lassa fever: with 50 years of study, hundreds of thousands of patients and an extremely high disease burden, what have we learned? Curr Opin Virol 2019;37:123–31.

55. Fisher-Hoch SP, Tomori O, Nasidi A, et al. Review of cases of nosocomial Lassa fever in Nigeria: the high price of poor medical practice. BMJ 1995;311(7009): 857–9.

56. Price ME, Fisher-Hoch SP, Craven RB, et al. A prospective study of maternal and fetal outcome in acute Lassa fever infection during pregnancy. BMJ 1988; 297(6648):584–7.

57. Paessler S, Walker DH. Pathogenesis of the viral hemorrhagic fevers. Annu Rev Pathol 2013;8:411–40.

58. Shao J, Liang Y, Ly H. Human hemorrhagic fever causing arenaviruses: molecular mechanisms contributing to virus virulence and disease pathogenesis. Pathogens 2015;4:283–306.
59. Andersen KG, Shylakhter I, Tabrizi S, et al. Genome-wide scans provide evidence for positive selection of genes implicated in Lassa fever. Philos Trans R Soc Lond B Biol Sci 2012;367:868–77.
60. Ehizibolo DO, Ehizibolo PO, Ehizibolo EE, et al. The control of neglected zoonotic diseases in Nigeria through animal intervention. Afr J Biomed Res 2011; 14:81–8.
61. Brown H, Kelly AH, Marí Sáez A, et al. Extending the "social": anthropological contributions to the study of viral haemorrhagic fevers. PLoS Negl Trop Dis 2015;9(4):e0003651.
62. Redding DW, Moses LM, Cunningham AA, et al. Environmental-mechanistic modelling of the impact of global change on human zoonotic disease emergence: a case study of Lassa fever. Methods Ecol Evol 2016. https://doi.org/ 10.1111/2041-210X.12549.
63. Tambo E, Adetunde OT, Olalubi OA. Re-emerging Lassa fever outbreaks in Nigeria: re-enforcing 'One Health' community surveillance and emergency response practice. Infect Dis Poverty 2018. https://doi.org/10.1186/s40249-018-0421-8.
64. Zumla A, Dar O, Kock R, et al. Taking forward a 'One Health' approach for turning the tide against the Middle East respiratory syndrome coronavirus and other zoonotic pathogens with epidemic potential. Int J Infect Dis 2016;47:5–9.
65. Ilori EA, Frank C, Dan-Nwafor CC, et al. Increase in Lassa Fever Cases in Nigeria, January-March 2018. Emerg Infect Dis 2019;25(5). https://doi.org/10. 3201/eid2505.181247.
66. Akpede GO, Asogun DA, Okogbenin SA, et al. Caseload and case fatality of Lassa fever in Nigeria, 2001-2018: a specialist center's experience and its implications. Front Public Health 2019;7:170.
67. Nigeria Center for Disease Control. An update of Lassa fever outbreak in Nigeria. 2019. Available at: https://ncdc.gov.ng/diseases/sitreps/?cat=5&name=An update of Lassa fever outbreak in Nigeria. Accessed March 27, 2019.
68. Grahn A, Bråve A, Lagging M, et al. Imported Case of Lassa Fever in Sweden With Encephalopathy and Sensorineural Hearing Deficit. Open Forum Infect Dis 2016;3(4):198.
69. Ehlkes L, George M, Samosny G, et al. Management of a Lassa fever outbreak, Rhineland-Palatinate, Germany, 2016. Euro Surveill 2017;22(39). https://doi.org/ 10.2807/1560-7917.ES.2017.22.39.16-00728.
70. Schoepp RJ, Rossi CA, Khan SH, et al. Undiagnosed acute viral febrile illnesses, Sierra Leone. Emerg Infect Dis 2014. https://doi.org/10.3201/eid2007. 131265.
71. Akpede GO, Adetunji AE, Udefiagbon EO, et al. Acute abdomen in pediatric patients with Lassa fever: prevalence and response to nonoperative management. J Pediatr Infect Dis Soc 2018. https://doi.org/10.1093/jpids/piy093.
72. Dongo AE, Kesieme EB, Iyamu CE, et al. Lassa fever presenting as acute abdomen: a case series. Virol J 2013;10:123.
73. Okokhere PO, Bankole IA, Iruolagbe CO, et al. Aseptic meningitis caused by Lassa virus: case series report. Case Rep Neurol Med 2016;2016:4.
74. Mateer EJ, Huang C, Shehu NY, et al. Lassa fever-induced sensorineural hearing loss: a neglected public health and social burden. PLoS Negl Trop Dis 2018; 12(2):e0006187.

75. Ibekwe TS, Okokhere PO, Asogun D, et al. Early-onset sensorineural hearing loss in Lassa fever. Eur Arch Otorhinolaryngol 2011;268(2):197–201.

76. Okokhere PO, Ibekwe TS, Akpede GO. Sensorineural hearing loss in Lassa fever: two case reports. J Med Case Rep 2009;3:36.

77. Cashman KA, Wilkinson ER, Zeng X, et al. Immune-mediated systemic vasculitis as the proposed cause of sudden-onset sensorineural hearing loss following lassa virus exposure in Cynomolgus Macaques. MBio 2018;9(5) [pii: e01896-18].

78. Walls B. Lassa fever and pregnancy. Midwives Chron 1985;1168(98):136–8.

79. Dahmane A, van Griensven J, Van Herp M, et al. Constraints in the diagnosis and treatment of Lassa fever and the effect on mortality in hospitalized children and women with obstetric conditions in a rural district hospital in Sierra Leone. Trans R Soc Trop Med Hyg 2014;108(3):126–32.

80. Shaffer JG, Grant DS, Schieffelin JS, et al. Lassa fever in post-conflict Sierra Leone. PLoS Negl Trop Dis 2014;8(3):e2748.

81. Okogbenin SA, Eigbefoh JO, Omorogbe F, et al. Eclampsia in Irrua Specialist Teaching Hospital: a five-year review. Niger J Clin Pract 2010;13(2):149–53.

82. WHO 2018. How to safely collect blood samples by phlebotomy from patients suspected to be infected with Lassa. Available at: https://www.who.int/emergencies/diseases/lassa-fever/collection-of-blood-samples-for-lassa.pdf?ua=1 -. Accessed March 22, 2019.

83. WHO 2018. How to safely ship human blood samples from Lassa cases within a country by road, rail and sea. Available at: https://www.who.int/emergencies/diseases/lassa-fever/shipment-of-blood-samples-lassa.pdf?ua=1. Accessed April 3, 2019.

84. Zhang Y, Gong Y, Wang C, et al. Rapid deployment of a mobile biosafety level-3 laboratory in Sierra Leone during the 2014 Ebola virus epidemic. PLoS Negl Trop Dis 2017;11(5):e0005622.

85. Wölfel R, Stoecker K, Fleischmann E, et al. Mobile diagnostics in outbreak response, not only for Ebola: a blueprint for a modular and robust field laboratory. Euro Surveill 2015;20(44). https://doi.org/10.2807/1560-7917.ES.2015.20.44.30055.

86. Raabe V, Koehler J. Laboratory diagnosis of Lassa fever. J Clin Microbiol 2017;55(6):1629–37.

87. Gabriel M, Adomeh DI, Ehimuan J, et al. Development and evaluation of antibody-capture immunoassays for detection of Lassa virus nucleoprotein-specific immunoglobulin M and G. PLoS Negl Trop Dis 2018;12(3):e0006361.

88. Mazzola LT, Kelly-Cirino C. Diagnostics for Nipah virus: a zoonotic pathogen endemic to Southeast Asia. BMJ Glob Health 2019;4(Suppl 2):e001118.

89. Boisen ML, Hartnett JN, Shaffer JG, et al. Field validation of recombinant antigen immunoassays for diagnosis of Lassa fever. Sci Rep 2018;8(1):5939.

90. Emperador DM, Yimer SA, Mazzola LT, et al. Diagnostic applications for Lassa fever in limited-resource settings. BMJ Glob Health 2019;4(Suppl 2):e001119.

91. Gootenberg JS, Abudayyeh OO, Kellner MJ, et al. Multiplexed and portable nucleic acid detection platform withCas13, Cas12a, and Csm6. Science 2018;360:439–44.

92. Dhillon RS, Srikrishna D, Garry RF. Early detection of Lassa fever: the need for point-of-care diagnostics. Lancet Infect Dis 2018;18(6):601–2.

93. Günther S, Weisner B, Roth A, et al. Lassa fever encephalopathy: Lassa virus in cerebrospinal fluid but not in serum. J Infect Dis 2001;184(3):345–9.

94. McCormick JB, Fisher-Hoch SP. Lassa fever. Curr Top Microbiol Immunol 2002; 262:75–109.
95. Rusnak JM. Experience with ribavirin for treatment and post-exposure prophylaxis of hemorrhagic fever viruses: Crimean Congo hemorrhagic fever, Lass fever, and Hantaviruses. Appl Biosaf 2011;16:67–87.
96. McCormick JB, King IJ, Webb PA, et al. Lassa fever. Effective therapy with ribavirin. N Engl J Med 1986;314(1):20–6.
97. Raabe VN, Kann G, Ribner BS, et al. Favipiravir and ribavirin treatment of epidemiologically linked cases of Lassa fever. Clin Infect Dis 2017;65:855–9.
98. Robinson JE, Hastie KM, Cross RW, et al. Most neutralizing human monoclonal antibodies target novel epitopes requiring both Lassa virus glycoprotein subunits. Nat Commun 2016;7:11544.
99. Mire CE, Cross RW, Geisbert JB, et al. Human-monoclonal antibody therapy protects nonhuman primates against advanced Lassa fever. Nat Med 2017; 23:1146–9.
100. Center for Disease Control and Prevention. Viral haemorrhagic fevers: infection control of viral haemorrhagic fevers in African health care setting. 2014. Available at: https://www.cdc.gov/vhf/abroad/vhf-manual.html. Accessed March 17, 2019.
101. Lukashevich IS, Paessler S, de la Torre JC. Lassa virus diversity and feasibility for universal prophylactic vaccine. F1000Res 2019;8 [pii:F1000 Faculty Rev-134].
102. Plotkin SA. Vaccines for epidemic infections and the role of CEPI. Hum Vaccin Immunother 2017;13(12):2755–62.
103. Warner BM, Safronetz D, Stein DR. Current research for a vaccine against Lassa hemorrhagic fever virus. Drug Des Devel Ther 2018;12:2519–27.

Ebola Virus Disease

Epidemiology, Clinical Features, Management, and Prevention

Emanuele Nicastri, PhD, MD[a], Gary Kobinger, PhD, MD[b],
Francesco Vairo, MD[a], Chiara Montaldo, MD[a],
Leonard E.G. Mboera, PhD, BVM[c], Rashid Ansunama, PhD[d],
Alimuddin Zumla, MD, PhD, FRCP, FRCPath, FAAS[e],
Giuseppe Ippolito, MD, FRCP[a],*

KEYWORDS

- Ebola • Ebola virus diseases • Ebola hemorrhagic fever • Epidemiology • Diagnosis
- Treatment • Prevention • Vaccines

KEY POINTS

- Ebola virus disease (EVD) is a severe zoonotic disease caused by the Ebola virus (EBOV), first discovered in 1976 near the Ebola River in the Democratic Republic of Congo.
- Bats are the most likely host reservoir of EBOV. Humans acquire infection through direct or indirect contact with blood, body fluids, and tissues.
- Human-to-human transmission of EBOV occurs via direct contact with an infected person. Sexual transmission has been described.
- Initial symptoms are nonspecific often misdiagnosed as influenza or malaria. Suspicion of EVD should prompt isolation and infection control measures.
- Outbreak control requires a multidisciplinary team effort applying case management, infection prevention and control practices, surveillance and contact tracing, good laboratory service, safe and dignified burials, social and community mobilization.

Conflicts of interest: All of the authors have an interest in global public health and emerging and reemerging infections. The authors have no other conflict of interest to declare.
[a] National Institute for Infectious Diseases, Lazzaro Spallanzani, IRCCS, Via Portuense, 292, Rome 00149, Italy; [b] Centre de Recherche en Infectiologie, Centre Hospitalier Universitaire de Québec, Université Laval, 2705, Boulevard Laurier, RC-709, Québec, Québec G1V 4G2, Canada; [c] SACIDS Foundation for One Health, Sokoine University of Agriculture, PO Box 3297, Chuo Kikuu, Morogoro, Tanzania; [d] Mercy Hospital Research Laboratory, School of Community Health Sciences, Njala University, Bo Campus, Kulanda Town, Bo, Sierra Leone; [e] Center for Clinical Microbiology, University College London, Royal Free Campus 2nd Floor, Rowland Hill Street, London NW3 2PF, UK
* Corresponding author.
E-mail address: giuseppe.ippolito@inmi.it

Infect Dis Clin N Am 33 (2019) 953–976
https://doi.org/10.1016/j.idc.2019.08.005
0891-5520/19/© 2019 Elsevier Inc. All rights reserved.

id.theclinics.com

INTRODUCTION

Ebola virus disease (EVD), also known as Ebola hemorrhagic fever or Ebola, is caused by the Ebola virus (EBOV). EBOV is a linear, nonsegmented, single negative-stranded RNA virus and is a member of the Filoviridae virus family, of which 6 species have been identified named after the region of discovery: Zaire EBOV, Bundibugyo EBOV, Sudan EBOV, Reston EBOV, Tai Forest EBOV, and Bombali EBOV. The Bundibugyo, Zaire, and Sudan EBOVs are the cause of the large outbreaks in Africa. The Zaire EBOV caused the 2014 to 2016 West African epidemic.[1] The high case fatality rates have endowed Ebola a reputation as one of the most deadly viral zoonotic diseases of humans. **Fig 1** shows the geographic distribution of Ebola in Africa.

The first human case of EVD was described in 1976 near the Ebola River in the Democratic Republic of Congo (DRC). The first outbreak of EBOV affected 284 people, with a mortality of 53%. This outbreak was followed a few months later by the second outbreak of EBOV in Yambuku, Zaire (now DRC). Until 2013, EBOV outbreaks consisted of small numbers of cases that were contained by basic public health and containment measures. The largest EVD epidemic occurred in West Africa between 2013 and 2016, and detection of EVD cases in the United Kingdom, Sardinia, Spain, and the United States focused global attention on the epidemic.

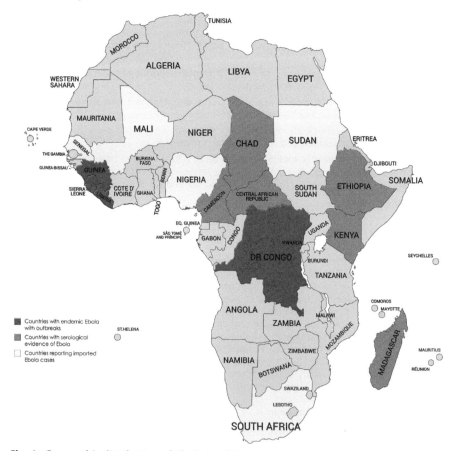

Fig. 1. Geographic distribution of Ebola in Africa.

On August 1, 2018, the Ministry of Health of the DRC declared a new outbreak of EVD in North Kivu Province. As of March 17, 2019, there have been a total of 867 confirmed cases, with 587 deaths.[1] The DRC outbreak shows that public health and surveillance efforts remain inadequate[2] and EVD remains an important public health threat to global health security. This article highlights the epidemiology, clinical features, diagnosis, management, and prevention of EVD. It also reviews emerging field-friendly and easy-to-use point-of-care rapid diagnostic technologies, viral characterization, geospatial mapping of EVD transmission in urban and rural areas, World Health Organization (WHO) standard-of-care and advanced clinical management of patients with EVD, use of investigational new drugs and vaccines within compassionate use or phase II and III clinical trials, and a WHO draft Ebola/Marburg research and development (R&D) roadmap to prioritize the development of countermeasures (diagnostics, therapeutics, and vaccines) that are most needed by EVD-affected countries.[3]

CASE DEFINITION OF EBOLA VIRUS DISEASE

In 1999 the WHO proposed the use of a case definition for hemorrhagic fever using the following clinical criteria: body temperature greater than or equal to 38.3°C (101°F) for less than 3 weeks'; severe illness and no predisposing factors for hemorrhagic manifestations; and at least 2 of the following: hemorrhagic symptoms of hemorrhagic or purple rash, epistaxis, hematemesis, hemoptysis, blood in stools, or other hemorrhagic signs; and no established alternative diagnosis.[4]

In 2009, a systematic review reported that only 58% of patients with EVD in the literature met the 2009 WHO case definition.[5] During the 2013 to 2016 West African outbreak, fever was absent in at least 10% of the cases with no major hemorrhagic manifestations.[6] This clinical presentation questions previous EVD case definitions, which, including fever and hemorrhagic manifestations, make it too specific, and not sensitive enough for case detection. Thus substantial changes have been proposed in the eleventh revision of the International Classification of Diseases (ICD-11), with an innovative EVD case definition that links epidemiologic and clinical perspective, including the presence of a severe disease with high case fatality and unusual prolonged disease manifestations.[7,8]

A confirmed case of EVD is now defined as a suspected case (patient with fever and no response to treatment of usual causes of fever in the area, with at least 1 of the following signs: bloody diarrhea, bleeding from gums, bleeding into skin [purpura], bleeding into eyes and urine) with laboratory EBOV confirmation (positive immunoglobulin M antibody, positive polymerase chain reaction [PCR] or viral isolation).

EPIDEMIOLOGY OF EBOLA VIRUS DISEASE
Historical

EVD was first recognized in 1976, when 2 separate outbreaks were identified in the DRC (then Zaire) and in South Sudan (then Sudan).[9] At that time, it was assumed that these outbreaks were a single event associated with an infected person traveling between the 2 regions. However, further investigations revealed that there were 2 genetically distinct viruses: Zaire EBOV and Sudan EBOV, which came from 2 different sources and spread independently in each of the affected areas.

The first case was reported on August 22, 1976. The patient was a 42-year-old headmaster of the Yambuku Mission School, Équateur Region, returned from a 2-week driving excursion to northern Zaire; along the route, he purchased antelope and smoked monkey meat. He presented on August 26 to the outpatient clinic of the 120-bed Yambuku Mission Hospital with chills and fever and was treated for malaria with apparent relief. One week later, he returned with severe headache, muscle pain, nausea, abdominal complaints, and intestinal bleeding. He died on September 6, after the occurrence of a severe hemorrhagic syndrome of unknown cause. The EBOV was first isolated in 1976 (isolate E718) from the blood sample of a 42-year-old Belgian nursing sister who was working at the Yambuku Mission Hospital, DRC.[10] Karl Johnson, the International Commission scientific director, suggested the name Ebola virus. Ebola is a river part of the Congo River network, about 60 km from the first EVD-affected area. It was chosen to ensure that the Yambuku community was not stigmatized. The name is a distortion of the local Ngbandi name Legbala, meaning white water or pure water.[10]

Ebola Virus Host Reservoir

The specific host reservoir for EBOV remains unknown. After the first discovery of EBOV, studies to find the host reservoir focused on animals, insects, and plants. Ebola seems to be introduced into the human population through close contact with the blood, secretions, meat, organs, or other bodily fluids of infected animals, such as bats, chimpanzees, gorillas, monkeys, forest antelope, and porcupines in rain forest. Although nonhuman primates and other mammals were implicated in the first cases of EVD, and the host reservoir is not yet confirmed, the candidate reservoir seems most likely to be African fruit bats.

Ebola Virus Disease Outbreaks in Africa Since 1976

Table 1 summarizes all EVD outbreaks recorded since the first discovery. Until the 2013 to 2016 EVD epidemic in West Africa, EVD outbreaks occurred in fairly isolated remote areas and were contained quickly. In contrast, the 2013 to 2016 EVD epidemic also involved major urban areas,[1] with a total of 28,646 suspected cases and 11,310 deaths (39.5% mortality). Approximately 20% of EVD cases occurred in children less than 15 years of age. A substantial portion of EBOV transmission events might have been undetected, particularly in the first phase of the 2013 to 2016 outbreak because there were cases of mild illness with minimal symptoms recorded.[11] These data bring new insight into the transmission dynamics and risk factors that underpin EBOV spill-over events.

During the ninth EVD outbreak in the first 2018 semester in Équateur Province in DRC, there was a total of 54 cases with 33 deaths (case fatality ratio [CFR], 61%). A vaccination strategy was successfully applied between May and June 2018, with a total of 3481 people vaccinated, targeting frontline health care workers (HCWs) as priority categories, and EVD primary and secondary contacts.[12]

Later, on August 1, 2018, the DRC Ministry of Health declared an outbreak of Zaire EBOV in the North Kivu province, the country's 10th outbreak since the discovery of EVD in 1976.[13] Since then, the EBOV epidemic has spread in the Ituri provinces. As of March 28, 2019, a total of 1044 cases (978 confirmed and 66 probable cases) and 652 deaths (586 confirmed and 66 probable) have been reported (**Fig 2**) (https://mailchi.mp/sante.gouv.cd/ebola_kivu_28mar19?e=2ee85af345).

CLINICAL FEATURES OF EBOLA VIRUS DISEASE

The clinical features of EVD are detailed in **Table 2**. The incubation period is between 5 and 9 days, with a range from 1 to 21 days. A range of clinical manifestations of EVD occur, from mild to the rapidly fulminant. Early symptoms of EVD may be similar to those of other causes of fever, such as malaria, dengue, Lassa fever, Marburg,

Table 1
Occurrence and distribution of Ebola virus disease outbreaks since 1976

	Date	Country	Virus	Cases (N)	Deaths (N)	CFR (%)	Description	Reference
1	Jun–Nov 1976	Sudan	SUDV	284	151	53	First outbreak in Sudan: index cases were workers in a cotton factory: 37% infected workers. Many medical care personnel infected	WHO,[71] 1978
2	Aug 1976	Zaire	EBOV	318	280	88	First outbreak in DRC, ex Zaire, in Équateur province in Yambuku and surrounding areas: 38% serologically confirmed survivors	WHO,[9] 1976
3	Jun 1977	Zaire	EBOV	1	1	100	Second outbreak in DRC, ex Zaire, with no known connection with the 1976 outbreak	Heymann et al,[72] 1980
4	Aug–Sep 1979	Sudan	SUDV	34	22	65	Second outbreak at the same site as the 1976 Sudan epidemic	Baron et al,[73] 1983
5	1989	Philippine	Reston	3	0	0	High mortality in the cynomolgus macaques with 3 asymptomatic infected individuals	Miranda et al,[74] 1991
6	1990	United States	Reston	4	0	0	Linked to monkeys imported from Philippines with 4 asymptomatic infected individuals	CDC,[75] 1990
7	1994	Cote d'Ivoire	Tai Forest	4	0	0	High mortality in the chimpanzee population in the Tai Forest, with 1 recovered scientist in Switzerland	Le Guenno et al,[76] 1995
8	Dec 1994 to Feb 1995	Gabon	EBOV	52	31	60	First outbreak in Gabon in Makoku in gold-mining camps in the rain forest along the Ivindo River, initially thought to be yellow fever	Georges et al,[77] 1999

(continued on next page)

Table 1
(continued)

	Date	Country	Virus	Cases (N)	Deaths (N)	CFR (%)	Description	Reference
9	May–Jul 1995	Zaire	EBOV	315	250	79	Third outbreak in DRC, ex Zaire, in Kikwit. Transmission was halted once PPE and other measures were used	Khan et al,[78] 1999
10	Jan–Apr 1996	Gabon	EBOV	60	45	75	Second outbreak in Gabon in the village of Mayibout and neighboring areas after eating a chimpanzee found dead	Georges et al,[77] 1999
11	Jul 1996 to Mar 1997	Gabon	EBOV	37	21	57	Third outbreak in Gabon in the Booué area with transport of patients to Libreville. The index patient was a hunter in a forest timber camp	Georges et al,[77] 1999
12	Oct 2000 to Jan 2001	Uganda	SUDV	425	224	53	First outbreak in Uganda, in the Gulu, Masindi, and Mbarara districts. Three main risk factors: attending funerals, having contact with affected patients, and providing medical care without PPE	Okware et al,[79] 2002
13	Oct 2001 to Jul 2002	Gabon, Republic of Congo	EBOV	124	96	77	Occurred on both sides of the border between Gabon (fourth outbreak) and the RC; first outbreak). Abnormal number of animals found dead in Gabon	WHO et al,[80] 2003
14	Dec 2002 to Apr 2003	Republic of Congo	EBOV	143	128	90	Second outbreak in RC in of Mbomo and Kéllé districts in the Cuvette Ouest Department	Formenty et al,[81] 2003

	Date	Country	Virus	Cases	Deaths	CFR	Description	Reference
15	Nov–Dec 2003	Republic of Congo	EBOV	35	29	83	Third outbreak in RC in Mbomo villages	WHO,[82] 2004
16	Apr–Jun 2004	Sudan	SUDV	17	7	41	Third outbreak in Yambio county concurrent with an outbreak of measles	WHO,[83] 2005
17	April 2005	Republic of Congo	EBOV	12	10	83	Fourth outbreak in RC in Etoumbi medical centers: most cases among hunters, caregivers, or funeral attendees	—
18	Aug–Nov 2007	DRC	EBOV	264	187	71	Fourth outbreak in DRC in the Kasai-Occidental province	WHO,[84] 2007
19	Dec 2007 to Jan 2008	Uganda	BDBV	149	37	25	Second outbreak in Uganda in the Bundibungyo district; this was the first identification of the BDBV	MacNeil et al,[85] 2011
20	Dec 2008 to Feb 2009	DRC	EBOV	32	15	47	Fifth outbreak in DRC in the Mweka and Luebo health zones in the Kasai-Occidental province	WHO,[86] 2009
21	May 2011	Uganda	SUDV	1	1	100	Third outbreak in Uganda in the Luwero district	Shoemaker et al,[87] 2012
22	Jun–Aug 2012	Uganda	SUDV	17	7	41	Fourth and fifth outbreaks in Uganda in 2 sites: Luwero, Jinja, and Nakasongola districts, and Orientale province	Albarino et al,[87] 2013

(continued on next page)

Table 1
(continued)

	Date	Country	Virus	Cases (N)	Deaths (N)	CFR (%)	Description	Reference
23	Jun–Nov 2012	DRC	BDBV	35	13	36	Sixth outbreak in DRC in the Orientale province. No epidemiologic link with 2012 outbreak in Uganda	Albarino et al,[88] 2013
24	Dec 2013 to Jan 2016	West Africa, mainly Liberia, Sierra Leone, and Guinea Conakry	EBOV	28,616	11,310	39	The largest Ebola outbreak in terms of human patients, fatalities, and multiple-site involvement in different countries in both urban and rural settings. It began in Guéckédou, Guinea, in December 2013	Baize et al.[89] 2014
25	Aug–Nov 2014	DRC	EBOV	66	49	74	Seventh outbreak in DRC in Équateur province	Maganga et al,[90] 2014
26	May 2017	DRC	EBOV	8	4	50	Eighth outbreak in DRC in the Likati health zone in Bas-Uélé province close to central African Republic	Nsio et al,[99] 2019
27	May–Jul 2018	DRC	EBOV	54	33	61	Ninth outbreak in DRC in the north-western towns of Bikoro and Mbandaka in Équateur province. VSV-ZEBOV vaccine has been used to contain the outbreak	Ebola outbreak team,[91] 2018
28	August 2018 to present	DRC	EBOV	3099	2074	66.9 ongoing	10th outbreak in DRC started on August 1, 2018: the second largest outbreak in North Kivu and, as of March 1, 2019, it is still ongoing	WHO, 2019[100]

Abbreviations: BDBV, Bundibungyo virus; CDC, US Centers for Disease Control and Prevention; CFR, case fatality ratio; PPE, personal protective equipment; RC, Republic of the Congo; SUDV, Sudan EBOV; VSV-ZEBOV, vesicular stomatitis virus–Zaire EBOV.

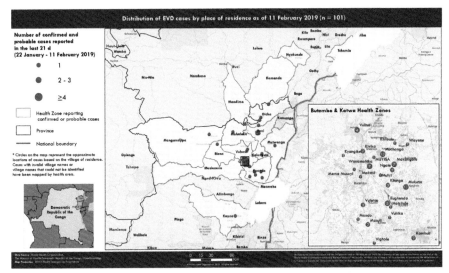

Fig. 2. Distribution of EVD cases by place of residence in the 2019 Ebola DRC outbreak. (*Courtesy of* the World Health Organization, Geneva, Switzerland, https://www.who.int/csr/don/08-august-2019-ebola-drc/en/ ; with permission.)

Crimean Congo hemorrhagic fever, typhoid, shigellosis, rickettsial diseases, borreliosis, leptospirosis, and viral hepatitis.

The clinical presentations of patients in the Zaire and Sudan EVD outbreaks in 1976 were similar and were characterized by initial unspecific febrile syndrome followed by vomiting, diarrhea, impaired kidney and liver functions, and internal and external bleeding.[9,10] The main differences involved the case fatality rates, with values of 88% (280 deaths from 318 cases) in Zaire and 53% (151 deaths from 284 cases) in Sudan, and the high frequency of chest pain (83%) and cough (49%) in Sudan.[1,9,10] In the 2013 to 2016 EVD outbreak in West Africa, severe presentations of EVD included severe gastroenteritis with dehydration,[14] severe sepsis, multiple organ failure (kidneys, liver, respiratory and coagulation systems),[15–18] and shock[19,20] (see **Table 2**). Bleeding was not commonly reported. EBOV viral load is an important prognostic factor. Patients who did not survive had 10-fold to 100-fold higher viral loads at the time of hospital admission compared with survivors.[21,22] Patients who survive seem to have lower average peak viremia levels, and show faster decay in viremia than those who did not survive.[6] In survivors, viremia decreases to less than the limit of reverse transcription (RT) PCR detection around 2 to 3 weeks after symptom's onset. The host immune response seems important in influencing the outcome of EVD. Early antibody responses to EBOV, and reduced lymphocyte depletion, are associated with effective EBOV viral clearance and survival.

CLINICAL MANAGEMENT OF EBOLA VIRUS DISEASE

There is no specific antiviral treatment of EVD, and recovery depends on supportive clinical care and treatment of complications (see **Table 2**). Management guidelines[23] from previous EVD outbreaks in 2013 were primarily focused on HCW safety and delivering treatment and care in rural areas with limited access to medical care. The management of patients with EVD was based on supportive therapy with oral hydration

Table 2
Clinical characteristics of Ebola virus disease

Phase of EVD	Duration	Clinical Disease Progression	Symptoms	Clinical Features	Treatment
Prodromal phase	1–3 d, following an incubation period of 5–9 d (range: 1–21 d)	Nonspecific febrile syndrome	Sudden onset of fever, tiredness, headaches, sore throat, muscular pain, weakness, loss of appetite, skin rash, cough	Feverish (<38°C) or remittent fever, lethargy, myalgia	Antipyretics, oral hydration
Systemic involvement	3–10 d	Gastrointestinal, liver, adrenal, pancreatic, and kidney involvement	Persistent fever, tiredness, abdominal pain, nausea, vomiting, profuse watery diarrhea, bruising and bleeding from gums Agitation and irritability	High temperature with pulse-temperature dissociation (relative bradycardia), progressive drowsiness, partial response to simple orders Patients unable to take care of themselves and may require intensive care Bleeding from gums and stools Hepatomegaly, splenomegaly Hematuria, proteinuria Low white cell count (lymphopenia), low platelet count, and abnormal liver and renal function tests. Both ALT and AST levels are increased (AST increases more than ALT) Urgent tests: malaria, Ebola RT-PCR, full blood count, serum creatinine and urea, liver function tests, arterial blood gases, coagulation studies, blood cultures	Early detection of systemic involvement and isolation with strict infection control measures. Use of PPE Instituting best supportive care measures Antipyretics, oral and aggressive intravenous hydration, antimalarials, antibiotics EBOV-specific therapy: Zmapp or REGN-1EB3 or mAb11
—		Neurologic involvement	Persistent high temperature with confusion, panic, seizures, hallucinations, agitation, and irritability Reduced or no response to simple orders with advancing disease	Deep prostration, mood alterations, rarely seizures, coma Completely dependent on caregivers in the community and acute/critical care setting in hospitals	Antipyretics, aggressive intravenous hydration, antimalarials, antibiotics with good CNS penetration EBOV-specific therapy: Zmapp or REGN-1EB3 or mAb11 plus remdesivir

Multiorgan failure (25%–90% mortality)	7–16 d	Systemic involvement	Nonresponsive and comatose, no response to simple orders. Bleeding from all mucous membranes and all orifices. Hiccups (sign of terminal illness)	Hypovolemic, severe sepsis or septic shock, acute renal insufficiency	Intensive care with circulatory/hemodynamic and ventilatory support, renal dialysis, transfusions. EBOV-specific therapy: Zmapp or REGN-1EB3 or mAb11 plus remdesivir
		Adult respiratory distress syndrome	Shortness and rapid breathing, cough, chest pain, and bluish skin coloration	Severe dyspnea at rest, central and peripheral cyanosis, drowsiness, jaundice	All previous therapy plus noninvasive or invasive mechanical ventilation

See **Table 3** for details on specific treatment of Ebola viral disease.

Abbreviations: ALT, alanine transaminase; AST, aspartate transaminase; RT-PCR, reverse transcription polymerase chain reaction; CNS, central nervous system.

and on the strict application of infection control measures to prevent transmission to HCWs, other patients and relatives, and to the community. High-level isolation and containment procedures hampered the implementation of standard clinical interventions for critically ill patients infected with other life-threatening pathogens in high-resources countries.[24]

Management of EVD is more challenging in both urban and rural settings. Management of EVD outbreaks requires strict and early implementation of infection prevention and control measures, assembly of multidisciplinary teams of trained staff, biocontainment units, and engagement of community leaders and community HCWs. Treating patients with EVD requires understanding of risk exposure of acquiring EBOV, training in infection prevention and control measures, and ability to work in difficult field conditions of extreme heat and humidity while wearing complete personal protective equipment (PPE).[19,24–26]

In the 2013 to 2016 West African EVD outbreak, aggressive supportive care and antiviral therapy improved patient outcomes. It is therefore likely that the dramatic decrease of CFR from around 75% in the first 2014 months to less than 40% at the end of the outbreak reflected both care enhancement and less severe case mix at presentation.[27–34] This lower CFR could gradually approximate the 18.5% CFR reported among HCWs evacuated to medical facilities in the United States and Europe.[30] However, despite the use of new high-level deployable infectious disease units, highly aggressive therapeutic strategies, and innovative antivirals and vaccines in first-line HCWs and EVD contacts in the 10th EVD outbreak in DRC, the CFR still reaches unacceptable levels (as high as 64%).

ADVANCED LEVELS OF CARE SETTING IN RESOURCE-LIMITED COUNTRIES

In 2014, many EVD care groups operating in the field[27,28] endorsed the need for more aggressive symptomatic treatment, early identification of severe cases, and prompt treatment of dehydration and related electrolyte imbalances and organ-supporting care. Human resources and funding, combined with experience from EVD treatment of patients transported to North America and Europe, strengthened the idea of critical care provision in resource-constrained settings.[30] The Italian nongovernmental organization EMERGENCY delivered care sequentially at 2 Ebola treatment centers (ETCs) in Sierra Leone: the first at Lakka, where general hospital medical care was provided to patients with EVD based on fluids, symptomatic drugs, antibiotics, and antimalarial treatment. In Goderich, a well-equipped intensive care unit (ICU), capable of providing 24-hour nursing and medical assessment and support, mechanical ventilation, intravenous vasoactive medications, and renal replacement therapy, was constructed to implement the first ever, dedicated ICU-ETC in Africa.[31] An ETC-ICU was set up in a very short time with limited resources and highly trained and skilled personnel. Intensive supportive treatment resulted in shorter time to discharge in survivors and survival advantage in patients with intermediate-severe EVD.[31] High-level optimized care seems to improve outcomes and needs to be promoted to overcome perceptions that EVD is always fatal. The added value and the feasibility of hemodialysis, artificial ventilation, or hemodynamic support in low-resource settings require further studies.[6]

EBOLA VIRUS–SPECIFIC TREATMENTS

The 2013 to 2016 EVD outbreak gave an opportunity to evaluate specific antiviral drugs, although the clinical trials evaluating favipiravir[32] and Zmapp[33] started too late in the outbreak to give any meaningful results. Most of the patients evacuated to Europe or to North America for medical treatment received investigational therapies and two-thirds of them received at least 2 experimental drugs under compassionate protocol.[30]

During the current 10th DRC EVD outbreak, DRC health regulatory authorities established a committee to review and recommend investigational use of therapeutics in individual patient's care under expanded access or compassionate use, based on the WHO ethical framework (monitored emergency use of unregistered and experimental interventions [MEURI], WHO 2016) until approved protocols for clinical trials are available (**Table 3**).

At present, 5 agents for compassionate use in the treatment of patients diagnosed with EVD have been approved. The monoclonal antibody MAb114 was the first agent to be approved for use, then additional biologics (REGN-EB3 and ZMapp) and the antivirals remdesivir and favipiravir completed the approval processes.[34–36] For most of these agents, efficacy studies involving EBOV challenges in nonhuman primates have been supportive. Very few data are available on the use of investigational new drugs during the 10th DRC EVD outbreak. At the end of 2018, a WHO situation report stated that investigational agents had been administered to 38 patients: MAb114 (22 patients), remdesivir (9 patients), and ZMapp (7 patients). Nineteen of these patients had been discharged, 12 had died, and 7 had remained hospitalized; those who died were in advanced stages of disease when treatment was initiated (WHO. Ebola situation reports: DRC; http://www.who.int/ebola/situation-reports/drc-2018/en/).

HIGH-LEVEL DEPLOYABLE INFECTIOUS DISEASE UNITS

The main function of the high-level infectious disease unit is to keep high-risk patients in 1 strictly selected and dedicated area. There are numerous challenges with implications for both staff safety and patient care in the plastic tents commonly used as high-level infectious disease units: daytime temperatures typically are high, with profuse sweating even before donning PPE to enter the high-risk zone; dehydration of staff is a constant concern; putting on PPE takes up to half an hour and each team member has to be carefully checked to ensure that there are no exposed skin areas at risk for infection. Every activity within the high-risk zone is performed according to written procedures and is strictly monitored. Different solutions to address these challenges have been proposed. Particularly, during the 10th DRC outbreak, a recent advance in patient care and management was the use by the Alliance for International Medical Action (ALIMA) of individual air-conditioned biosecure cubicles, Cube (manufactured by Securotec in France, http://www.securotec.fr/), in ETCs.[37] With such cubicles, HCWs can provide intravenous fluids and therapeutics through specialized ports and are thus free from the burdensome PPE used during the 2013 to 2016 West African outbreak and able to spend more time with their patients.[37] However, the role of the cubicle strategy is mostly recognized in the early phase of an EVD outbreak or in patients with EVD without severe clinical presentations.

EBOLA VIRUS VACCINES

As of December 31, 2018, 58 clinical trials on Ebola vaccine are registered on ClinicalTrials.gov: of them, 40 trials are completed, 7 are active and not recruiting, and 7 are recruiting.[38] However, clinical efficacy data are only reported in the Ebola Ça Suffit vaccination trial in Guinea.[39] This trial evaluated vaccine effectiveness in EVD contacts, randomized for immediate or delayed vaccination with the recombinant, replication-competent, vesicular stomatitis virus–based vaccine expressing the glycoprotein of a Zaire EBOV (rVSV-ZEBOV). Investigators estimated a 100% vaccine efficacy in individuals vaccinated in the immediate group compared with those

Table 3
Newer treatments for Ebola virus disease

Ebola Treatment	Mode of Action	Protection	Human Use	EVD Clinical Phase	Drug Company	Web Site	Bibliography
Convale-scence sera	Human serum obtained from EVD survivors	Ebola NtAb titer increases in survivors compared with deceased patients; also in vitro data	Used since the KiKwit outbreak but no efficacy in 2016 clinical trial	Phase III	NA	http://www.who.int/bloodproducts/brn/ brn_positionpaperconvplasmafiloviruses_ finalweb14august2014.pdf	Van Griensven et al,[92,93] 2016
Zmapp[a]	Human/mouse chimeric triple monoclonal antibody mixture (c13C6, h-13F6, and c6D8) produced on cellular lines obtained from tobacco plants	Postexposure protection in NHP up to day 5	It seems beneficial but no significant efficacy in PREVAIL trial	Phase II	Mapp Biopharma-ceuticals	www.mappbio.com	Qiu et al,[94] 2014; PREVAIL II Writing Group; Multi-National PREVAIL II Study Team,[33] 2016
REGN-1EB3	Specific anti- EBOV triple antibody mixture by immunizing VelocImmune mice	Postexposure protection by IV single dose in NHP up to day 5	Anecdotal use	Phase I-II	Regeneron	https://www.regeneron.com/perspectives/ making-ebola-drug	Pascal et al,[95] 2018

mAb114	Single human monoclonal antibody identified from a survivor of the 1995 Kikwit outbreak, approximately 11 y after infection	Postexposure protection by IV single dose in NHP	Anecdotal use. Safe and well tolerated in humans	Phase I	Ridgeback Biotherapeutics by US NIAID license	http://www.ridgebackcap.com	Corti et al,[36] 2016; Gaudinski et al,[96] 2019
Remdesivir, GS-5734,	A monophosphoramidate prodrug of adenosine analogues, inhibits EBOV RNA-dependent RNA polymerase	Postexposure protection by IV infusion in all NHP at day 3–15	Anecdotal use and use in survivors with viral persistence in semen	Phase II	Gilead Sciences	www.gilead.com/science-and-medicine/pipeline	Warren et al,[97] 2016; Jacobs et al,[51] 2016
Favipiravir, T-705	Influenza viral RNA polymerase inhibitor, could share antiviral activity against other RNA viruses such as Ebola	Postexposure protection in laboratory mouse up to day 6	Stockpile available, limited efficacy in low to moderate viremia, well tolerated	Phase III	MediVector per Fujifilm	http://www.medivector.com/	Furuta et al,[98] 2013; Sissoko et al,[32] 2016

Abbreviations: IV, intravenous; NA, not available; NHP, non-human primate; NIAID, National Institute of Allergy and Infectious Diseases; NtAb, neutralizing antibody.

[a] In a few anecdotal cases, ZMab (a murine monoclonal Ab mixture) and Mil 77 (a monoclonal antibody produced by MabWorks in China) was used in the 2013 to 2016 outbreak. The preliminary data of the WHO/NIAID/INRB multi-drug randomized control trial (PALM study) to evaluate the safety and efficacy of four drugs (ZMapp, remdesivir, mAb114 and REGN-EB3) used for treatment of Ebola patients in the Democratic Republic of the Congo (DRC) have been released on August 12, 2019. The data and safety monitoring board (DSMB) recommended that the study be stopped and that all future patients be randomized to receive either REGN-EB3 or mAb114 in what is being considered an extension phase of the study. This recommendation was based on the fact that an early stopping criterion in the protocol had been met by one of the products, REGN-EB3. The preliminary results in 499 study participants indicated that individuals receiving REGN-EB3 or mAb114 had a greater chance of survival compared to participants in the other two arms.[101]

The reported mortality was 49% in patients receiving ZMapp, 53% in those who received remdesivir, 34%, in the group that received mAb114, 29% in those on REGN-EB3. In the patients who sought treatment early after infection and had lower viremia the mortality was 6% in the Regeneron antibody group and 11% with mAb114, versus 24% and 33% in patients treated with ZMapp and remdesivir respectively.[102]

eligible and randomized to the delayed group. However, on days 0 to 9, incident cases occurred in vaccine recipients at a similar rate to that in controls. The magnitude of this efficacy has been widely debated, but a likely substantial protection to immediate recipients seems to be warranted.[40] Vaccination-related adverse events are a major concern for rVSV-ZEBOV recipients. In a Swiss cohort study, despite a significant dose vaccine reduction strategy, 10 (19%) of 53 vaccine recipients experienced arthritis.[41] Female gender (odds ratio [OR], 2.2, 95% confidence interval [CI], 1.1–4.1) and a medical history of arthritis (OR, 2.8; 95% CI, 1.3–6.2) were independent risk factors for the development of arthritis after vaccination.[41] Soon after the announcement of the 10th EVD outbreak in DRC, vaccination with rVSV-ZEBOV began on August 8, 2018, implementing a ring protocol strategy. A cumulative total of 92,502 people have been vaccinated as of March 18, 2019 (Ministère de la Santé, DRC; see https://mailchi.mp/sante.gouv.cd/ebola_kivu_28mar19?e=2ee85af345).

CLINICAL SEQUELAE AND EBOLA VIRUS PERSISTENCE IN SURVIVORS

In EVD survivors, clinical sequelae such as uveitis, arthralgia, and fatigue are common and can affect up to the two-thirds of survivors.[42] All studies from the 2013 to 2016 outbreak are consistently finding no association with EBOV viral load in plasma during the acute phase. However in a single longitudinal study in Port Loko, a higher EBOV viral load at presentation was independently associated with uveitis (adjusted OR [aOR], 3.33; 95% CI, 1.87–5.91) and with new ocular symptoms or ocular diagnoses (aOR, 3.04; 95% CI, 1.87–4.94).[43] However, this finding was not confirmed in subsequent studies,[44] and EBOV was not identified by RT-PCR in ocular fluid or conjunctivae in 50 EVD survivors with ocular disease.[45] Clinical and laboratory evidence suggests that pathogenesis of eye disease involves blood-ocular barrier breakdown and the potential for EBOV to persist in monocytes, macrophages, and retinal pigment epithelium.[46]

PERSISTENCE OF EBOLA VIRUS IN SURVIVORS

The EBOV can persist in selected body compartments of EVD survivors, most notably in semen. EBOV has been isolated from the semen of an EVD survivor on day 83 after symptom onset,[47] and EBOV RNA has been detected in the semen of 4 of 38 (11%) survivors up to month 15, and in 1 of 25 survivors (4%) up to month 18.[48] Although the potential contribution of sexual transmission to the scale of the epidemic is largely unknown, a case report has been published on EBOV sexual transmission about 470 days after symptoms onset in a survivor from Guinea with EBOV persistence in semen up to day 531.[49] In addition, of 5 male-to-female events associated with EBOV transmission from survivors, 1 of them, with at least 4 generations of secondary cases, was reported.[50] Understanding the duration of EBOV shedding in EVD survivors and preventing further transmission is essential for promoting infection control public health measures and for controlling the Ebola epidemic. In addition, the central nervous system might also be a reservoir for EBOV, as described in the case of a patient who developed meningoencephalitis with EBOV detection 9 months after initial recovery from acute EVD.[51]

POSTEXPOSURE PROPHYLAXIS

The most effective method of protecting HCWs and laboratory workers from acquiring EBOV when managing patients with EVD is the implementation of strict infection control measures with the use of appropriate PPE. However, even when optimal measures are taken, accidental exposures to EBOV have occurred.[52] In these cases, postexposure prophylaxis has been considered.

Antiviral Drugs

In the antiviral portfolio, favipiravir is reported to have a weak antiviral activity against EBOV at low viral load.[32] This result can preclude its efficacy as a therapeutic agent but not as postexposure prophylaxis characterized by presumed low viremia settings. Favipiravir was used as postexposure prophylaxis in few HCWs during the 2013 to 2016 West Africa outbreak, with no secondary cases.[53] Two of them received additional monoclonal antibody therapy. Other small-molecule inhibitors are under development, including the nucleoside analogue BCX4430 and the nucleotide analogue GS-5734, but, although promising, only in vivo data are available.

Prophylactic Vaccines

Development of the rVSV-ZEBOV vaccine offered the first opportunity for use of EVD postexposure prophylaxis. It has been used in 8 HCWs with different EBOV exposures, 7 of them during the West African outbreak.[52] However, there are a few concerns about the use of vaccines as postexposure prophylaxis. First, when considering the 7-day to 10-day EBOV incubation period, vaccine-induced immunity could be insufficiently rapid to prevent the disease, and might only attenuate or delay the symptom onset. Second, current vaccines are specific for Zaire EBOV and might offer less or no protection against other species.

EBOLA VIRUS DIAGNOSTIC TESTS

During an outbreak, empiric EVD diagnosis is usually made based on unspecific febrile syndrome. It is the most frequently used clinical diagnostic tool used in low-resource settings and is not discriminatory in areas with a high incidence of malaria, Lassa fever virus, yellow fever, and other arbovirus infections.

Laboratory diagnosis of EBOV infection plays a critical role in patent management and outbreak response efforts. However, establishing safe testing strategies for this high-biosafety-level pathogen in resource-poor environments remains extremely challenging.

Over the past decade, 3 basic methods for diagnosing EBOV infection have been developed: (1) serologic tests that detect anti-EBOV antibodies, (2) antigen tests that detect EBOV viral proteins, and (3) molecular tests that detect viral RNA sequences.

There are 2 types of diagnostic test for Ebola. Rapid diagnostic tests detect a viral protein[54] and those based on PCR identify the virus's genomic material.[55]

Serologic testing for antiviral antibodies is generally not used because antibodies can persist for many months after recovery, and antibody responses during acute illness are variable. However, EBOV antigen detection and molecular tests have proved very effective for acute diagnosis, because virus levels in the blood typically increase to high levels within the first few days of infection. Some antigen diagnostic tests are designed to broadly detect EBOV infection, whereas others distinguish among the 5 known EBOV species. No tests have yet shown the ability to detect Ebola antigen before the onset of symptoms.

During recent EVD outbreaks, the WHO approved an in vitro RT-PCR diagnostic product, RealStar Filovirus Screen RT-PCR Kit 1.0 (Altona Diagnostics GmbH), which was assessed under an emergency quality assessment mechanism established by the WHO to address the lack of Ebola tests, and to fast track countries' access to reliable testing options.

This product was successfully used to diagnose EBOV infections. However, its deployment and clinical impact were limited because of the infrastructure and training required to accurately run the assay. Capillary blood samples could serve as an alternative to venous blood samples for EBOV diagnosis by RT-PCR even in cases in which venipuncture is difficult to perform; for example, with newborns and infants or when adult patients reject venipuncture for cultural or religious reasons.[56] These limitations highlight the need for portable diagnostics with ambient temperature–stable reagents that can be deployed in low-resource settings. To bridge this gap, several diagnostic platforms and assays compatible with austere environments have been designed and approved as Emergency Use Assessment and Listing procedures by the WHO.[57]

At present, 14 tests for EBOV are under development and evaluation as point-of-care portable and fully automated tests. HCWs and public health groups have not been able to access them quickly because of high costs and it takes staff at laboratories or health centers 2 to 8 weeks to obtain the tests. The recently developed DPP Ebola Antigen System (Chembio Diagnostic Systems Inc.) is used with blood specimens, including capillary fingerstick whole blood, and has been approved by the US Food and Drug Administration.[55]

PREVENTION, SURVEILLANCE, AND CONTROL
Early Case Detection and Isolation

Early case diagnosis and isolation of patients with EVD during outbreaks is important.[58] A surveillance system is essential in guiding the control measures required to reduce morbidity and mortality caused by EVD.[59] Control strategies during an Ebola outbreak include proactive case detection, contact tracing and management, safe and dignified burials, and prevention of new infections.[60,61]. Successful contact tracing requires skills in the assessment of EVD symptoms, interviewing techniques, and counseling. Persons who conduct contact tracing should have investigative skills to find and track all potential contacts and the ability to analyze the evidence,[62] and their success is determined by the level of trust between the community and the public health system and the quality of the diagnostic and treatment services.[63]

Community Engagement and Education

Control strategy efforts might be improved with data on the knowledge, attitudes, and practices in EVD-affected populations.[64] Health communication and social mobilization efforts to improve the public's knowledge, attitudes, and practices regarding EVD were important in controlling the 2013 to 2016 outbreak.[65] The 2018 to 2019 outbreak in eastern DRC differed from the 2013 to 2016 outbreak in several ways, including multiple previous EVD outbreaks in the country, long-standing violent conflict, large numbers of internally displaced persons living in temporary camps, and availability of the new rVSV-ZEBOV vaccine.[64] Despite the knowledge that transmission via infected corpses was high, 8% of Congolese people involved in the survey would wash or touch the body if a family member died of suspected EVD. It suggests that an important minority of Congolese people might also engage in high-risk burial practices.[64]

During an EVD epidemic, prevention and control measures include mandatory prompt and safe burial of the dead. The burial team refer to guidelines for dignified burial of Muslim and Christian patients. A safe burial can be accomplished by a trained burial team using appropriate PPE, placing the body in a puncture-resistant and leak-resistant plastic body bag and burying the body in a grave. Ideally, used burial team PPE should be incinerated.[66]

Preventing Infection in Health Care Workers

HCWs can be exposed to health care–related EBOV infection when caring for patients with EVD. During the 2014 EVD outbreak in DRC, all 8 HCWs died, whereas during the

2013 to 2016 West African epidemic more than 890 HCWs were infected, with a case fatality rate of 57%.[67] Before working with patients with EVD, all HCWs involved in the care of patients with EVD must receive training and show competency in performing all Ebola-related infection control practices and procedures, specifically in proper donning and doffing PPE.[68] PPE should include double gloves; gown or coverall and apron; facemask (N95 mask) or powered, air-purifying respirator (PAPR); eye protection (goggles or face shield); head cover; and boots. PAPR may be preferable to the N95 mask during procedures that generate aerosols of body fluids. Use of PAPR, compared with the N95 mask, is more comfortable for the HCWs, but it could increase the contamination risk.[69,70]

ACKNOWLEDGMENTS

This study was supported by the Italian Ministry of Health. E. Nicastri, F. Vairo, C. Montaldo, and G. Ippolito acknowledge support from the Italian Ministry of Health, grants to Ricerca Corrente linea 1 to National Institute for Infectious Diseases Lazzaro Spallanzani, IRCCS. L. Mboera, R. Ansumana, F. Vairo, C. Montaldo, A. Zumla, and G. Ippolito acknowledge support from the PANDORA-ID-NET Consortium, which is funded by the European and Developing Countries Clinical Trials Partnership (EDCTP2) programme (EDCTP Grant RIA2016E-1609), which is supported under Horizon 2020, the European Union's Framework Programme for Research and Innovation. E. Nicastri, F. Vairo, and G. Ippolito are Professors at Saint Camillus International University of Health and Medical Sciences in Rome.

REFERENCES

1. World Health Organization. Ebola virus disease. 2018. Available at: https://www.who.int/news-room/fact-sheets/detail/ebola-virus-disease. Accessed April 1, 2019.
2. Lamontagne F, Clément F, Kojan R, et al. The evolution of supportive care for Ebola virus disease. Lancet 2019;393(10172):620–1.
3. World Health Organization. WHO. Ebola/Marburg Research and development (R&D) roadmap. 2018. Available at: https://www.who.int/blueprint/priority-diseases/key-action/Ebola-Marburg_Draft_Roadmap_publiccomment_MAY2018.pdf?ua=1. Accessed February 1, 2019.
4. World Health Organization. WHO recommended surveillance standards, second edition 1999. Available at: http://www.who.int/csr/resources/publications/surveillance/WHO_CDS_CSR_ISR_99_2_EN/en/. Accessed February 1, 2019.
5. Pittalis S, Fusco FM, Lanini S, et al. Case definition for Ebola and Marburg haemorrhagic fevers: a complex challenge for epidemiologists and clinicians. New Microbiol 2009;32(4):359–67.
6. Malvy D, McElroy AK, de Clerck H, et al. Ebola viral disease. Lancet 2019;393(10174):936–48.
7. World Health Organization. WHO international classification of diseases – 11. 2018. Available at: https://www.who.int/classifications/icd/en/. Accessed February 1, 2019.
8. Kuhn JH, Adachi T, Adhikari NKJ, et al. New filovirus disease classification and nomenclature. Nat Rev Microbiol 2019. https://doi.org/10.1038/s41579-019-0187-4.
9. World Health Organization. Ebola haemorrhagic fever in Zaire, 1976. Bull World Health Organ 1978;56(2):271–93.

10. Breman JG, Heymann DL, Lloyd G, et al. Discovery and description of ebola zaire virus in 1976 and relevance to the west african epidemic during 2013-2016. J Infect Dis 2016;214(suppl 3):S93–101.

11. Timothy JWS, Hall Y, Akoi-Boré J, et al. Early transmission and case fatality of Ebola virus at the index site of the 2013–16 west African Ebola outbreak: a cross-sectional seroprevalence survey. Lancet 2019;19(4):429–38.

12. World Health Organization. Situation report: declaration of the end of the Ebola outbreak in Équateur Province. 2018. Available at: http://apps.who.int/iris/bit stream/handle/10665/273348/SITREP_EVD_DRC_20180725-eng.pdf?ua=1. Accessed February 1, 2019.

13. Democratic Republic of Congo – Ministere dela Santé. Declaration of 10th outbreak, August 1, 2018. Available at: https://us13.campaign-archive.com/? u=89e5755d2cca4840b1af93176&id=24b904b316. Accessed September 14, 2019.

14. Liddell AM, Davey RT Jr, Mehta AK, et al. Characteristics and clinical management of a cluster of 3 patients with Ebola virus disease, including the first domestically acquired cases in the United States. Ann Intern Med 2015;163: 81–90.

15. Petrosillo N, Nicastri E, Lanini S, et al. Ebola virus disease complicated with viral interstitial pneumonia: a case report. BMC Infect Dis 2015;15:432.

16. Hunt L, Gupta-Wright A, Simms V, et al. Clinical presentation, biochemical, and haematological parameters and their association with outcome in patients with Ebola virus disease: an observational cohort study. Lancet Infect Dis 2015;15: 1292–9.

17. Schieffelin JS, Shaffer JG, Goba A, et al. Clinical illness and outcomes in patients with Ebola in Sierra Leone. N Engl J Med 2014;371:2092–100.

18. Nicastri E, Brucato A, Petrosillo N, et al. Acute rhabdomyolysis and delayed pericardial effusion in an Italian patient with Ebola virus disease: a case report. BMC Infect Dis 2017;17:597.

19. Fowler RA, Fletcher T, Fischer WA, et al. Caring for critically ill patients with Ebola virus disease. Perspectives from West Africa. Am J Respir Crit Care Med 2014;190:733–7.

20. West TE, von Saint Andre-von Arnim A. Clinical presentation and management of severe Ebola virus disease. Ann Am Thorac Soc 2014;11:1341–50.

21. de La Vega MA, Caleo G, Audet J, et al. Ebola viral load at diagnosis associates with patient outcome and outbreak evolution. J Clin Invest 2015;125:4421–8.

22. Lanini S, Portella G, Vairo F, et al. Blood kinetics of Ebola virus in survivors and nonsurvivors. J Clin Invest 2015;125:4692–8.

23. Sterk E, Borchert M, Coeur C, et al. Filovirus haemorrhagic fever guideline Medicines Sans Frontières. 2008. Available at: https://www.medbox.org/ebola-guidelines/ filovirus-haemorrhagic-fever-guideline/preview. Accessed December 1, 2018.

24. Ippolito G, Feldmann H, Lanini S, et al. Viral hemorrhagic fevers: advancing the level of treatment. BMC Med 2012;10:31.

25. Lamontagne F, Clement C, Fletcher T, et al. Doing today's work superbly well-treating Ebola with current tools. N Engl J Med 2014;371:1565–6.

26. Leligdowicz A, Fischer WA, Uyeki TM, et al. Ebola virus disease and critical illness. Crit Care 2016;20:217.

27. Bah EI, Lamah MC, Fletcher T, et al. Clinical presentation of patients with Ebola virus disease in Conakry, Guinea. N Engl J Med 2015;372:40–7.

28. Haaskjold YL, Bolkan HA, Krogh KO, et al. Clinical features of and risk factors for fatal Ebola virus disease, Moyamba District, Sierra Leone, December 2014–February 2015. Emerg Infect Dis 2016;22:1537–44.

29. Qin E, Bi J, Zhao M, et al. Clinical features of patients with Ebola virus disease in Sierra Leone. Clin Infect Dis 2015;61:491–5.

30. Uyeki TM, Mehta AK, Davey RT Jr, et al. Clinical management of ebola virus disease in the United States and Europe. N Engl J Med 2016;374(7):636–46.

31. Langer M, Portella G, Finazzi S, et al. Intensive care support and clinical outcomes of patients with Ebola virus disease (EVD) in West Africa. Intensive Care Med 2018;44(8):1266–75.

32. Sissoko D, Laouenan C, Folkesson E, et al. Experimental treatment with favipiravir for Ebola virus disease (the JIKI Trial): a historically controlled, single-arm proof-of concept trial in Guinea. PLoS Med 2016;13:e1001967.

33. PREVAIL II Writing Group, Multi-National PREVAIL II Study Team. A randomized, controlled trial of ZMapp for Ebola virus infection. N Engl J Med 2016;375(15):1448–56.

34. Keusch G, McAdam K, Cuff PA, et al, editors. Integrating clinical research into epidemic response: the Ebola experience. Washington, DC: National Academies Press; 2017. Available at: https://www.nap.edu/catalog/24739/integrating-clinical-research-into-epidemic-response-the-ebola-experience.

35. World Health Organization. Ebola/Marburg research and development (R&D) roadmap. Available at: https://www.who.int/blueprint/priority-diseases/key-action/Ebola-Marburg_Draft_Roadmap_publiccomment_MAY2018.pdf?ua=1. Accessed April 1, 2019.

36. Corti D, Misasi J, Mulangu S, et al. Protective monotherapy against lethal Ebola virus infection by a potently neutralizing antibody. Science 2016;351:1339–42.

37. Damon IK, Rollin PE, Choi MJ, et al. New tools in the ebola arsenal. N Engl J Med 2018;379(21):1981–3.

38. Lévy Y, Lane C, Piot P, et al. Prevention of Ebola virus disease through vaccination: where we are in 2018. Lancet 2018;392(10149):787–90.

39. Henao-Restrepo AM, Camacho A, Longini IM, et al. Efficacy and effectiveness of an rVSV-vectored vaccine in preventing Ebola virus disease: final results from the Guinea ring vaccination, open-label, cluster-randomised trial (Ebola Ça Suffit!). Lancet 2017;389:505–18.

40. Metzger WG, Vivas-Martínez S. Questionable efficacy of the rVSV-ZEBOV Ebola vaccine. Lancet 2018;391:1021.

41. Agnandji ST, Huttner A, Zinser ME, et al. Phase 1 trials of rVSV Ebola vaccine in Africa and Europe. N Engl J Med 2016;374:1647–60.

42. Vetter P, Kaiser L, Schibler M, et al. Sequelae of Ebola virus disease: the emergency within the emergency. Lancet Infect Dis 2016;16(6):e82–91.

43. Mattia JG, Vandy MJ, Chang JC, et al. Early clinical sequelae of Ebola virus disease in Sierra Leone: a cross-sectional study. Lancet Infect Dis 2016;16(3):331–8.

44. Wing K, Oza S, Houlihan C, et al. Surviving Ebola: a historical cohort study of Ebola mortality and survival in Sierra Leone 2014-2015. PLoS One 2018;13(12):e0209655.

45. Shantha JG, Mattia JG, Goba A, et al. Ebola virus persistence in ocular tissues and fluids (EVICT) study: reverse transcription-polymerase chain reaction and cataract surgery outcomes of Ebola survivors in Sierra Leone. EBioMedicine 2018;30:217–24.

46. Smith JR, Todd S, Ashander LM, et al. retinal pigment epithelial cells are a potential reservoir for Ebola virus in the human eye. Transl Vis Sci Technol 2017; 6(4):12.

47. Rodriguez LL, De Roo A, Guimard Y, et al. Persistence and genetic stability of Ebola virus during the outbreak in Kikwit, Democratic Republic of the Congo, 1995. J Infect Dis 1999;179(Suppl 1):S170–6.

48. Deen GF, Broutet N, Xu W, et al. Ebola RNA persistence in semen of Ebola virus disease survivors - final report. N Engl J Med 2017;377(15):1428–37.

49. Diallo B, Sissoko D, Loman NJ, et al. Resurgence of Ebola virus disease in guinea linked to a survivor with virus persistence in seminal fluid for more than 500 days. Clin Infect Dis 2016;63(10):1353–6.

50. Den Boon S, Marston BJ, Nyenswah TG, et al. Ebola virus infection associated with transmission from survivors. Emerg Infect Dis 2019;25(2):249–55.

51. Jacobs M, Rodger A, Bell DJ, et al. Late Ebola virus relapse causing meningo-encephalitis: a case report. Lancet 2016;388(10043):498–503.

52. Fischer WA, Vetter P, Bausch DG, et al. Ebola virus disease: an update on post-exposure prophylaxis. Lancet Infect Dis 2018;18(6):e183–92.

53. Jacobs M, Aarons E, Bhagani S, et al. Post-exposure prophylaxis against Ebola virus disease with experimental antiviral agents: a case-series of health-care workers. Lancet Infect Dis 2015;15:1300–4.

54. Wonderly B, Jones S, Gatton ML, et al. Comparative performance of four rapid Ebola antigen-detection lateral flow immunoassays during the 2014-2016 Ebola epidemic in West Africa. PLoS One 2019;14(3):e0212113.

55. Tembo J, Simulundu E, Changula K, et al. Recent advances in the development and evaluation of molecular diagnostics for Ebola virus disease. Expert Rev Mol Diagn 2019. https://doi.org/10.1080/14737159.2019.1595592.

56. Strecker T, Palyi B, Ellerbrok H, et al. Field evaluation of capillary blood samples as a collection specimen for the rapid diagnosis of ebola virus infection during an outbreak emergency. Clin Infect Dis 2015;61(5):669–75.

57. World Health Organization. Ebola emergency use assessment and listing status after PHEIC termination. Available at: https://www.who.int/diagnostics_laboratory/procurement/purchasing/en/. Accessed February 1, 2019.

58. Lamontagne F, Fowler RA, Adhikari NK, et al. Evidence-based guidelines for supportive care of patients with Ebola virus disease. Lancet 2018;391(10121): 700–8.

59. Kouadio KI, Clement P, Bolongei J, et al. Epidemiological and Surveillance Response to Ebola Virus Disease Outbreak in Lofa County, Liberia (March-September, 2014); Lessons Learned. PLoS Curr 2015;7.

60. Jiang H, Shi GQ, Tu WX, et al. Rapid assessment of knowledge, attitudes, practices, and risk perception related to the prevention and control of Ebola virus disease in three communities of Sierra Leone. Infect Dis Poverty 2016;5(1):53.

61. Chowell D, Safan M, Castillo-Chavez C. Modeling the case of early detection of ebola virus disease. In: Chowell G, Hyman J, editors. Mathematical and statistical modeling for emerging and re-emerging infectious diseases. Cham(Switzerland): Springer; 2016. p. 57–70.

62. World Health Organization. Contact tracing during an outbreak of Ebola virus disease: disease surveillance and response programme area disease prevention and control cluster. (Republic of Congo): WHO press; 2014.

63. Saurabh S, Prateek S. Role of contact tracing in containing the 2014 Ebola outbreak: a review. Afr Health Sci 2017;17(1):225–36.

64. Claude KM, Underschultz J, Hawkes MT. Ebola epidemic in war torn eastern DR Congo. Lancet 2018. https://doi.org/10.1016/S0140-6736(18)32419-X.

65. Jalloh MF, Robinson SJ, Corker J, et al. Knowledge, attitudes, and practices related to Ebola virus disease at the end of a national epidemic - Guinea, 2015. MMWR Morb Mortal Wkly Rep 2017;66(41):1109–15.

66. World Health Organization. New WHO safe and dignified burial protocol-key to reducing Ebola transmission. Geneva (Switzerland): World Health Organization; 2017. Available at: www.who.int/csr/resources/publications/ebola/safe-burial-protocol/en/.

67. Ngatu NR, Kayembe NJ, Phillips EK, et al. Epidemiology of ebolavirus disease (EVD) and occupational EVD in health care workers in sub-Saharan Africa: need for strengthened public health preparedness. J Epidemiol 2017;27(10):455–61.

68. CDC Centers for Disease Control and Prevention Guidance for Donning and Doffing Personal Protective Equipment (PPE) during management of patients with Ebola Virus Disease in U.S. Hospitals. Available at: www.cdc.gov/vhf/ebola/hcp/ppe-training/index.html. Accessed March 1, 2019.

69. Mumma JM, Durso FT, Ferguson AN, et al, Centers for Disease Control and Prevention Epicenters Program, Division of Healthcare Quality Promotion. Human factors risk analyses of a doffing protocol for Ebola-level personal protective equipment: mapping errors to contamination. Clin Infect Dis 2018;66(6):950–8.

70. Roberts V. To PAPR or not to PAPR? Can J Respir Ther 2014;50(3):87–90.

71. World Health Organization. Ebola haemorrhagic fever in Sudan, 1976. Report of a WHO/International Study Team. Bull World Health Organ 1978;56(2):247–70.

72. Heymann DL, Weisfeld JS, Webb PA, et al. Ebola hemorrhagic fever: Tandala, Zaire, 1977-1978. J Infect Dis 1980;142:372–6.

73. Baron RC, McCormick JB, Zubeir OA. Ebola virus disease in southern Sudan: hospital dissemination and intrafamilial spread. Bull World Health Organ 1983; 61(6):997–1003.

74. Miranda ME, White ME, Dayrit MM, et al. Seroepidemiological study of filovirus related to Ebola in the Philippines. Lancet 1991;337:425–6.

75. Centers for Disease Control. Update: filovirus infection in animal handlers. MMWR Morb Mortal Wkly Rep 1990;39(13):221.

76. Le Guenno B, Formenty P, Wyers M, et al. Isolation and partial characterisation of a new strain of Ebola virus. Lancet 1995;345:1271–4.

77. Georges AJ, Leroy EM, Renaud AA, et al. Ebola hemorrhagic fever outbreaks in Gabon, 1994-1997: epidemiologic and health control issues. J Infect Dis 1999; 179:S65–75.

78. Khan AS, Tshioko FK, Heymann DL, et al. The reemergence of Ebola hemorrhagic fever, democratic Republic of the Congo, 1995. J Infect Dis 1999;179: S76–86.

79. Okware SI, Omaswa FG, Zaramba S, et al. An outbreak of Ebola in Uganda. Trop Med Int Health 2002;7:1068–75.

80. World Health Organization. Outbreak(s) of Ebola haemorrhagic fever, Congo and Gabon, October 2001- July 2002. Wkly Epidemiol Rec 2003;78(26):223–5.

81. Formenty P, Libama F, Epelboin A, et al. Outbreak of Ebola hemorrhagic fever in the Republic of the Congo, 2003: a new strategy? Med Trop (Mars) 2003;63(3): 291–5.

82. World Health Organization. Ebola haemorrhagic fever in the Republic of the Congo – update 6. 6 January 2004. Disease Outbreak Reported. Available at: https://www.who.int/csr/don/2004_01_06/en/. Accessed September 14, 2019.

83. World Health Organization. Outbreak of Ebola haemorrhagic fever in Yambio, south Sudan, April-June 2004. Wkly Epidemiol Rec 2005;80(43):370–5.
84. World Health Organization. Ebola virus haemorrhagic fever, democratic Republic of the Congo – Update. Wkly Epidemiol Rec 2007;82(40):345–6.
85. MacNeil A, Farnon EC, Morgan OW, et al. Filovirus outbreak detection and surveillance: lessons from Bundibugyo. J Infect Dis 2011;204:S761–7.
86. World Health Organization. End of the Ebola outbreak in the Democratic Republic of the Congo. Press release, February 17 2019. Available at: https://www.who.int/csr/don/2009_02_17/en/. Accessed September 14, 2019.
87. Shoemaker T, MacNeil A, Balinandi S, et al. Reemerging Sudan Ebola Virus Disease in Uganda, 2011. Emerg Infect Dis 2012;18(9):1480–3.
88. Albarino CG, Shoemaker T, Khristova ML, et al. Genomic analysis of filoviruses associated with four viral hemorrhagic fever outbreaks in Uganda and the Democratic Republic of the Congo in 2012. Virology 2013;442(2):97–100.
89. Baize S, Pannetier D, Oestereich L, et al. Emergence of Zaire Ebola virus disease in Guinea. N Engl J Med 2014;371(15):1418–25.
90. Maganga GD, Kapetshi J, Berthet N, et al. Ebola virus disease in the democratic Republic of Congo. N Engl J Med 2014;371(22):2083–91.
91. Ebola Outbreak Epidemiology Team. Outbreak of Ebola virus disease in the Democratic Republic of the Congo, April-May, 2018: an epidemiological study. Lancet 2018;392(10143):213–21.
92. Van Griensven J, Edwards T, de Lamballerie X, et al. Evaluation of convalescent plasma for Ebola virus disease in guinea. N Engl J Med 2016;374(1):33–42.
93. Van Griensven J, De Weiggheleire A, Delamou A, et al. The use of Ebola convalescent plasma to treat Ebola virus disease in resource-constrained settings: a perspective from the field. Clin Infect Dis 2016;62(1):69–74.
94. Qiu X, Wong G, Audet J, et al. Reversion of advanced Ebola virus disease in nonhuman primates with ZMapp. Nature 2014;514(7520):47–53.
95. Pascal KE, Dudgeon D, Trefry JC, et al. Development of clinical-stage human monoclonal antibodies that treat advanced ebola virus disease in nonhuman primates. J Infect Dis 2018;218(suppl_5):S612–26.
96. Gaudinski MR, Coates EE, Novik L, et al. Safety, tolerability, pharmacokinetics, and immunogenicity of the therapeutic monoclonal antibody mAb114 targeting Ebola virus glycoprotein (VRC 608): an open-label phase 1 study. Lancet 2019;393(10174):889–98.
97. Warren TK, Jordan R, Lo MK, et al. Therapeutic efficacy of the small molecule GS-5734 against Ebola virus in rhesus monkeys. Nature 2016;531(7594):381–5.
98. Furuta Y, Gowen BB, Takahashi K, et al. Favipiravir (T-705), a novel viral RNA polymerase inhibitor. Antiviral Res 2013;100(2):446–54.
99. Nsio J, Kapetshi J, Makiala S, et al. 2017 Outbreak of ebola virus disease in northern democratic republic of Congo. J Infect Dis 2019. in press.
100. WHO 2019. Available at: https://www.who.int/emergencies/diseases/ebola/drc-2019. Accessed September 14, 2019.
101. Available at: https://www.nih.gov/news-events/news-releases/independent-monitoring-board-recommends-early-termination-ebola-therapeutics-trial-drc-because-favorable-results-two-four-candidates.
102. Kupferschmidt K. Finally, some good news about Ebola: Two new treatments dramatically lower the death rate in a trial. Available at: https://www.sciencemag.org/news/2019/08/finally-some-good-news-about-ebola-two-new-treatments-dramatically-lower-death-rate.

Viral Hemorrhagic Fevers Other than Ebola and Lassa

Marco Iannetta, MD, PhD[a], Antonino Di Caro, MD[a], Emanuele Nicastri, MD, PhD[a],
Francesco Vairo, MD[a], Honorati Masanja, PhD[b], Gary Kobinger, MD, PhD[c],
Ali Mirazimi, MD, PhD[d], Francine Ntoumi, PhD, FRCP[e,f],
Alimuddin Zumla, MBChB, MSc, PhD, MD, FRCP(Lond), FRCP(Edin), FRCPath(UK), FAAS[g],
Giuseppe Ippolito, MD, FRCP[a],*

KEYWORDS

- Viral hemorrhagic fever • Flavivirus • Arenavirus • Bunyavirus • Hantavirus
- Filovirus • Marburg

KEY POINTS

- Viral hemorrhagic fevers represent a group of lethal zoonotic diseases of humans caused by enveloped RNA viruses belonging to 6 taxonomic families: filoviruses, arenaviruses, hantaviruses, nairoviruses, phenuiviruses, and flaviviruses.
- Viral hemorrhagic fevers are severe febrile illnesses characterized by vascular abnormalities with plasma leakage and widespread bleeding in tissues and organs.
- Rapid identification of the viruses causing hemorrhagic fevers is fundamental for patient management, outcome improvement, and limitation of disease propagation, particularly in health care settings.
- There are no specific treatments or vaccines and management of viral hemorrhagic fevers is essentially supportive.

INTRODUCTION

The first definition of viral hemorrhagic fever (VHF) was given by Soviet investigators in the 1930s, while studying hantaviral hemorrhagic fever with renal syndrome (HFRS).[1]

Author Declarations: All authors have an interest in global public health and emerging and re-emerging infections. All authors have no other conflict of interest to declare.
[a] National Institute for Infectious Diseases, Lazzaro Spallanzani, IRCCS, Via Portuense 292, Rome 00149, Italy; [b] Ifakara Health Institute, Ifakara Health Research and Development Centre, Kiko Avenue, Plot N 463, Mikocheni, Dar es Salaam, Tanzania; [c] Centre de Recherche en Infectiologie, Centre Hospitalier Universitaire de Québec, Université Laval, 2325 Rue de l'Université, Quebec City, Quebec G1V 0A6, Canada; [d] Division of Clinical Microbiology, Department of Laboratory Medicine, Karolinska Institutet, Alfred Nobels Alle 8 Plan 7, Stockholm 14183, Sweden; [e] Université Marien NGouabi, Fondation Congolaise pour la Recherche Médicale (FCRM), Villa D6, Campus OMS//AFRO Djoué, Brazzaville, Congo; [f] Institute for Tropical Medicine, University of Tübingen, Germany; [g] Center for Clinical Microbiology, University College London, Royal Free Campus 2nd Floor, Rowland Hill Street, London NW3 2PF, United Kingdom
* Corresponding author.
E-mail address: giuseppe.ippolito@inmi.it

Infect Dis Clin N Am 33 (2019) 977–1002
https://doi.org/10.1016/j.idc.2019.08.003
0891-5520/19/© 2019 Elsevier Inc. All rights reserved.

id.theclinics.com

Currently, VHFs represent a group of diseases caused by enveloped single-stranded RNA viruses belonging to 6 taxonomic families:

- Filoviruses (Ebola and Marburg virus [MARV]);
- Arenaviruses (Lassa and other Old World [OW] arenaviruses and New World [NW] arenaviruses);
- Hantaviruses, nairoviruses, and phenuiviruses, formerly included in the prior bunyaviridae family (Congo-Crimean Hemorrhagic Fever, Rift Valley fever [RVF], Huaiyangshan virus [alternatively known as severe fever with thrombocytopenia syndrome virus], and hantaviruses);
- Flaviviruses (dengue, yellow fever, Omsk hemorrhagic fever, Kyasanur Forest disease, and Alkhumra viruses).[2,3]

The epidemiology of VHFs is broadly variable, ranging from geographically localized and sporadic infections to more diffuse outbreaks or endemic diseases.[1] A general overview on VHF agents, their reservoir and eventual arthropod vector is summarized in **Table 1**.

Considering that several experimental attempts demonstrated the possibility of infecting nonhuman primates through aerosolized viruses, in the twentieth century different countries tried to weaponize VHF viruses.[4]

The agents of these infections are classified in risk groups 3 and 4; therefore, their manipulation can be performed only in laboratories at the highest level of biocontainment (biosafety levels 3 and 4). In contrast, the diagnostic activities, although hampered by the scarcity of commercially available diagnostic methods, can be carried out, with due exceptions, in laboratories with lower levels of biocontainment. However, these diagnostic methods are often complex, afflicted by cross-reactivity, and need confirmation by specialized reference laboratories, especially for sporadic infections or at the beginning of an epidemic. Although molecular methods are of primary importance in laboratory diagnosis, serologic methods for IgG and IgM detection assay can be helpful for the diagnosis of acute VHF, especially in case of short viremic period and viral shedding.[5] Treatment of VHF is essentially supportive, consisting of administration of fluids, electrolytes, and blood products. Although no antiviral drugs are currently approved by the US Food and Drug Administration for VHFs, small published trials described the use of intravenous ribavirin to treat Congo-Crimean Hemorrhagic fever and other VHFs with significant reduction in mortality.[6,7] Favipiravir, alone or in combination with ribavirin, seems to be active against different species of RNA viruses causing VHFs.[6] The treatment of VHF-infected patients should be performed, maintaining appropriate barrier controls to prevent exposure of health care providers and laboratory personnel. For some of these infections, effective human vaccines are available (such as yellow fever) and for others development and/or validation are ongoing (Dengue, Marburg), or relevant animal vaccines have been developed (RVF virus [RVFV]). A list of recent VHF outbreaks (from January 2017 to April 2019) is presented in **Table 2**.

In this article, we focus attention on yellow fever and VHFs other than Ebola and Lassa virus diseases that have been described elsewhere in this issue.

YELLOW FEVER AND OTHER FLAVIVIRUSES CAUSING VIRAL HEMORRHAGIC FEVERS (DENGUE, OMSK HEMORRHAGIC FEVER, KYASANUR FOREST DISEASE, AND ALKHUMRA VIRUSES)

Flaviviruses are enveloped viruses characterized by a single stranded positive sense RNA molecule, which encodes for several nonstructural and 3 structural proteins, envelope, precursor of membrane/membrane, and capsid proteins.[8]

Table 1
Reservoirs and modes of transmission for selected hemorrhagic fever viruses

VHF Agent	Reservoir	Arthropod Vector	Modes of Transmission
Flaviviridae			
Yellow fever virus	Primates	*Aedes* in Africa *Haemagogus* and *Sabethes* in South America mosquito species	Bite of infected mosquito Laboratory infections
Dengue virus	Unknown	*Aedes* species	Bite of infected mosquito Peripartum vertical transmission
Omsk hemorrhagic fever virus	Rodents, including muskrats (*Ondatra zibethica*)	*Dermacentor pictus* *Dermacentor reticulatus*	Bite of infected tick Direct contact with infected animals (muskrats)
Kyasanur Forest disease virus	Rodents, bats, other small mammals; monkeys	*Haemaphysalis spinigera*	Bite of infected tick Laboratory infections
Alkhumra viruses	Camels, goats, and sheep	*Ornithodoros savignyi* soft ticks *Hyalomma dromedarii* hard ticks	Bite of infected tick
Filoviridae			
Marburg virus	Fruit bat (*Rousettus aegypticus*)	Unknown	Contact with blood, tissues, or tissue cultures from infected monkeys Person-to-person (contact with blood or body fluids, sexual transmission, mucosal exposure to infectious droplets, aerosols) Percutaneous (accidental needle sticks) Laboratory infections
New Word *Arenaviridae*			
Junin virus	*Calomys musculinus* (drylands vesper mouse)	None	Airborne (contact with infected aerosols of rodent excreta)
Machupo virus	*Calomys callosus* (large vesper mouse)	None	Airborne (contact with infected aerosols of rodent excreta) Person-to-person (nosocomial outbreaks)
Guanarito virus	*Zygodontomys brevicauda* (cane mouse)	None	Presumably airborne, through aerosolized rodent excreta

(*continued on next page*)

Table 1			
(continued)			
VHF Agent	**Reservoir**	**Arthropod Vector**	**Modes of Transmission**
Sabia virus	Unknown	None	Unknown Laboratory transmission (infected aerosols)
Chapare	Unknown	Unknown	Unknown
Whitewater Arroyo virus	*Neotoma* species (woodrats)	None	Presumably airborne, through aerosolized rodent excreta
Hantaviridae, Nairoviridae, and *Phenuiviridae* (formerly *Bunyaviridae*)			
Rift Valley virus	Ruminants (cattle, sheep) Rats in some areas (Egypt) Wild animals	*Aedes* and *Culex* mosquitoes	Bite of infected mosquito Contact with blood or amniotic fluid of infected animals Mother-to-child transmission Laboratory transmission (through infected aerosols)
Crimean-Congo hemorrhagic fever	*Ixodidae* ticks (reservoir) Cattle, goats, sheep, hares (amplifying hosts)	*Ixodidae* ticks (*Hyalomma* genus is the most effective vector)	Bite of infected tick Human-to-human transmission (almost in hospital settings)
Hantaviruses	Rodents: deer mouse, white-footed mouse, cotton rat, yellow- necked mouse, striped field mouse, bank vole, shrews, rats	None	Airborne (contact with infected aerosols of rodent excreta: urine, feces, saliva)

Among Flaviviruses, yellow fever virus (YFV) and dengue virus (DENV) can cause VHF. Besides, other flaviviruses can be responsible of hemorrhagic diseases in very limited areas of the world, such as Omsk hemorrhagic fever, Kyasanur Forest disease, and Alkhumra viruses.[2]

Yellow Fever

YFV is considered the prototype member of *Flavivirus* genus. YFV is endemic in tropical and subtropical regions of South America and Africa, and is transmitted by mosquitoes of the *Haemogogus*, *Sabethes*, and *Aedes* genera.[9] The virus was introduced in South America from Africa with the slave trade in the sixteenth century **(Fig. 1)**.[10]

The zoonotic cycle involving sylvatic mosquitoes (*Haemogogus* and *Sabethes* in South America, *Aedes* in Africa) and nonhuman primates occurs in tropical forests, where humans can be accidently bitten by sylvatic mosquitoes that previously fed on a viremic monkey (jungle yellow fever). Infected humans can introduce the virus in an urban cycle, where the main vector is represented by *Aedes aegypti* (urban yellow fever). Noteworthy, in Africa YFV transmission can be sustained also by a mixed cycle (usually in the savannah), involving both sylvatic and domestic vector species and humans living or working in jungle border areas.[2,9] YFV is also maintained in

Table 2
Reported VHF outbreaks (January 2017–April 2019)

Year	Hemorrhagic Disease	Country
2019	Ebola virus disease	Democratic Republic of the Congo
2019	Rift Valley fever	Mayotte (France)
2019	Yellow fever	Brazil
2019	Lassa fever	Nigeria
2019	Dengue fever	Jamaica
2019	Hantavirus cardiopulmonary syndrome	Argentine Republic
2019	Yellow fever	Nigeria
2019	Hantavirus cardiopulmonary syndrome	Republic of Panama
2018	Yellow fever	Kingdom of the Netherlands
2018	Yellow fever	Republic of the Congo
2018	Yellow fever	French Guyana (France)
2018	Rift Valley fever	Kenya
2018	Dengue Fever	Réunion, France
2018	Ebola virus disease	Democratic Republic of the Congo
2018	Lassa Fever	Nigeria
2018	Yellow fever	Brazil
2018	Rift Valley fever	Gambia
2018	Lassa Fever	Liberia
2017	Yellow fever	Nigeria
2017	Yellow fever	Brazil
2017	Marburg virus disease	Uganda and Kenya
2017	Yellow fever	French Guyana (France)
2017	Dengue fever	Côte d'Ivoire
2017	Dengue fever	Sri Lanka
2017	Lassa fever	Nigeria
2017	Ebola virus disease	Democratic Republic of the Congo
2017	Yellow fever	Suriname
2017	Lassa fever	Benin, Togo and Burkina Faso
2017	Hantavirus hemorrhagic fever with renal syndrome (Seoul virus)	United States of America and Canada

Data from WHO Emergencies preparedness, response Disease Outbreak News (DONs) Disease outbreaks by year, 2017, 2018 and 2019, (at: www.who.int/csr/don/archive/year/en/); with permission.

mosquito populations through vertical (transovarial) transmission.[9] Approximately 80,000 to 200,000 YFV cases are reported worldwide every year, with a case fatality rate ranging from 20% to 60%.[11]

After an incubation period of 3 to 6 days after the bite of an infected mosquito, yellow fever classical picture is characterized by 3 clinical stages. The disease begins with flulike symptoms (viremic period), lasting for 3 to 5 days and characterized by fever, headache, malaise, photophobia, myalgia, irritability, nausea, and vomiting. During this period, the blood is infectious to biting mosquitoes. The viremic period is followed by a remission period of 1 to 2 days. Subsequently, some patients (20%–60%) progress to the third phase (period of intoxication), in which the patients become severely ill with signs of liver and renal failure. This phase is characterized by

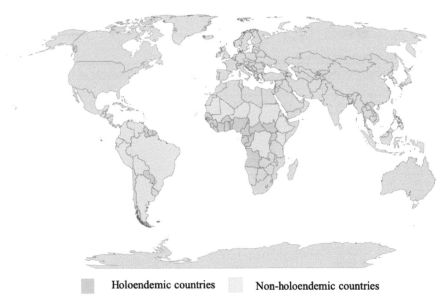

Holoendemic countries   Non-holoendemic countries

Fig. 1. Countries at risk of yellow fever transmission. In the map, countries at risk of yellow fever transmission are represented in shades of yellow. Light yellow has been used for countries in which only some areas are endemic for yellow fever transmission (nonholoendemic), and dark yellow has been used for countries totally at risk of yellow fever transmission (holoendemic). (*Data from* Virus Families | Viral Hemorrhagic Fevers (VHFs) | CDC. Available at: https://www.cdc.gov/vhf/virus-families/index.html. Accessed April 25, 2019; and Yellow Fever - Chapter 3 - 2018 Yellow Book | Travelers' Health | CDC. Available at: https://wwwnc.cdc.gov/travel/yellowbook/2018/infectious-diseases-related-to-travel/yellow-fever#9972. Accessed May 2, 2019.)

hemorrhages, jaundice, and thrombocytopenia, and the disease can progress to more generalized multiorgan dysfunction, vasculopathy, and even death.[12] This final stage is characterized by thrombocytopenia, coagulation abnormalities, deficiency of liver clotting factors, and elevated levels of fibrin split products, which indicate disseminated intravascular coagulation (DIC).[12]

According to current models, YFV is transmitted from the mosquito salivary glands to the host's dermis, where the virus infects dendritic cells and is transported to the lymph nodes. In the lymph nodes, YFV replicates and spreads through the peripheral blood, reaching the liver, where the virus infects Kupffer cells and hepatocytes, and induces apoptosis and necrosis, which results in the liver damage observed during the toxic phase of the infection.[11] Other organs can also be involved, as reported in humans[13] and in animal models.[14]

YFV pathogenesis relies on hepatocyte apoptosis induced by the virus itself and indirectly by host immunity, via an unbalanced cytokine production and $CD4^+$ and $CD8^+$ T-lymphocyte immune response.[15] Moreover, tumor necrosis factor-α, interferon-γ, and transforming growth factor-β are increased in the liver of fatal human cases, suggesting their pathogenetic role.[12,15]

Diagnostic procedures are based on IgM and IgG detection through different methods, such as enzyme-linked immunosorbent assay (ELISA), immunofluorescence assay (IFA), and serum neutralization tests (which remain the gold standard reference for detecting specific IgM and IgG).[16] Molecular diagnostic is based on reverse transcriptase polymerase chain reaction (RT-PCR), which can detect YFV in clinical specimens (whole blood, serum, and urine[17]) at a low virus concentration. New approaches are based on loop-mediated isothermal amplification and recombinase polymerase amplification assays. NS1 antigen detection by ELISA represents a promising test with high sensitivity and specificity for the diagnosis of acute yellow fever.[18] Virus isolation can be achieved with cell culture (using Vero cells or C6/36 *Aedes albopictus* cells) or by inoculation of infected samples in suckling mice or hamsters.[18,19]

No approved antiviral drugs against YFV are currently available. An effective vaccine based on the live attenuated YFV-17D virus confers long-lasting protection against the disease in immunocompromised and healthy individuals.[20] In 2014, the World Health Organization (WHO) indicated that a single dose of YFV-17D vaccine provides sustained immunity and lifelong protection.[21]

Dengue Fever

There are 4 antigenically distinct DENVs, which are named DENV 1, 2, 3, and 4. Dengue infection is transmitted by *Aedes* mosquitoes in the intertropical regions worldwide.[1] In dengue-endemic countries, DENV serotypes cocirculate in the same area at the same time, causing concurrent infections.[22] Little is known about the role of possible animal reservoirs for dengue transmission.[23] Autochthonous cases of DENV infections sustained by *A albopictus* have been described in Europe (France and Spain)[24] and in some states of the United States (Florida, Hawaii, and Texas)[25] (**Fig. 2**). In *Aedes* mosquitoes, natural vertical transmission of DENV from infected adults to some part of their offspring has been described, representing an important phenomenon for explaining endemicity.[26]

The incidence of dengue infections is estimated to be around 400 million per year, of which about 25% are symptomatic. Asia accounts for 75% of the dengue disease burden.[27] The 2009 WHO dengue case classification identified symptomatic individuals as having dengue without major complications, or as having severe dengue if

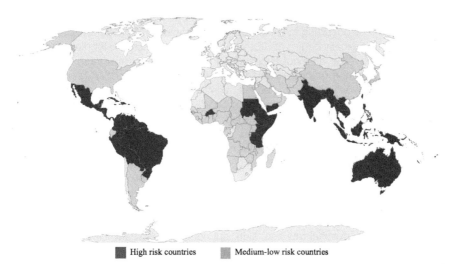

■ High risk countries   ■ Medium-low risk countries

Fig. 2. Countries at risk of dengue fever transmission. In the map, countries at risk of dengue fever transmission are represented in shadow of blue. Light and dark blue have been used for countries at medium to low risk and high risk of dengue fever transmission, respectively. (*Data from* Refs.[1,2,24,25])

they experienced complications in any of 3 categories: (1) plasma leakage causing shock syndrome or respiratory distress, (2) severe bleeding, or (3) severe organ impairment.[28] Severe dengue occurs more frequently during reinfection (with a heterologous infecting serotype compared with the primary infection) and in infants from mothers who have previously had dengue during pregnancy, in the phase in which maternal antibodies wane to subneutralizing titers.[29,30] In hyperendemic areas, the risk for severe disease is also high in pregnant women, especially during the third trimester.[31] Additionally, in regions with low endemicity, severe clinical disease is reported more frequently among adults with underlying comorbidities.[32]

Dengue is transmitted by the bite of an infected female mosquito. Nonvector transmission is also possible, through blood transfusion, organ transplantation, needle stick injuries, and mucosal splashes.[33] Although DENV has been detected in the semen[34] and vaginal secretions[35] of human beings, sexual transmission has not been reported so far. Vertical transmission is common among mothers who are viremic at delivery; no cases of transmissions through maternal milk have been reported.[36]

Both viral and host factors contribute to dengue infection pathogenesis. Among viral factors, NS1 protein seems to play a crucial role, interacting with several host proteins, being secreted from infected cells with the function of protecting the virus from complement and lectin-mediated neutralization. Moreover, NS1 may disrupt the endothelial glycocalyx increasing vascular permeability and contributing to vascular leakage.[37] Considering host factors, the adaptive immune response after infection with any serotype of DENV provides long-term immunity to the homologous virus, but protection against heterologous DENVs is short lived. Previous infection with one DENV serotype increases the risk of severe dengue upon secondary infection with a heterologous virus (original antigenic sin).[38] This phenomenon has been explained with the theory of the antibody-dependent enhancement: cross-reactive antibodies at subneutralizing concentrations bind heterologous DENV and facilitate virus entry through Fc receptors expressed on target cells.[30] However, only a fraction of infections occurring in the presence of non-neutralizing IgG progresses to severe dengue, indicating that appropriate antibody-to-virus ratios are required for antibody-dependent enhancement.[37]

DENV infections occurring in childhood are mostly asymptomatic. In adults, symptomatic dengue typically begins abruptly and follows 3 phases: the febrile, critical, and recovery phases. After an incubation period of 4 to 7 days (maximum of 14 days), symptomatic infection manifests and is characterized by a sudden onset of fever, myalgia, retroorbital headache, nausea, vomiting, conjunctival congestion, and a maculopapular rash with generalized lymphadenopathy. This phase lasts for 2 to 7 days. Complications can develop around the time of defervesence, marking the onset of the critical phase. During this phase, vascular permeability is increased and progression to dengue shock syndrome can occur. Conventionally, hemoconcentration of 20% or more marks the condition of dengue associated plasma leakage. Moreover, volume depletion causes the narrowing of the pulse pressure (the difference between the systolic and diastolic blood pressure). A pulse pressure equal to or less than 20 mm Hg, defines the state of dengue shock syndrome.[37,39] During the critical phase, hemorrhagic manifestations are often observed. Hemorrhages involve the gastrointestinal mucosa, skin, pulmonary alveoli, and serosal surfaces.[39] Severe organ impairment can also be observed during the critical phase, especially in individuals with underlying diseases. Even in patients who develop complications, good supportive care can ensure full recovery, within 1 to 2 weeks.[1,37]

During the first 5 days, DENV infection can be diagnosed by virus isolation in cell culture, detection of viral RNA by RT-PCR, or detection of viral antigens such as

NS1 by ELISA or rapid tests from blood and urine. DENV-RNA amplification and sequencing allow also for serotype identification. After 4 to 5 days from symptom onset, specific IgM and IgG antibodies can be detected with serologic assays (ELISA, IFA, hemagglutination inhibition test). In patients with a past dengue (or other flaviviruses) infection, dengue IgG titers increase rapidly within the first week of illness. Serologic assays require paired (acute and convalescent) samples and neutralization assay to confirm specificity.[28] Currently, the combination of NS1 antigen, IgM, and IgG testing at the point of care has improved the diagnosis of dengue.[37]

No antiviral drugs able to reduce DENV viral load or prevent complications are currently available. Ivermectin is under evaluation as an anti-DENV molecule in a clinical trial, still in progress (ClinicalTrials.gov number NCT02045069). NS4B inhibitors are under development. Steroid use is controversial.[37] In 2015, Sanofi Pasteur licensed the first recombinant, live attenuated, tetravalent vaccine, based on the yellow fever 17D backbone (CYD-TDV or Dengvaxia).[40] Postmarketing analyses revealed an excess risk of severe dengue in seronegative vaccine recipients, compared with seronegative nonvaccinated individuals.[41] In 2018 WHO recommended prevaccination screening to vaccinate only dengue-seropositive persons.[42] Two chimeric live attenuated dengue vaccines are currently in phase 3 trials.[37]

Other Flaviviruses Causing Hemorrhagic Fevers (Omsk Hemorrhagic Fever, Kyasanur Forest Disease, and Alkhumra Viruses)

Omsk hemorrhagic fever virus (OHFV) was first isolated from a patient in 1947, and later from ticks belonging to the species *Dermacentor reticulatus*, muskrats, and other vertebrates and arthropods in the rural region of Omsk (Siberia). Although antigenically and genetically distinct, OHFV is strictly related to tick born encephalitis virus. OHFV can be found in the forest–steppe of western Siberia (**Fig. 3**).[43,44]

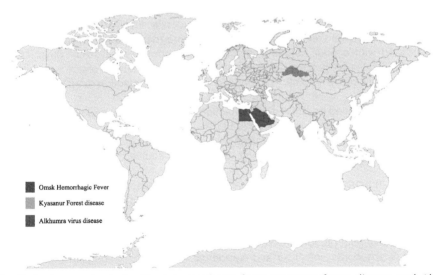

Fig. 3. Regions endemic for Omsk hemorrhagic fever, Kyasanur forest disease, and Alkhumra virus disease. In the map regions endemic for Omsk hemorrhagic fever, Kyasanur Forest disease, and Alkhumra virus disease are represented in blue, green, and red, respectively. Some cases have also been described outside endemic regions in travelers. (*Data from* Refs.[2,43,44,47–50])

The classic route of transmission is a tick bite in the endemic regions. *D reticulatus* is the natural reservoir, and OHFV is transmitted trans-stadially and transovarially. Recently, most human cases have been related to direct contact with infected musk-rats (*Ondatra zibethica*) in which the virus has been isolated from urine and feces.[43]

After an incubation period of 3 to 7 days, clinical manifestations of OHFV infection are characterized by fever, headache, myalgia, cough, and sometimes a petechial rash. This phase lasts for 5 to 12 days, followed by recovery or a more severe second febrile phase, during which meningeal signs can occur without neurologic involvement. In this phase, hemorrhagic manifestations are frequent but not severe, and are due to vascular and circulatory capillary damage. Mortality rates range from 0.5% to 3.0%.[43,45]

Diagnosis relies on OHFV-RNA detection through RT-PCR and specific IgM and IgG detection in patients' sera through ELISA or the hemagglutination inhibition test.[43] There is some evidence that a tick born encephalitis vaccine could confer cross-protection against OHFV, although this has not yet been formally demonstrated. An OHFV formalin-inactivated vaccine was developed in 1948, but its use was abandoned because of neurologic side effects.[43,45]

Kyasanur Forest disease virus (KFDV) was first isolated in the Indian state of Karnataka in 1957, after an outbreak involving monkeys in Kyasanur Forest and people living near the forest (see **Fig. 3**). Transmission of KFDV is mainly due to the bites of infected ticks from the genus *Haemaphysalis*. Natural hosts of KFDV are the Blanford rat (*Rattus blanfordi*), the striped forest squirrel (*Funambulus tristriatus tristriatus*), and the house shrew (*Suncus murinus*).[46] The annual incidence of KFD in India is estimated to be around 400 to 500 cases with seasonal outbreaks.[44]

The incubation period of KFDV in humans is 3 to 8 days. The clinical presentation of KFD is usually biphasic. In the first phase, patients usually present with sudden onset of fever, headache and generalized body pain. Conjunctivitis and gastrointestinal symptoms (vomiting, abdominal pain, and diarrhea) occur in the majority of patients in this phase. Hemorrhagic manifestations may begin 3 to 4 days after symptom onset and are characterized by mucosal bleeding, ocular involvement, hematemesis, epistaxis, and rectal bleeding. Persistence of hemorrhagic manifestations is usually associated with a poor outcome. Most patients recover in 10 to 14 days. Up to 20% of patients may present with biphasic illness and the second phase is characterized by neurologic symptoms. The mortality rate of KFDV infection ranges from 2% to 10%.[47]

Diagnosis is based on KFDV-RNA detection through RT-PCR and specific IgM and IgG detection in patients' sera through ELISA.

A formalin-inactivated KFDV vaccine derived from infected cell cultures has been produced and used in India. However, the current vaccine protocol showed limited efficacy.[44,47]

In 1994 in Saudi Arabia, a genetic variant of KFDV caused several outbreaks. This genetic variant was named Alkhumra (or Alkurma) hemorrhagic fever virus (see **Fig. 3**).[48] This disease was mainly found in sheep handlers, butchers, and meat consumers. Alkhumra (or Alkurma) hemorrhagic fever virus can be transmitted through direct contact with blood or secretions of infected animals or eventually through the bite of *Ornithodoros* soft ticks and *Hyalomma* hard ticks,[49] mosquito bites.[50] Oral transmission via camel milk has also been reported.[46]

Clinical characteristics of Alkhumra (or Alkurma) hemorrhagic fever virus infection are an acute febrile flulike illness with hepatitis, hemorrhagic manifestations, and encephalitis. The mortality rate is 25%.[50,51] Geographic distribution includes Arabic peninsula and east Africa (Djibouti and the border region between Egypt and Sudan).[49]

In Europe imported cases affecting travelers have been reported[52] and Alkhumra virus has been detected in ticks collected from migrating birds.[49]

FILOVIRUSES: MARBURG VIRUS DISEASE

Filoviruses show a filamentous morphology and are characterized by 3 distinct genera: Ebolavirus, Marburgvirus, and Cuevavirus.[53]

MARV was first identified in 1967, when laboratory workers in Germany and Yugoslavia (now Serbia) were infected with a previously unknown infectious agent. The source of infection was traced back to African green monkeys (*Chlorocebus aethiops*) that had been imported from Uganda.[54]

Marburgvirus genus consists of a single species, *Marburg Marburgvirus,* with 2 variants: MARV and Ravn virus, and causes disease in human and nonhuman primates. MARV has been isolated from Egyptian fruit bats (*Rousettus aegypticus*), which represents the major natural reservoir. Insectivorous bats and the urban-dwelling straw-colored bat may also represent viral carriers.[53] The virus is not known to be native in counties outside of the African continent.[53] MARV is transmitted to humans by contact with infected animals (nonhuman primates or fruit bats) or their body fluids or tissues. However, human-to-human infection occurs with direct contact with droplets or body fluids from infected persons, or contact with equipment and other objects contaminated with infectious blood or tissues.[1]

The viruses enter the body through small skin lesions or mucosal membranes. Cells of the mononuclear phagocyte system have been identified as early targets in human patients. Early sites of virus replication are the lymph nodes, liver, and spleen where the most severe necrotic lesions are observed. Lymphatic circulation and the bloodstream contribute to the dissemination of the virus to multiple organs, resulting in a systemic infection. Hepatocytes, adrenal cortical and medullary cells and fibroblasts are permissive to MARV infection, as well as endothelial cells during late stages of MARV infection. Despite a high viral load, only minor inflammation is observed in infected tissues, indicating a dysregulation in the immune response. Liver involvement is characterized by an impairment in the production of coagulation factors. Although lymphocytes are not susceptible to MARV infection, bystander lymphocyte apoptosis is a characteristic of MARV infection.[54]

Marburg disease has an incubation period ranging from 3 to 21 days (typically 5–10 days). The disease manifests abruptly with nonspecific flulike symptoms (chills, fever, myalgia, general malaise), followed by lethargy, nausea, vomiting, abdominal pain, anorexia, diarrhea, coughing, headache, hypotension, and a maculopapular rash. Hemorrhagic manifestations do not occur in all cases and vary in severity. Early symptoms are similar in survivors and nonsurvivors, although bloods test revealed 100- to 1000-fold higher levels of viremia in nonsurvivors compared with survivors. Fatal cases progress to more severe symptoms by days 7 to 14 after the onset of the disease. Survivors experience a prolonged convalescence.[54–56] The fatality rate has been estimated to be 82% in low-income countries, and 24% in patients receiving care in Europe and in the United States.[1]

Diagnosis is based on RNA viral detection by RT-PCR (on blood samples and tissues) and serologic assays for IgG and IgM detection. Recently an isothermal assay for RNA amplification has been developed (loop-mediated isothermal amplification), with the potential of improving MARV infections diagnosis.

No approved treatments for MARV infection are available so far. Supportive care represents the primary treatment. There are currently no licensed vaccines available against MARV; however, several vaccines obtained from different platforms have shown potential to protect nonhuman primates from MARV infection, including DNA vectors, virus-like particles, recombinant adenovirus vectors, and recombinant vesicular stomatitis virus vectors.[57,58]

NEW WORLD ARENAVIRUSES

The family *Arenaviridae* (of the *Bunyavirales* order) consists of 3 separated genera: *Mammarenavirus*, *Reptarenavirus*, and *Hartmanivirus*. The genus *Mammarenavirus*, encompassing viruses that infect mammals, is further divided into the OW and NW arenaviruses.[59] All members of the family have a negative sense, bisegmented single-strand RNA genome consisting of a large and small segment.[60]

The natural host for OW arenaviruses is represented by rodents belonging to the subfamily *Murinae* of the *Muridae* family of mice. OW arenavirus species include lymphocytic choriomeningitis virus, Lassa virus, and the newly emerged Lujo virus. The OW arenaviruses are geographically confined to the African continent, with the exception of lymphocytic choriomeningitis virus.[61] The NW arenaviruses are geographically distributed in South and North America (**Fig. 4**). The natural host for the NW arenaviruses is the *Sigmodontinae* subfamily of *Muridae* family mice with the exception of Tacaribe virus, which is found in *Artibeus* bats. The NW arenaviruses are further divided into 4 clades: A, B, C, and D (also known as A/Rec). The human hemorrhagic pathogens Junin virus (JUNV; Argentine hemorrhagic fever), Chapare and Machupo viruses (Bolivian hemorrhagic fever), Guanarito virus (Venezuelan hemorrhagic fever), Sabia, Cupixi, and Amapari viruses (Brazilian hemorrhagic fever), cluster in clade B together with the prototypic nonpathogenic Tacaribe virus (identified in bats in Trinidad and ticks in Florida). North American viruses Whitewater Arroyo, Bear Canyon, and Tamiami viruses belong to clade D (A/Rec).[61,62] Of these viruses, JUNV is the most relevant pathogen, with approximately 300 to 1000 cases per year (before the development of the Candid#1 vaccine).[63] Humans become

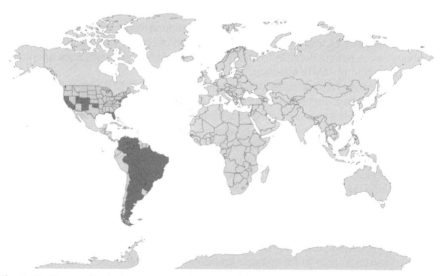

Fig. 4. Regions endemic for NW arenaviruses. In the map, regions endemic for NW hemorrhagic arenaviruses are presented. NW arenaviruses-related diseases are Argentine hemorrhagic fever, Bolivian hemorrhagic fever, Venezuelan hemorrhagic fever, Brazilian hemorrhagic fever, and North American viruses causing outbreaks in California, Colorado, Florida, New Mexico, Oklahoma, and Utah. (*Data from* Refs.[2,59–62])

infected through contact with infected rodents, or inhalation of their urine or feces.[62] Although rare, human-to-human transmission of NW arenaviruses has been described and may occur via direct contact with infected body fluids of viremic patients.[64]

The clade B pathogenic NW arenaviruses use transferrin receptor 1 to infect human cells. Transferrin receptor 1 is expressed in several human cell types; thus, NW arenavirus can infect a large number of target sells.[65] Studies in humans and animal models showed that macrophages and dendritic cells represent the main targets for NW arenavirus after airborne infection, causing aberrant cytokine production and bystander effects on endothelial cells.[61–63] Specifically, NW arenaviruses proteins have been shown to block type I interferon production.[66] Moreover, patients with NW arenaviruses showed high levels tumor necrosis factor-α, and other inflammatory mediators that correlate with the severity of disease.[67]

Among the NW arenaviruses, Chapare virus and Sabia virus infections have been identified as single cases, whereas JUNV, Machupo virus, and Guanarito virus have been associated with larger outbreaks.[62]

In the setting of JUNV infection and Argentine hemorrhagic fever, incubation ranges from 1 to 2 weeks. Argentine hemorrhagic fever manifests with fever, asthenia, muscular pain, dizziness, skin and mucosal rashes, and lymph node swelling. After 6 to 10 days from symptom onset, disease worsens with cardiovascular, gastrointestinal, renal, and neurologic involvement, associated with coagulation abnormalities and hemorrhages. Similarly, patients infected with Machupo virus may exhibit gingival hemorrhage, nausea, gastrointestinal bleeding, thrombocytopenia, hematuria, tremor, anorexia, and respiratory distress.[67] Hemorrhages observed in NW arenavirus infections are caused by coagulation abnormalities and marked thrombocytopenia; DIC has not been observed, like in other VHF.[62,67]

Diagnosis relies on arenavirus RNA detection by RT-PCR from serum, plasma, urine, and throat wash samples and from several human tissues. The identification of the specific arenavirus causing the disease can be performed through viral RNA sequencing. Serologic diagnosis is based on the detection of specific IgG and IgM antibodies by immunofluorescence tests and ELISA. Virus isolation can be achieved by propagation in cell culture (Vero cells).[68] NW arenaviruses are considered risk group 4 pathogens.[62]

Supportive therapy is essential during NW arenaviral infections. Ribavirin showed some efficacy in reducing fatality rates during Lassa fever and other arenaviral diseases, although few data are currently available for NW arenaviruses. New drugs are currently under development, such as polymerase and viral budding inhibitors, and small interfering RNA. Convalescent serum from JUNV-infected patients was effective in decreasing the fatality rate of Argentine hemorrhagic fever in a double-blind trial.[69] However, little is known about cross-protection against other NW arenaviruses.[68,70]

A live attenuated JUNV vaccine (Candid#1) is currently available. Its efficacy was proven in a double-blind trial and was able to significantly decrease the incidence of Argentine hemorrhagic fever.[62,70]

ORDER *BUNYAVIRALES*: *HANTAVIRIDAE*, *NAIROVIRIDAE*, AND *PHENUIVIRIDAE*

Viruses belonging to the *Hantaviridae*, *Nairoviridae*, and *Phenuiviridae* families (formerly encompassed in the unique *Bunyaviridae* family) have been associated to VHF and include RVFV, Crimean-Congo hemorrhagic fever virus (CCHFV), and several hantaviral agents causing hantavirus cardiopulmonary syndrome (HCPS) and HFRS.[71]

Recently, an emerging tick-borne infection, owing to a *Banyangvirus* (of the *Phenuiviridae* family) known as Huaiyangshan banyangvirus, which causes severe fever with thrombocytopenia syndrome, has been identified in China, South Korea, and Japan.[3,72]

Rift Valley Fever Virus

RVF was first described in 1930, during an outbreak characterized by high abortion rate among pregnant ewes associated to a high mortality rate of newborn lambs, in the Rift Valley region of Kenya (**Fig. 5**). The causative agent of RVF was then identified in South Africa in 1951.[73]

RVFV belongs to the *Phlebovirus* genus (of the *Phenuiviridae* family) and its viral genome contains 3 single-stranded, negative-polarity RNA segments.[74]

The epidemiology of RVFV is complex and involves mosquitoes, wild animals, domesticated livestock, and humans. RVFV has been isolated from a wide range of mosquito genera (*Aedes, Culex, Anopheles*, and *Mansonia*).[75] *Aedes* mosquitos maintain RVFV in nature by transovarial transmission.[76] RVFV alternates between mosquitoes and vertebrate hosts. Evidence of RVFV infection has been found in many wild mammalian species in Africa causing mild or inapparent illness in these species. Conversely, RVFV is highly pathogenic in domesticated ruminants, in which the virus replicates with high viral loads.[77] Humans can be infected by the bite of a mosquito, although mucous membrane exposure or inhalation of viral particles during the handling of infected animals represent the primary means of transmission of the virus to humans. There is no documented human-to-human transmission.[77,78] Women with acute RVFV infection during pregnancy have a higher rate of miscarriage and a vertical transmission has been reported.[79]

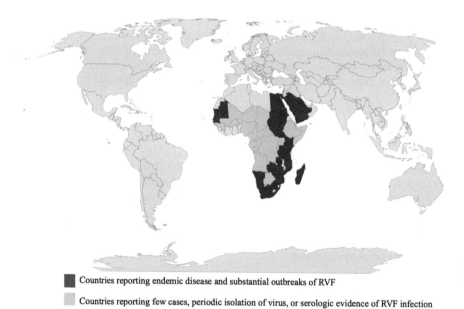

■ Countries reporting endemic disease and substantial outbreaks of RVF

▨ Countries reporting few cases, periodic isolation of virus, or serologic evidence of RVF infection

Fig. 5. Countries reporting RVF cases. In the map, countries reporting endemic disease and substantial outbreaks of RVF are presented in blue and countries reporting few cases, periodic isolation of the virus, or serologic evidence of RVF virus infection are presented in green. (*Data from* Refs.[2,73–75])

The nonstructural protein encoded by the small and medium RNA segments of the virus seem to be the major virulence factors, counteracting immune response and modulating host cell apoptosis.[80] The factors determining disease severity are still unknown. Genetic polymorphisms involving genes of the innate immunity may contribute to RVF severity.[65] Comorbidities can influence disease outcome and complication onset. HIV infection seems to be associated with a higher incidence of neurologic complications and death.[79]

Most infected people develop uncomplicated RVF, which is characterized by flulike symptoms, sometimes with a biphasic fever. Symptoms can be debilitating, and convalescence may take several weeks.[77] Complicated RFV usually manifests with ocular complications ($\leq$10% and characterized by uveitis, retinitis, vasculitis retinal hemorrhages)[81]; severe hepatic disease (1%–2%, jaundice and hemorrhagic manifestations, including gastrointestinal bleeding)[77,82]; and neurologic disease, typically with a delayed onset (severe headache, hallucination, disorientation, vertigo, excessive salivation, and weakness or partial paralysis).[82]

Blood samples from acutely infected people can be tested for the presence of RVFV-RNA by RT-PCR, multiplex PCR-based microarray assay, isothermal amplification methods (loop-mediated isothermal amplification), and recombinase polymerase amplification. Antigen detection can be performed by ELISA. Isolation of live virus can be performed in suckling mice or in cell cultures. Serologic tests for the detection of specific IgG and IgM by ELISA, IFA, and hemagglutination inhibition assay are available.[73,77,82]

There are no specific treatments for RVF. Ribavirin is considered a potential antiviral drug for RVF because of its in vitro efficacy. Although no licensed vaccine preparations for use in humans are available so far, 3 licensed veterinary vaccines are being used to protect ruminant populations. Inactivated, live attenuated, and innovative vaccines are currently under development.[73]

Crimean-Congo Hemorrhagic Fever

The CCHFV is an *Orthonairovirus* of the *Nairoviridae* family, with a genome consisting of 3 negative-sense single-stranded RNA molecules.[43] It was first identified in 1944 in the Crimean Peninsula and then isolated in the Congo in 1956.[83] CCHFV is widely distributed in Africa, the Middle East, and central and southwestern Asia. It has also been found in different European countries.[84] CCHFV is endemic in the Balkans, and Bulgaria regularly reports a small number of cases occurring every years. Most of the cases in last 15 years has been reported from Turkey. In 2016, for the first time, autochthonous human cases were reported in southwestern Europe (Spain). The primary case most likely became infected through contact with a tick while hiking in Avila Province. The secondary case was a health care worker who looked after the patient while in the intensive care unit (**Fig. 6**).[85] In 2018, a second report of human CCHF case was reported in Spain in a 74-year-old man who died during hospitalization.[86]

CCHF is a thick-born VHF. The virus has been detected in at least 30 species of tick (28 *Ixodidae* and 2 *Argasidae*). However, *Argasidae* are not capable of serving as vectors. Many *Ixodidae* tick species can transmit the virus to humans, but the genus *Hyalomma* represent the most effective vector.[43] CCHFV is maintained in nature by *Ixodidae* species by trans-stadial and transovarial transmission.[83] Human-to-human transmission is also reported, especially in health care settings.[87]

The mechanism behind the pathogenesis of CCHF is majorly unknown; however, data from in vitro and in vivo studies suggested that the disease is related to a cytokine storm initiated by virus replication. CCHFV dysregulates the immune response

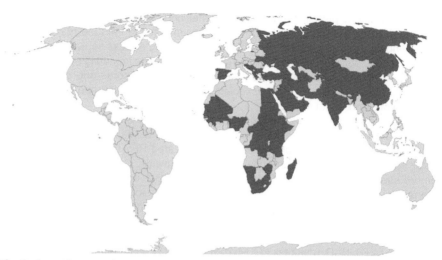

Fig. 6. Countries reporting Crimean-Congo hemorrhagic fever cases. In the map, countries reporting cases of CCHFV infection are presented in red. (*Data from* Refs.[2,83–86])

with the consequence of a marked viral replication, vascular system alterations, and lymphoid organs involvement. It has also been suggested that infection of the endothelium plays a crucial role in CCHFV pathogenesis. The endothelium is directly targeted by viral infection and replication, and indirectly affected by host-derived soluble factors, which can cause endothelial activation and dysfunction. Endothelial damage contributes to platelet degranulation, with consequent activation of the intrinsic coagulation cascade, consumption of coagulation factors, and DIC.[88,89]

After an incubation period of 2 to 7 days, early signs of the disease include fever, hypotension, conjunctivitis, headache, dizziness, neck pain, nuchal rigidity, photophobia, retro-orbital pain, myalgia and arthralgia, skin rash, nausea, vomiting, diarrhea, and abdominal pain (prehemorrhagic period). Later (after 4–5 days from symptom onset), patients may develop hemorrhagic manifestations (petechial rash, ecchymoses, hematemesis and melena), DIC, and circulatory shock (hemorrhagic period). Hepatomegaly and splenomegaly represent common features of CCHFV infection. Survivors enters in the convalescent period usually after 10 days from symptom onset.[89] The mortality rate of CCHF is between 3% and 30%.[43,89]

Early diagnosis is essential for patient survival and nosocomial infection prevention.[89] Classic RT-PCR is considered the method of choice for rapid laboratory diagnosis of CCHFV infection on blood and urine samples.[90] IgG and IgM antibodies can be detected with ELISA and IFA from about day 7 after the onset of the disease. Viral isolation can be achieved by intrathecal inoculation of viremic blood or urine in newborn mice or in cell culture.[91] A consensus document on laboratory management of CCHFV infection has been recently published.[92]

Ribavirin is the only available drug with a demonstrated antiviral effect against CCHFV in vitro and in animal models,[93,94] although its effectiveness in humans is controversial.[95] A vaccine for CCHFV derived from inactivated virus obtained from mouse brain is used in Bulgaria. Its efficacy has not been well-established. New potential antiviral compounds and therapeutic approach are under evaluation.[89,91]

Hantavirus Cardiopulmonary Syndrome and Hemorrhagic Fever with Renal Syndrome

Hantaviruses are negative-sense single-stranded RNA viruses, with a genome consisting of 3 distinct RNA segments.[96] In humans, OW hantaviruses can cause HFRS (including also a milder form, called nephropathia epidemica and caused by Puumala virus), and NW hantavirus can cause HCPS. Currently, 150,000 to 200,000 cases of hantavirus disease occur yearly, the majority being reported in Asia, with fewer infections reported in the Americas and Europe (**Fig. 7**).[97]

Hantaviruses are directly transmitted to humans by small rodents, which represent the natural reservoir and influence hantavirus geographic distribution.[98,99] Transmission to humans occurs via inhalation of aerosols derived from the urine, feces, or saliva of infected animals, but can also be due to infected rodent bites. In the environment, virus particles remain infectious for several weeks.[100] **Table 3** summarizes pathogenic hantaviruses and their geographic distribution.

The primary target of hantavirus infection is the endothelium of different organs and tissue, including the lung and the kidneys. The main endothelial receptor for pathogenic hantaviruses is β3-integrin. Although hantavirus infection of endothelial cell is noncytolytic, this event is followed by impairment of the barrier function, fluid extravasation, and organ failure. One hypothesis is that the host cellular immune response, sustained by cytotoxic $CD8^+$ T cells, may cause endothelial disfunction.[96,101] However, an animal model did not confirm this hypothesis.[102] Some studies showed a higher frequency of hantavirus-specific $CD8^+$ T cells in patients with a severe outcome, as compared with those with a mild or moderate

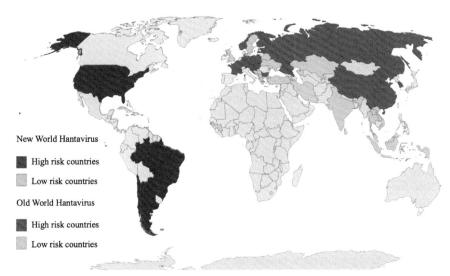

New World Hantavirus

■ High risk countries

▢ Low risk countries

Old World Hantavirus

■ High risk countries

▢ Low risk countries

Fig. 7. Countries reporting Hantavirus-related diseases. OW hantaviruses associated to HFRS are presented in red in the map. Specifically, high- and low-risk countries for OW hantavirus infections are represented in dark and light red, respectively. NW hantaviruses associated to HCPS are presented in shades of blue in the map. Specifically, high- and low-risk countries for NW hantavirus infections are presented in dark and light blue, respectively. (*Data from* Refs.[2,97–99])

Table 3
Human pathogenic hantaviruses and their geographic distribution

Virus (Abbreviation)	Disease	Rodent Host	Geographic Distribution
Amur virus (AMRV)	HFRS	*Apodemus peninsulae*	Russia, China, Korea
Dobrava-Belgra (DOBV)		*Apodemus flavicollis*	Europe
Hantaan Virus (HTNV)		*Apodemus agrarius*	China, South Korea, Russia
Puumala virus (PUUV)		*Clethrionomys glareolus* *Myodes glareolus*	Europe
Saaremaa virus (SAAV)		*A agrarius*	Europe
Seoul virus (SEOV)		*Rattus norvegicus*	Worldwide
Thailand hantavirus (THAIV)		*Bandicota indica*	Thailand
Tula virus (TULV)		*Microtus arvalis*	Europe
Andes Virus (ANDV)	HCPS	*Oligoryzomys longicaudatus*	Argentina, Chile
Araraquara Virus (ARAV)		*Necromys lasiurus*	Brazil
Bayou virus (BAYV)		*Oryzomys palustris*	North America
Bermejo virus (BMJV)		*Oligoryzomys chacoensis* *Oligoryzomys flavescens*	Argentina, Bolivia
Black Creek Canal virus (BCCV)		*Sigmodon hispidus*	North America
Castelo Dos Sonhos virus (CASV)		*Oligoryzomys spp.*	Brazil
Choclo virus (CHOV)		*Oligoryzomys fulvescens*	Panama
Juquitiba virus (JUQV)		*Oligoryzomys nigripes*	Argentina, Brazil
Laguna Negra virus (LANV)		*Calomys callosus*	Argentina, Paraguay, Bolivia
Lechiguanas virus (LECV)		*O flavescens*	Argentina
Maciel virus (MCLV)		*Bolomys obscurus*	Argentina
Monongahela virus (MGLV)		*Peromyscus leucopus*	North America
Muleshoe virus (MULEV)		*S hispidus*	North America
New York virus (NYV)		*P leucopus*	North America
Oran virus (ORNV)		*O chacoensis*	Argentina
Sin Nombre virus (SNV)		*Peromyscus maniculatus*	North America

Adapted from Jiang H., Zheng X., Wang L., et al. Hantavirus infection: a global zoonotic challenge. Virol Sin 2017;32(1):32–43. https://doi.org/10.1007/s12250-016-3899-x; with permission.

outcome.[97,103] Host factor such as HLA B*35 have been associated to an increased risk for severe HCPS outcomes.[104] During convalescence in patients with severe HCPS, the viral genome can be detected up to 90 days after the onset of clinical symptoms.[97]

Hantaviruses can cause 2 zoonotic diseases in humans: HFRS or HCPS.[97] For HFRS, after an incubation period ranging from 10 days to 6 weeks, clinical symptoms occur and are characterized by a first febrile phase (1–7 days) with fever accompanied by nonspecific signs (myalgia, headache, abdominal pain, and malaise). Neurologic, ocular, cardiovascular, and gastrointestinal symptoms can also be present at this stage. Conjunctival and mucosal hemorrhages can occur. Subsequently, patients enter a hypotensive phase (1–3 days) characterized by vascular leakage, associated with thrombocytopenia, shock and mental confusion. The following oliguric phase (2–6 days) is characterized by a decrease in urine output, with possible hypertension, pulmonary edema, and renal insufficiency. Approximately 50% of all fatalities occur in this phase. Survivors enter in the polyuric phase (lasting for several weeks), which is followed by the convalescent phase (3–6 months) characterized by residual fatigue and weakness. Severity and case fatality rates of HFRS depend on the specific causative agent.[101]

In the setting of HCPS, the incubation period is widely variable, ranging from 7 to 39 days.[105] Symptoms first manifest with a flulike syndrome (febrile phase), which may last for up to 5 days and be characterized by fever, myalgia, headache, malaise, and arthralgia. Gastrointestinal and neurologic signs may also occur. Laboratory tests show thrombocytopenia, leukocytosis or leukopenia, a high hematocrit, peripheral immunoblasts, lymphocytosis, abnormal liver enzyme levels, a mild increase in creatinine, hyponatremia, and proteinuria. One-half of infections evolve to the cardiopulmonary phase, characterized by capillary leakage and low cardiac output progressing to pulmonary edema with dyspnea, cough, tachycardia, and hypotension. Cardiogenic shock represents the main cause of death. Thrombocytopenia and intravascular coagulation can occur in this phase and cause hemorrhagic manifestations (hematuria, intestinal bleeding, metrorrhagia). Renal failure may occur in up to 50% of the patients. The case fatality rate ranges from 10% to 40%, according to the causative agent.[96]

IgG and IgM responses against 3 structural proteins of hantaviruses (Gn, Gc, and N) represent the standard diagnostic tool. ELISA, IFA, immunoblot assay, focus reduction neutralization test represent the methods of choice. Viral genome can be detected with sensitive and specific RT-PCR in blood and urine. Viral isolation of hantaviruses is usually performed only for research purposes. Samples should be handled in a biosafety level 3 facility if viral culture techniques are used.[106]

No antiviral drugs are currently available for hantaviral diseases. Data on ribavirin efficacy are controversial, considering that it seems to decrease morbidity mortality in patients with HFRS,[107] but not in patients with acute HCPS.[108] Passive immunotherapy could represent a promising treatment for acute HCPS. Currently, different vaccines are under development.[97,109]

SUMMARY

VHFs represent a challenging problem for the global health, considering that effective treatments or vaccines are currently unavailable for the majority of the viruses causing VHFs. Moreover, the clinical management of patients with VHF requires highly specialized personnel and, in many cases, specific isolation precautions, to reduce the risk of human-to-human transmission in the health care setting, as well as accidental exposition in the diagnostic laboratories. Besides, mortality rates associated with VHFs are significantly high. Because of all these elements, the WHO is currently considering VHF as a research priority. Although some viruses causing VHFs are present in high-income countries, most of them are endemic in low-income countries, thus limiting private research investments for developing new antiviral drugs or vaccines. In this scenario, funding from public institutions, nonprofit organizations, and supranational organizations is of paramount importance to sustain the research for developing new diagnostic tools, such as a rapid test for case identification and contact tracing; finding new molecules with direct antiviral activity, by using high-throughput screening methods; and developing effective and safe vaccines. Considering the mobility of increasing numbers of people owing to migrations, travel, climate changes, VHFs could become a relevant health issue in larger areas of the world, involving previously unaffected countries. For this reason, the preparedness for possible VHF outbreaks outside classical endemic areas should

Table 4
Clinical and pathologic aspects of some VHFs

VHF Agent	Jaundice	Liver Involvement	Kidney Involvement	Lung Involvement	CNS Involvement	Heart Involvement	DIC
Flaviviridae							
YFV	+++	+++	+	+	++	++	-
DENV	+	+	-	+	+	-	-
OHFV	-	-	-	++	+++	-	-
KFDV	-	+	+	++	+++	-	-
AHFV	+	+	+	+	+++	-	-
Filoviridae							
Marburg virus	+++	+++	+	+	+	+	+
NW Arenaviridae							
JUNV	-	+	+	+	++	+	-
Machupo virus	-	+	+	+	++	+	-
Guanarito virus	-	+	+	+	++	+	-
Bunyaviridae							
RVFV	+++	++	++	+	+++	-	+
CCHFV	-	+	+	+	++	+	+
Hantaviruses (HFRS)	-	+	+++	+	++	+	-
Hantavirus (HCPS)	-	+	+	+++		+++	-

Abbreviations: -, not observed or anecdotic description; +, less frequently observed; ++, commonly observed; +++, frequently observed and severe; AHFV, Alkhumra (or Alkurma) hemorrhagic fever virus; CCHFV, Crimean-Congo hemorrhagic fever; CNS, central nervous system.

be reinforced. Suspect case identification, differential diagnosis, and case confirmation represent the essential steps for the correct management of possible VHF cases. A knowledge of the epidemiology and clinical presentation can help in identifying patients with suspect VHF, either naturally acquired or because of bioterrorism attacks. **Table 4** summarizes some clinical and pathologic aspects of the VHFs described in the text.

VHFs represent also the ideal setting for a "One Health" approach, in which optimal health outcomes can be achieved by integrating physicians, epidemiologists, virologists, veterinarians, and ecologists aiming to realize a transdisciplinary approach. Indeed, an effective intervention for limiting or preventing VHF outbreaks should take into account the population at risk, the animal reservoir, the eventual arthropod vector and the environmental factors.

ACKNOWLEDGMENTS

This study has been supported by the Italian Ministry of Health. M. Iannetta, A. Di Caro, E. Nicastri, F. Vairo, and G. Ippolito received financial support from the Italian Ministry of Health, grants to Ricerca Corrente linea 1 to National Institute for Infectious Diseases Lazzaro Spallanzani, IRCCS. G. Ippolito, F. Vairo, F. Ntoumi and A. Zumla acknowledge support from the PANDORA-ID-NET consortium grant, funded by the European, and Developing Countries Clinical Trials Partnership (EDCTP2) programme (EDCTP Reg/Grant RIA2016E-1609), which is supported under Horizon 2020, the European Union's Framework Programme for Research and Innovation. A. Zumla is in receipt of a UK NIHR Senior Investigator Award. A. Di Caro, E. Nicastri, F. Vairo, and G. Ippolito are Professors at Saint Camillus International University of Health and Medical Sciences in Rome.

REFERENCES

1. Paessler S, Walker DH. Pathogenesis of the viral hemorrhagic fevers. Annu Rev Pathol 2013;8:411–40.
2. Virus Families | Viral Hemorrhagic Fevers (VHFs) | CDC. Available at: https://www.cdc.gov/vhf/virus-families/index.html. Accessed April 25, 2019.
3. Zhang Y-Z, Xu J. The emergence and cross species transmission of newly discovered tick-borne Bunyavirus in China. Curr Opin Virol 2016;16:126–31.
4. Borio L, Inglesby T, Peters CJ, et al. Hemorrhagic fever viruses as biological weapons: medical and public health management. JAMA 2002;287(18):2391–405.
5. Racsa LD, Kraft CS, Olinger GG, et al. Viral Hemorrhagic Fever Diagnostics. Clin Infect Dis 2016;62(2):214–9.
6. Westover JB, Sefing EJ, Bailey KW, et al. Low-dose ribavirin potentiates the antiviral activity of favipiravir against hemorrhagic fever viruses. Antiviral Res 2016;126:62–8.
7. Keshtkar-Jahromi M, Kuhn JH, Christova I, et al. Crimean-Congo hemorrhagic fever: current and future prospects of vaccines and therapies. Antiviral Res 2011;90(2):85–92.
8. Heinz FX, Stiasny K. Flaviviruses and their antigenic structure. J Clin Virol 2012;55(4):289–95.
9. Barrett AD, Monath TP. Epidemiology and ecology of yellow fever virus. Adv Virus Res 2003;61:291–315.
10. Bryant JE, Holmes EC, Barrett ADT. Out of Africa: a molecular perspective on the introduction of yellow fever virus into the Americas. PLoS Pathog 2007;3(5):e75.

11. Douam F, Ploss A. Yellow Fever virus: knowledge gaps impeding the fight against an old foe. Trends Microbiol 2018;26(11):913–28.

12. Quaresma JAS, Pagliari C, Medeiros DBA, et al. Immunity and immune response, pathology and pathologic changes: progress and challenges in the immunopathology of yellow fever. Rev Med Virol 2013;23(5):305–18.

13. De Brito T, Siqueira SA, Santos RT, et al. Human fatal yellow fever. Immunohistochemical detection of viral antigens in the liver, kidney and heart. Pathol Res Pract 1992;188(1–2):177–81.

14. Meier KC, Gardner CL, Khoretonenko MV, et al. A mouse model for studying viscerotropic disease caused by yellow fever virus infection. PLoS Pathog 2009; 5(10):e1000614.

15. Quaresma JAS, Barros VLRS, Pagliari C, et al. Revisiting the liver in human yellow fever: virus-induced apoptosis in hepatocytes associated with TGF-beta, TNF-alpha and NK cells activity. Virology 2006;345(1):22–30.

16. Niedrig M, Kürsteiner O, Herzog C, et al. Evaluation of an indirect immunofluorescence assay for detection of immunoglobulin M (IgM) and IgG antibodies against yellow fever virus. Clin Vaccin Immunol 2008;15(2):177–81.

17. Reusken CBEM, Knoester M, GeurtsvanKessel C, et al. Urine as sample type for molecular diagnosis of natural Yellow fever virus infections. J Clin Microbiol 2017;55(11):3294–6.

18. Domingo C, Charrel RN, Schmidt-Chanasit J, et al. Yellow fever in the diagnostics laboratory. Emerg Microbes Infect 2018;7. https://doi.org/10.1038/s41426-018-0128-8.

19. Monath TP, Vasconcelos PFC. Yellow fever. J Clin Virol 2015;64:160–73.

20. Wieten RW, Goorhuis A, Jonker EFF, et al. 17D yellow fever vaccine elicits comparable long-term immune responses in healthy individuals and immune-compromised patients. J Infect 2016;72(6):713–22.

21. Yellow Fever - Chapter 3 - 2018 Yellow Book | Travelers' Health | CDC. Available at: https://wwwnc.cdc.gov/travel/yellowbook/2018/infectious-diseases-related-to-travel/yellow-fever#9972. Accessed May 2, 2019.

22. Andrade EHP, Figueiredo LB, Vilela APP, et al. Spatial–temporal co-circulation of dengue virus 1, 2, 3, and 4 associated with coinfection cases in a hyperendemic area of Brazil: a 4-week survey. Am J Trop Med Hyg 2016;94(5):1080–4.

23. Thongyuan S, Kittayapong P. First evidence of dengue infection in domestic dogs living in different ecological settings in Thailand. PLoS One 2017;12(8): e0180013.

24. Rapid risk assessment: local transmission of dengue fever in France and Spain. European Centre for Disease Prevention and Control. Available at: http://ecdc.europa.eu/en/publications-data/rapid-risk-assessment-local-transmission-dengue-fever-france-and-spain. Accessed May 18, 2019.

25. Dengue in the US States and Territories | Dengue | CDC. Available at: https://www.cdc.gov/dengue/areaswithrisk/in-the-us.html. Accessed May 18, 2019.

26. Ferreira-de-Lima VH, Lima-Camara TN. Natural vertical transmission of dengue virus in Aedes aegypti and Aedes albopictus: a systematic review. Parasit Vectors 2018;11(1):77.

27. Bhatt S, Gething PW, Brady OJ, et al. The global distribution and burden of dengue. Nature 2013;496(7446):504–7.

28. Special Programme for Research and Training in Tropical Diseases., World Health Organization. Dengue: guidelines for diagnosis, treatment, prevention, and control. New edition. Geneva (Switzerland): TDR : World Health Organization; 2009.

29. Halstead SB, Lan NT, Myint TT, et al. Dengue hemorrhagic fever in infants: research opportunities ignored. Emerg Infect Dis 2002;8(12):1474–9.

30. Katzelnick LC, Gresh L, Halloran ME, et al. Antibody-dependent enhancement of severe dengue disease in humans. Science 2017;358(6365):929–32.

31. Nascimento LB, Siqueira CM, Coelho GE, et al. Symptomatic dengue infection during pregnancy and livebirth outcomes in Brazil, 2007-13: a retrospective observational cohort study. Lancet Infect Dis 2017. https://doi.org/10.1016/S1473-3099(17)30169-X.

32. Rowe EK, Leo Y-S, Wong JGX, et al. Challenges in dengue fever in the elderly: atypical presentation and risk of severe dengue and hospital-acquired infection [corrected]. PLoS Negl Trop Dis 2014;8(4):e2777.

33. Chen LH, Wilson ME. Update on non-vector transmission of dengue: relevant studies with Zika and other flaviviruses. Trop Dis Travel Med Vaccines 2016; 2:15.

34. Lalle E, Colavita F, Iannetta M, et al. Prolonged detection of dengue virus RNA in the semen of a man returning from Thailand to Italy, January 2018. Euro Surveill 2018;23(18). https://doi.org/10.2807/1560-7917.ES.2018.23.18.18-00197.

35. Iannetta M, Lalle E, Musso M, et al. Persistent detection of dengue virus RNA in vaginal secretion of a woman returning from Sri Lanka to Italy, April 2017. Euro Surveill 2017;22(34). https://doi.org/10.2807/1560-7917.ES.2017.22.34.30600.

36. Arragain L, Dupont-Rouzeyrol M, O'Connor O, et al. Vertical transmission of dengue virus in the peripartum period and viral kinetics in newborns and breast milk: new data. J Pediatr Infect Dis Soc 2017;6(4):324–31.

37. Wilder-Smith A, Ooi E-E, Horstick O, et al. Dengue. Lancet 2019;393(10169): 350–63.

38. Rothman AL. Immunity to dengue virus: a tale of original antigenic sin and tropical cytokine storms. Nat Rev Immunol 2011;11(8):532–43.

39. Morra ME, Altibi AMA, Iqtadar S, et al. Definitions for warning signs and signs of severe dengue according to the WHO 2009 classification: systematic review of literature. Rev Med Virol 2018;28(4):e1979.

40. Wilder-Smith A, Vannice KS, Hombach J, et al. Population perspectives and World Health Organization recommendations for CYD-TDV Dengue vaccine. J Infect Dis 2016;214(12):1796–9.

41. Sridhar S, Luedtke A, Langevin E, et al. Effect of dengue serostatus on dengue vaccine safety and efficacy. N Engl J Med 2018;379(4):327–40.

42. Dengue vaccine: WHO position paper, September 2018 - Recommendations. Vaccine 2018. https://doi.org/10.1016/j.vaccine.2018.09.063.

43. Charrel RN, Attoui H, Butenko AM, et al. Tick-borne virus diseases of human interest in Europe. Clin Microbiol Infect 2004;10(12):1040–55.

44. Lani R, Moghaddam E, Haghani A, et al. Tick-borne viruses: a review from the perspective of therapeutic approaches. Ticks Tick Borne Dis 2014;5(5):457–65.

45. Růžek D, Yakimenko VV, Karan LS, et al. Omsk haemorrhagic fever. Lancet Lond Engl 2010;376(9758):2104–13.

46. Dobler G. Zoonotic tick-borne flaviviruses. Vet Microbiol 2010;140(3–4):221–8.

47. Munivenkatappa A, Sahay RR, Yadav PD, et al. Clinical & epidemiological significance of Kyasanur forest disease. Indian J Med Res 2018;148(2):145–50.

48. Zaki AM. Isolation of a flavivirus related to the tick-borne encephalitis complex from human cases in Saudi Arabia. Trans R Soc Trop Med Hyg 1997;91(2): 179–81.

49. Hoffman T, Lindeborg M, Barboutis C, et al. Alkhurma Hemorrhagic fever virus RNA in hyalomma rufipes ticks infesting migratory birds, Europe and Asia Minor. Emerg Infect Dis 2018;24(5):879–82.
50. Madani TA. Alkhumra virus infection, a new viral hemorrhagic fever in Saudi Arabia. J Infect 2005;51(2):91–7.
51. Madani TA, Azhar EI, Abuelzein E-TME, et al. Alkhumra (Alkhurma) virus outbreak in Najran, Saudi Arabia: epidemiological, clinical, and laboratory characteristics. J Infect 2011;62(1):67–76.
52. Carletti F, Castilletti C, Di Caro A, et al. Alkhurma hemorrhagic fever in travelers returning from Egypt, 2010. Emerg Infect Dis 2010;16(12):1979–82.
53. Emanuel J, Marzi A, Feldmann H. Filoviruses: ecology, molecular biology, and evolution. Adv Virus Res 2018;100:189–221.
54. Brauburger K, Hume AJ, Mühlberger E, et al. Forty-five years of Marburg virus research. Viruses 2012;4(10):1878–927.
55. Hartman AL, Towner JS, Nichol ST. Ebola and Marburg hemorrhagic fever. Clin Lab Med 2010;30(1):161–77.
56. Gear JS, Cassel GA, Gear AJ, et al. Outbreak of Marburg virus disease in Johannesburg. Br Med J 1975;4(5995):489–93.
57. Reynolds P, Marzi A. Ebola and Marburg virus vaccines. Virus Genes 2017; 53(4):501–15.
58. Marzi A, Menicucci AR, Engelmann F, et al. Protection against Marburg Virus using a recombinant VSV-vaccine depends on T and B cell activation. Front Immunol 2018;9:3071.
59. Maes P, Alkhovsky SV, Bào Y, et al. Taxonomy of the family Arenaviridae and the order Bunyavirales: update 2018. Arch Virol 2018;163(8):2295–310.
60. Morin B, Coutard B, Lelke M, et al. The N-terminal domain of the arenavirus L protein is an RNA endonuclease essential in mRNA transcription. PLoS Pathog 2010;6(9):e1001038.
61. Hallam SJ, Koma T, Maruyama J, et al. Review of mammarenavirus biology and replication. Front Microbiol 2018;9:1751.
62. Sarute N, Ross SR. New world arenavirus biology. Annu Rev Virol 2017;4(1): 141–58.
63. McLay L, Liang Y, Ly H. Comparative analysis of disease pathogenesis and molecular mechanisms of New World and Old World arenavirus infections. J Gen Virol 2014;95(Pt 1):1–15.
64. Kilgore PE, Peters CJ, Mills JN, et al. Prospects for the control of Bolivian hemorrhagic fever. Emerg Infect Dis 1995;1(3):97–100.
65. Flanagan ML, Oldenburg J, Reignier T, et al. New world clade B arenaviruses can use transferrin receptor 1 (TfR1)-dependent and -independent entry pathways, and glycoproteins from human pathogenic strains are associated with the use of TfR1. J Virol 2008;82(2):938–48.
66. Fan L, Briese T, Lipkin WI. Z proteins of New World arenaviruses bind RIG-I and interfere with type I interferon induction. J Virol 2010;84(4):1785–91.
67. Moraz M-L, Kunz S. Pathogenesis of arenavirus hemorrhagic fevers. Expert Rev Anti Infect Ther 2011;9(1):49–59.
68. Charrel RN, de Lamballerie X. Arenaviruses other than Lassa virus. Antiviral Res 2003;57(1–2):89–100.
69. Maiztegui JI, Fernandez NJ, de Damilano AJ. Efficacy of immune plasma in treatment of Argentine haemorrhagic fever and association between treatment and a late neurological syndrome. Lancet Lond Engl 1979;2(8154):1216–7.

70. Charrel RN, Coutard B, Baronti C, et al. Arenaviruses and hantaviruses: from epidemiology and genomics to antivirals. Antiviral Res 2011;90(2):102–14.
71. Gowen BB, Hickerson BT. Hemorrhagic fever of bunyavirus etiology: disease models and progress towards new therapies. J Microbiol 2017;55(3):183–95.
72. Li P, Tong Z-D, Li K-F, et al. Seroprevalence of severe fever with thrombocytopenia syndrome virus in China: a systematic review and meta-analysis. PLoS One 2017;12(4):e0175592.
73. Mansfield KL, Banyard AC, McElhinney L, et al. Rift Valley fever virus: a review of diagnosis and vaccination, and implications for emergence in Europe. Vaccine 2015;33(42):5520–31.
74. Ferron F, Li Z, Danek EI, et al. The hexamer structure of Rift Valley fever virus nucleoprotein suggests a mechanism for its assembly into ribonucleoprotein complexes. PLoS Pathog 2011;7(5):e1002030.
75. Linthicum KJ, Britch SC, Anyamba A. Rift Valley fever: an emerging Mosquito-Borne disease. Annu Rev Entomol 2016;61:395–415.
76. Linthicum KJ, Davies FG, Kairo A, et al. Rift Valley fever virus (family Bunyaviridae, genus Phlebovirus). Isolations from Diptera collected during an interepizootic period in Kenya. J Hyg (Lond) 1985;95(1):197–209.
77. Hartman A. Rift Valley fever. Clin Lab Med 2017;37(2):285–301.
78. Al-Hamdan NA, Panackal AA, Al Bassam TH, et al. The risk of nosocomial transmission of Rift Valley fever. PLoS Negl Trop Dis 2015;9(12):e0004314.
79. McMillen CM, Hartman AL. Rift Valley fever in animals and humans: current perspectives. Antiviral Res 2018;156:29–37.
80. Jansen van Vuren P, Shalekoff S, Grobbelaar AA, et al. Serum levels of inflammatory cytokines in Rift Valley fever patients are indicative of severe disease. Virol J 2015;12:159.
81. Al-Hazmi A, Al-Rajhi AA, Abboud EB, et al. Ocular complications of Rift Valley fever outbreak in Saudi Arabia. Ophthalmology 2005;112(2):313–8.
82. Madani TA, Al-Mazrou YY, Al-Jeffri MH, et al. Rift Valley fever epidemic in Saudi Arabia: epidemiological, clinical, and laboratory characteristics. Clin Infect Dis 2003;37(8):1084–92.
83. Mourya DT, Yadav PD, Shete AM, et al. Detection, isolation and confirmation of Crimean-Congo hemorrhagic fever virus in human, ticks and animals in Ahmadabad, India, 2010-2011. PLoS Negl Trop Dis 2012;6(5):e1653.
84. Leblebicioglu H. Crimean-Congo haemorrhagic fever in Eurasia. Int J Antimicrob Agents 2010;36(Suppl 1):S43–6.
85. Negredo A, de la Calle-Prieto F, Palencia-Herrejón E, et al. Autochthonous Crimean-Congo Hemorrhagic Fever in Spain. N Engl J Med 2017;377(2):154–61.
86. ProMED-mail. Available at: https://www.promedmail.org/index.php. Accessed May 22, 2019.
87. Leblebicioglu H, Sunbul M, Guner R, et al. Healthcare-associated Crimean-Congo haemorrhagic fever in Turkey, 2002-2014: a multicentre retrospective cross-sectional study. Clin Microbiol Infect 2016;22(4):387.e1-4.
88. Schnittler H-J, Feldmann H. Viral hemorrhagic fever–a vascular disease? Thromb Haemost 2003;89(6):967–72.
89. Ergönül O. Crimean-Congo haemorrhagic fever. Lancet Infect Dis 2006;6(4):203–14.
90. Drosten C, Kümmerer BM, Schmitz H, et al. Molecular diagnostics of viral hemorrhagic fevers. Antiviral Res 2003;57(1–2):61–87.

91. Flick R, Whitehouse CA. Crimean-Congo hemorrhagic fever virus. Curr Mol Med 2005;5(8):753–60.
92. Bartolini B, Gruber CE, Koopmans M, et al. Laboratory management of Crimean-Congo haemorrhagic fever virus infections: perspectives from two European networks. Euro Surveill 2019;24(5). https://doi.org/10.2807/1560-7917. ES.2019.24.5.1800093.
93. Watts DM, Ussery MA, Nash D, et al. Inhibition of Crimean-Congo hemorrhagic fever viral infectivity yields in vitro by ribavirin. Am J Trop Med Hyg 1989;41(5): 581–5.
94. Tignor GH, Hanham CA. Ribavirin efficacy in an in vivo model of Crimean-Congo hemorrhagic fever virus (CCHF) infection. Antiviral Res 1993;22(4):309–25.
95. Koksal I, Yilmaz G, Aksoy F, et al. The efficacy of ribavirin in the treatment of Crimean-Congo hemorrhagic fever in Eastern Black Sea region in Turkey. J Clin Virol 2010;47(1):65–8.
96. Macneil A, Nichol ST, Spiropoulou CF. Hantavirus pulmonary syndrome. Virus Res 2011;162(1–2):138–47.
97. Manigold T, Vial P. Human hantavirus infections: epidemiology, clinical features, pathogenesis and immunology. Swiss Med Wkly 2014;144:w13937.
98. Kruger DH, Figueiredo LTM, Song J-W, et al. Hantaviruses–globally emerging pathogens. J Clin Virol 2015;64:128–36.
99. Jiang H, Zheng X, Wang L, et al. Hantavirus infection: a global zoonotic challenge. Virol Sin 2017;32(1):32–43.
100. Hardestam J, Simon M, Hedlund KO, et al. Ex vivo stability of the rodent-borne Hantaan virus in comparison to that of arthropod-borne members of the Bunyaviridae family. Appl Environ Microbiol 2007;73(8):2547–51.
101. Jiang H, Du H, Wang LM, et al. Hemorrhagic fever with renal syndrome: pathogenesis and clinical picture. Front Cell Infect Microbiol 2016;6:1.
102. Prescott J, Safronetz D, Haddock E, et al. The adaptive immune response does not influence hantavirus disease or persistence in the Syrian hamster. Immunology 2013;140(2):168–78.
103. Mori M, Rothman AL, Kurane I, et al. High levels of cytokine-producing cells in the lung tissues of patients with fatal hantavirus pulmonary syndrome. J Infect Dis 1999;179(2):295–302.
104. Borges AA, Donadi EA, Campos GM, et al. Polymorphisms in human leukocyte antigens, human platelet antigens, and cytokine genes in hantavirus cardiopulmonary syndrome patients from Ribeirão Preto, Brazil. J Med Virol 2014;86(11): 1962–70.
105. Vial PA, Valdivieso F, Mertz G, et al. Incubation period of hantavirus cardiopulmonary syndrome. Emerg Infect Dis 2006;12(8):1271–3.
106. Mattar S, Guzmán C, Figueiredo LT. Diagnosis of hantavirus infection in humans. Expert Rev Anti Infect Ther 2015;13(8):939–46.
107. Huggins JW, Hsiang CM, Cosgriff TM, et al. Prospective, double-blind, concurrent, placebo-controlled clinical trial of intravenous ribavirin therapy of hemorrhagic fever with renal syndrome. J Infect Dis 1991;164(6):1119–27.
108. Mertz GJ, Miedzinski L, Goade D, et al. Placebo-controlled, double-blind trial of intravenous ribavirin for the treatment of hantavirus cardiopulmonary syndrome in North America. Clin Infect Dis 2004;39(9):1307–13.
109. Hjelle B. Vaccines against hantaviruses. Expert Rev Vaccines 2002;1(3):373–84.

Chikungunya

Epidemiology, Pathogenesis, Clinical Features, Management, and Prevention

Francesco Vairo, MD[a],*, Najmul Haider, Vet PhD[b],
Richard Kock, MA, VetMB, Vet MD, MRCVS[b], Francine Ntoumi, PhD, FRCP[c,d,e],
Giuseppe Ippolito, MD, MSc, FRCP[a],
Alimuddin Zumla, MBChB, MSc, PhD, MD, FRCP(Lond), FRCP(Edin), FRCPath(UK), FAAS[f]

KEYWORDS

- Chikungunya • Arbovirus • Epidemic • Diagnosis, prevention, and treatment
- Zoonoses • Mosquito • *Aedes* spp

KEY POINTS

- Chikungunya (CHIK) is a disabling and debilitating zoonotic disease of humans caused by the Chikungunya virus (CHIKV); it is transmitted by infected *Aedes* spp mosquitoes, which sustain sylvatic and human rural and urban CHIK cycles.
- Chikungunya is listed on the WHO Blueprint priority pathogens because in the past 5 years an alarming and unprecedented increase in spread to over 100 countries across Asia, Africa, Europe, and the Americas.
- The incubation period of between 1 and 12 days is followed by symptoms similar to dengue, Zika, parvovirus, enterovirus, malaria, with an abrupt onset of high fever, nausea, polyarthralgia, myalgia, widespread skin rash, and conjunctivitis.
- Serious complications include myocarditis, uveitis, retinitis, hepatitis, acute renal disease, severe bullous lesions, meningoencephalitis, Guillain-Barré syndrome, myelitis, and cranial nerve palsies. Severe disease occurs in neonates exposed during pregnancy, the elderly, and those with comorbid diabetes, renal, liver, and heart disease.
- Treatment is supportive and there is no specific antiviral treatment and no effective vaccines.

Disclosure: See last page of article.
[a] National Institute for Infectious Diseases, "Lazzaro Spallanzani"Istituto di ricovero e cura a carattere scientifico - IRCCS, Via Portuense 292, 00149, Rome, Italy; [b] The Royal Veterinary College, University of London, Hawkshead Lane, North Mymms, Hatfield, Hertfordshire AL9 7TA, UK; [c] Fondation Congolaise pour la Recherche Médicale (FCRM), Brazzaville, Congo; [d] Faculty of Sciences and Techniques, University Marien Ngouabi, PO Box 69, Brazzaville, Congo; [e] Institute for Tropical Medicine, University of Tübingen, Wilhelmstraße 27 72074, Tübingen, Germany; [f] Center for Clinical Microbiology, University College London, Royal Free Campus 2nd Floor, Rowland Hill Street, London NW3 2PF, United Kingdom
* Corresponding author.
E-mail address: francesco.vairo@inmi.it

Infect Dis Clin N Am 33 (2019) 1003–1025
https://doi.org/10.1016/j.idc.2019.08.006
0891-5520/19/© 2019 Elsevier Inc. All rights reserved.

id.theclinics.com

INTRODUCTION

Chikungunya (CHIK) is a disabling and debilitating zoonotic disease of humans caused by the Chikungunya virus (CHIKV), which is transmitted by CHIKV-infected *Aedes* spp mosquitoes (**Fig 1**). The primary CHIKV reservoir hosts are nonhuman primates.[1] Chikungunya is listed on the WHO Blueprint priority pathogens (https://www.who.int/blueprint/en/) because in the past 5 years, an alarming and unprecedented increase in spread has occurred with cases reported from more than 100 countries across the Americas, Africa, Europe, and Asia, affecting millions of people (**Fig. 2**).

HISTORICAL

CHIKV most likely originated in East and central Africa where the virus is endemic to a sylvatic cycle between mosquitoes and nonhuman primates living in forests. In 1952, CHIK was described during an outbreak on the Makonde plateau in southern Tanzania on the border with Mozambique.[2] CHIKV was isolated from the serum of a febrile patient during an outbreak of an exanthematous febrile disease. Soon after in 1953, CHIKV was isolated in mosquitoes of the *Aedes aegypti* (*Ae aegypti*), and the virus was placed in arbovirus group A.[3] There are remarkable similarities between the clinical syndromes caused by dengue virus and CHIKV.[4] Before the discovery of CHIKV, cases were mostly diagnosed and treated as malaria or dengue. The actual name Chikungunya is derived from the Makonde tribe (Kimakonde language) meaning "that which bends up" or "to become contorted," which describes the stooped bent posture of patients with CHIKV who develop joint pain (Virusnet.com). The virus is maintained in a complex sylvatic and rural cycle, progressing to an urban cycle every 5 to 20 years, causing global pandemics (**Fig. 3**). Following discovery of CHIK in Tanzania, it was identified in Uganda and subsequently in many other sub-Saharan African countries[5] with global spread in the ensuing years (see **Fig. 2**). These CHIKV strains were grouped in a single lineage and named after the geographic location as East, Central and South Africa (ECSA) CHIKV lineage. A different monophyletic group was identified during outbreaks in Asia from 1958 to 1973 and called Asian CHIKV lineage.[6,7] These different geographic genotypes exhibit differences in their transmission cycles. In Asia, the CHIKV seems to be maintained in an urban cycle with *Ae aegypti* mosquito vectors, whereas CHIKV transmission in Africa involves a sylvatic cycle, primarily with *Ae furcifer* and *Ae africanus* mosquitoes. A distinct CHIKV clade, the West Africa lineage, was isolated from West Africa, and this

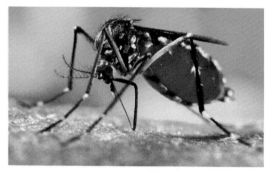

Fig. 1. Mosquito vector of CHIKV: female *Aedes aegypti* mosquito. A close-up lateral view of the female *Aedes aegypti* mosquito from a left lateral perspective, feeding on the human host with distended abdomen filled with host blood. (*Courtesy of* US-CDC, Public Health Image Library (PHIL) https://phil.cdc.gov/Details.aspx?pid=9260.)

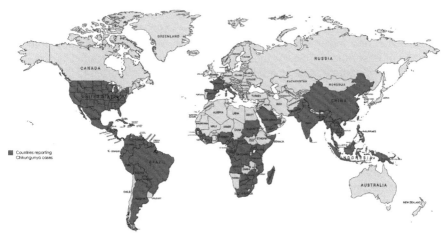

Fig. 2. World map showing countries and territories reporting CHIKV. (*Data from* The Centers for Disease Control: https://www.cdc.gov/chikungunya/geo/index.html.)

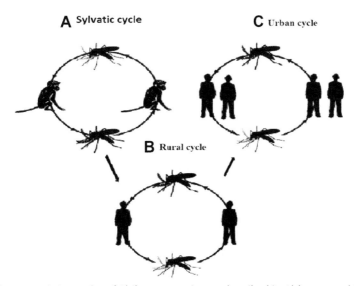

Fig. 3. The transmission cycles of Chikungunya virus as described in Althouse et al (2018). A) The sylvatic cycles of Chikungunya virus exists primarily in Africa between non-human primates, rodents and possibly in bats and forest-dwelling *Aedes species* (*Ae. albopictus, Ae. furcifer, Ae africanus, Ae. taylori*). B) The rural transmission occur when rural population bitten by infected forest-dwelling mosquitoes, especially by *Ae albopictus*. C) Movement of infected humans can result in establishment of a large urban transmission through urban *Aedes mosquitoes* (*Ae. aegypti and Ae. albopictus*), where a human-mosquito-human cycle is established. *Ae. albopictus* feeds on a range of hosts including humans and wild mammals whereas *Ae. aegypti* primarily feeds on human, and most forest dwelling *Aedes species* (*Ae. furcifer, Ae africanus, Ae. taylori*) feeds primarily on animals. (*Date from* Althouse, B. M. *et al*. Role of monkeys in the sylvatic cycle of chikungunya virus in Senegal. *Nat. Commun.* (2018); and adapted from Petersen, L. R., Stramer, S. L. & Powers, A. M. Chikungunya Virus: Possible Impact on Transfusion Medicine. *Transfus. Med. Rev.* (2010); with permission.)

has been circulating in the past 30 years. The 2 major enzootic CHIKV lineages in Africa were introduced from eastern Africa into Asia between 1920 and 1950. The more recent Indian Ocean and Indian epidemic CHIKV strains emerged independently from the mainland of East Africa.[8] This lineage has been called the Indian Ocean Lineage (IOL) and has been repeatedly associated with outbreaks from 2005 to 2014.[8,9]

EPIDEMIOLOGY
The Chikungunya Virus

Phylogenetic analysis has shown 4 different genotypes of CHIKV based on geographic regions: the west African genotype (Senegal and Nigeria), the ECSA genotype, the Asian genotype, and the IOL genotype.[4,6,7,10] CHIKV is an enveloped, spherical, single-stranded positive-sense RNA alphavirus belonging to the family Togaviridae. It has a genome size of ~12 kb, and it consists of 2 open reading frames cleaved into 4 nonstructural proteins (nsP1, nsP2, nsP3, and nsP4)[11] and 5 structural proteins (C, E3, E2, 6K, and E1).[12] E1 and E2 are surface glycoproteins, 439 and 423 amino acids long, respectively.[13] E1 and E2 carry the major viral epitopes and participate in the attachment and the entry of the virus into target cells, where E2 is responsible for receptor binding and E1 for membrane fusion.[14] E3 consists of 64 amino acids that are required for E3-E2-6K-E1 or E3-E2-TF polyprotein translocation into the endoplasmic reticulum for virus spike formation.[15] The 6K protein is a cation-selective ion channel that causes increased cell permeability to monovalent cations and virion budding during infection.[16] Transframe protein TF is produced as a result of C-terminal extension of 6K protein in the −1 frame.[17] It retains ion-channel activity similar to that of 6K and seems to be important for assembly and release of the virus particle.[17] Although the nonstructural proteins nsP1-nsP4 are primarily associated with the viral replication process,[18,19] they have additional functions during the viral infection, just like in other alphaviruses.[20] Nonstructural proteins are not packaged into the final virions, and hence the structural proteins (mainly surface glycoproteins E2 and E1) are the key targets of the host humoral immune response and of most CHIK vaccines.[21]

Global Distribution, Transmission, and Chikungunya Virus Outbreaks

Human cases of CHIK have been reported from all continents affecting males and females of all age groups. The CHIKV circulates between mosquitoes and naive human hosts in cyclical form similar to dengue viruses. Until 5 years ago, most CHIK cases were reported from Africa, Asia, Europe, and the Indian and Pacific Oceans. International travel led to the spread of CHIKV to Europe and focused global attention.[22] The first local transmission of CHIKV in the Americas was identified in Caribbean countries and territories in 2013 and subsequently spread rapidly throughout the Americas[23] (see **Fig. 2**). To date, human cases of CHIK have been found in more than 100 countries (**Table 1**).

Large outbreaks were reported in Comoros in 2005 with approximately 215,000 cases[24] and in Reunion Island between March 2005 and April 2006 with 255,000 cases.[25] The spread of CHIKV to the islands of the Indian Ocean, India, and Southeast Asia after a large outbreak in Kenya in 2004 has been a key factor in focusing global attention. Selected outbreaks in various countries are listed in **Table 2**. CHIKV subsequently spread beyond its original tropical locations in Africa and the Indian subcontinent, becoming a serious emerging issue in temperate regions of Europe and the Americas with autochthonous small outbreaks occurring as a consequence of spillover from endemic tropical areas in continental Europe: Italy in 2007, and in France in 2010, in 2014, and 2017.[26–29] In 2017, a major outbreak in Italy was concentrated

Table 1
Countries where CHIKV human infections have been reported

Continent	Country	
Africa	• Angola • Benin • Burundi • Cameroon • Central African Republic • Comoros • Cote d'Ivoire • Democratic Republic of the Congo • Djibouti • Equatorial Guinea • Gabon • Guinea • Kenya • Madagascar • Malawi	• Mauritius • Mayotte • Mozambique • Nigeria • Republic of the Congo • Reunion • Senegal • Seychelles • Sierra Leone • South Africa • Somalia • Sudan • Tanzania • Uganda • Zimbabwe
Asia	• Bangladesh • Bhutan • Cambodia • China • India • Indonesia • Laos • Malaysia • Maldives • Myanmar (Burma)	• Nepal • Pakistan • Philippines • Saudi Arabia • Singapore • Sri Lanka • Thailand • Timor-Leste • Vietnam • Yemen
Europe	• France • Italy • Spain	
Americas	• Anguilla • Antigua and Barbuda • Argentina • Aruba • Bahamas • Barbados • Belize • Bolivia • Brazil • British Virgin Islands • Cayman Islands • Colombia • Costa Rica • Cuba • Curacao • Dominica • Dominican Republic • Ecuador • El Salvador • French Guiana • Grenada • Guadeloupe • Guatemala • Guyana	• Haiti • Honduras Jamaica • Martinique • Mexico • Montserrat • Nicaragua • Panama • Paraguay • Peru • Puerto Rico • Saint Barthelemy • Saint Kitts and Nevis • Saint Lucia • Saint Martin • Saint Vincent and the Grenadines • Sint Maarten • Suriname • Trinidad and Tobago • Turks and Caicos Islands • Venezuela • United States • US Virgin Islands

(continued on next page)

Table 1 (continued)		
Continent	**Country**	
Oceania/Pacific Islands	• American Samoa • Cook Islands • Federal States of Micronesia • Fiji • French Polynesia • Kiribati	• Marshall Islands • New Caledonia • Papua New Guinea • Samoa • Tokelau • Tonga

(*Courtesy of* The Centers for Disease Control: https://www.cdc.gov/chikungunya/geo/index.html.)

around 3 main foci (Anzio, Rome, Guardavalle Marina) in 2 different regions, Lazio (Anzio, Rome) and Calabria (Guardavalle Marina), in Central and Southern Italy.[30] Phylogenetic analysis showed that the CHIKV from the Lazio outbreak belonged to the ECSA clade and clusters within the IOL.[31]

In Africa, CHIKV epidemics have been reported from Central African Republic, Guinea, Burundi, Angola, Uganda, Malawi, Nigeria, Democratic Republic of the Congo, South Africa, and Nigeria. In June 2004 in an outbreak that occurred in Lamu Atoll, Kenya, and spread to Mauritius, Seychelles, Comoros, and Reunion Island, almost half a million cases were reported. Several other epidemics occurred in all southwestern Indian Ocean islands except Madagascar from 2005 to 2007. In 2011, a CHIKV epidemic occurred in the Democratic Republic of the Congo (317 cases), Pool (460 cases), and Brazzaville (7014 cases).

Table 2 Major global outbreaks of CHIKV	
Year	**Country**
1954	United Republic of Tanzania
1999–2000	Democratic Republic of Congo
2005 to date	Islands of the Indian Ocean Maldives India Myanmar Thailand
2006–2007	India
2007	Gabon
2007	Italy
2011	Republic of Congo
2013	France
2014	Pacific Islands (Cook, Marshall, and others)
2015	Americas
2016	Pakistan
2017	Italy
2017	Kenya
2019	Republic of Congo
2019	Democratic Republic of Congo

Mosquito Vectors

In Africa, CHIKV circulates in an enzootic cycle between forest-dwelling *Aedes* spp mosquitoes (*Ae furcifer*, *Ae taylori*, *Ae africanus*, *Ae luteocephalus*) and is maintained in nonhuman primates and other vertebrate reservoirs such as rodents and bats (see **Figs. 1** and **3**).[1,32,33] The primary CHIKV reservoir hosts are nonhuman primates, and the 5- to 10-year periodicity of CHIKV transmission may depend on oscillations in monkey herd immunity.[1] In Senegal, enzootic strains of CHIKV have been isolated from diverse species of mosquito including *Ae (Diceromyia) furcifer*, *Ae (Diceromyia) taylori*, *Ae (Stegomyia) luteocephalus*, *Ae (Stegomyia) africanus*, and *Ae (Stegomyia) neoafricanus*.[1] Sporadic spillover of enzootic CHIKV into urban interhuman transmission cycles is amplified by the involvement of anthropophilic mosquito species such as *Ae (Stegomyia) aegypti* and *Ae (Stegomyia) albopictus*.[34]

The behavior and ecology of *Ae aegypti* makes it an ideal vector during epidemic cycles because of its anthropophilic nature. Moreover, adult females often take several blood meals during a single gonotrophic cycle, and artificial containers are preferred larval sites.[35] *Ae albopictus* mosquitoes are both zoophilic and anthropophilic and are active throughout the day. In Asia, CHIKV is maintained in an urban transmission cycle vectored by the mosquito *Ae aegypti* and *Ae albopictus*.[8]. *Ae albopictus*, the Asian tiger mosquito, was discovered in 1894 in India and is endemic to Southeast Asia. *Ae albopictus* mosquitoes have successfully colonized all 5 continents throughout both temperate and tropical regions.[36] It has successfully spread because of its ability to thrive in arid and cold conditions, undergo periods of adult diapause, and overwinter by laying desiccation-resistant eggs. Although these mosquitoes do not have a specific ecological niche, distinct temperate and tropical populations have arisen. CHIKV circulation typically coincides with periods of heavy rains and increased density of mosquito.[37] The urbanization and human migration from rural to urban areas has led to the introduction of *Ae aegypti* and *Ae albopictus* living around human habitations, sustaining CHIKV transmission in a mosquito-human cycle.

Chikungunya Virus Mutations and Infectivity

The E1-A226V mutation has resulted in a dramatic increase in the infectivity of CHIKV, and the transmission of CHIKV has spread to Europe and the Americas facilitated by widespread distribution of the *Aedes* spp vectors. The nonsynonymous mutation in the E1 glycoprotein of the viral envelope (E1-A226V) was identified in 90% of isolates during the outbreak in Reunion Island in 2006.[38] This mutation is important for viral fitness in *Ae albopictus*, although the mutation does not affect viral replication in *Ae aegypti*.[39,40] This adapted variant was involved in outbreaks in north-eastern Italy in 2007 and in south-eastern France in 2014 and 2017, where *Ae albopictus* is widespread.[27,41,42] Thus, although *Ae aegypti* was widely recognized as the main urban vector of CHIKV in tropical areas, *Ae albopictus* is considered able to transmit CHIKV in temperate climate areas too. Mosquito studies highlighted the role of *Ae albopictus* as a CHIKV vector during the European outbreaks [26, 27], and experimental infection confirmed a high susceptibility of local European *Ae albopictus* populations to the mutated ECSA CHIKV strain. Other less widespread mutations are believed to increase initial infection in *Ae albopictus* midgut cells, all of them in the IOL lineage. E2-K252Q, E2-K233E, E2/E3-R198Q/S18F, and E2-L210Q affect the initial infection of the *Ae albopictus* midgut cells with major effects on infection of *Ae aegypti*.[43] The same mutations are predicted to affect CHIKV Asian lineages circulating in the

Americas as a result of a so-called founder effect and resultant epistasis. The amino acid mutation A98T in E1 protein in the Asian lineage prevents penetrance for *Ae albopictus* infection.[8,44]

MODES OF CHIKUNGUNYA VIRUS TRANSMISSION

There are several ways in which CHIKV is acquired by humans.[45]

CHIKV is transmitted to people through bites from *Ae aegypti*, *Ae albopictus*, and *Ae polynesienses* mosquitoes, the same mosquitoes that transmit the dengue virus. These mosquitoes breed in or near human habitations and prefer to feed on humans during the daytime in shady areas and early in the evening. Horizontal transmission in *Aedes* spp can occur and contribute to the maintenance of CHIKV cycles.[46] Vertical transmission is rare but has been observed under natural and experimental conditions.[47–49] In Africa, CHIKV circulates primarily in an enzootic cycle, with occasional spillover infections of humans.

Coinfection with dengue virus and CHIKV,[50] and CHIKV with dengue virus, Zika virus, yellow fever virus, and West Nile virus have been described.[51]

Iatrogenic Transmission

To date, no studies on transfusion-transmitted CHIKF from viremic donors to recipients has been published. There is increasing concern that CHIKV might be transmitted by way of transfusions given its high-level viremia attack rate during outbreaks and a significant proportion of asymptomatic infections. Viremic asymptomatic[52] CHIKV-infected cases have shown high potential as disseminators of transfusion-associated CHIKF, because CHIKV levels capable of inducing CHIKF were found in the blood of asymptomatic cases during the 2009 epidemic in Songkhla, Thailand.[52] As with other arboviruses, several factors determine the impact of CHIKV on transfusion medicine: (1) prevalence of viremia among blood donors, (2) proportion of components derived from viremic donations that transmit infection to recipients, (3) clinical impact on infected transfusion recipients, (4) availability of measures to reduce transfusion transmission when required, and (5) the cost and disruption incurred by those measures. Several models have been applied to estimate the risk of transfusion-associated HIKV transmission. Model results from Reunion Island[53] and Thailand[52] indicate a significant short-term risk of transfusion-associated CHIKV transmission during large outbreaks, whereas the Italian model suggests a small, but quantifiable risk that may exceed accepted safety standards during smaller, focal outbreaks[54] that may occur in temperate areas.

Few cases of CHIKV infection in solid-organ transplant (SOT) recipients have been reported.[55–57] In a case series from Brazil, 13 SOT recipients (9 kidney, 4 liver) infected with CHIKV showed similar clinical presentation to immunocompetent hosts, including chronic joint symptoms in 46%. However, there were no complications or deaths, and these transplant patients experienced no apparent damage to the graft. In addition, infectious CHIKV can be isolated from corneal grafts from both symptomatic and asymptomatic donors, although no cases transmitted by corneal transplant have been reported to date.[58] SOT recipients who travel to or live in CHIKV endemic areas are at high risk of acquiring the disease.

Maternal-fetal transmission has been reported. Intrapartum contamination without actual placental infection has been well documented for CHIKV virus, which is not able to infect the placenta.[59,60] CHIKV is not transmitted to the fetus in the absence of placental breaches, which allow transfer of maternal blood to the fetal circulation.[59] A recent meta-analysis[61] estimated a pooled mother-to-child transmission risk across the analyzed cohorts of 15.5%, with the highest risk among infections in the intrapartum period (+2 days from delivery). During intrapartum viremia, the vertical transmission rate of CHIKV is reported as 48.7%. Mothers who have a high viral load in their placenta are more likely to transmit the virus.[59] There is no evidence of CHIKV transmission by way of breast milk to infants.[62]

CHIKV has been detected in semen 30 days after symptom's onset,[63] indicating possible sexual transmission. No evidence of sexual transmission between humans has been reported so far.

PATHOGENESIS

During the first week of infection, CHIKV can be found in the blood and can be passed from an infected person to a mosquito through mosquito bites. CHIKV has certain cell types that are particularly susceptible to infection; these include human epithelial and endothelial cells, primary fibroblasts, and monocyte-derived macrophages.[64] Lymphoid and monocytoid cells, primary lymphocytes and monocytes, and monocyte-derived dendritic cells did not demonstrate CHIKV replication.[65] The human skin is the first site of viral replication, mainly in the dermal fibroblasts. From here, the virus enters the lymph nodes and the circulatory system, disseminating to all organs.[66] During the acute and subacute phases, CHIKV reaches muscle and joint compartments: primary muscle fibroblasts and skeletal muscle fibroblasts, and both have been found to be permissive.[60,67]

Chikungunya clinical syndrome is characterized by arthralgia, which is usually symmetric and affects distal synovial joints more than proximal joints.[68] In patients, during acute and persistent arthralgia CHIKV RNA and proteins have been found in synovial tissue and fluids, with synovial fibroblasts and macrophages susceptible to the infection.[60,68,69] Infected macrophages are the preferred site for viral replication, contributing to viral persistence and chronic symptoms.[68] The presence of increased levels of cartilage bioproducts in urine[70] and low plasma levels of hepatocyte growth factor in chronic patients[71] indicate connective tissue alterations and cartilage damage. CHIKV replicates actively and persists in the osteoblasts.[69,72] Bone loss is a characteristic of CHIK-associated arthritis. The pathogenesis of persistent symptoms after CHIK infection is still unclear. CHIKV proteins have been detected in macrophages and muscle cells of patients with relapse of chronic pain, suggesting that low replicative viruses or nonreplicative CHIKV debris may persist. A persistent immune activation has been detected in mouse models.[73,74] Immune and inflammatory responses to CHIKV infection may also contribute to pathogenesis.[75,76]

Neurologic manifestations have often been reported in several outbreaks, with an increasing number of cases with neurologic complications after the reemergence of CHIKV in the Indian Ocean in 2005. The virus has frequently been isolated from cerebrospinal fluid (CSF).[77] The target cells for CHIKV in the human brain remain unknown. In vitro infection of human cells have demonstrated the susceptibility of neuroblastoma cells,[78] microglial cells,[79] and glial cells, such as astrocytes,[80] showing signs of apoptosis. Nevertheless, it is still unclear if the pathogenesis of the nervous system is directly connected with the infection of the neurons and glial cells or is indirectly connected triggering the immune-mediated effects.

CLINICAL FEATURES
Incubation Period

The incubation period can vary from 1 to 12 days (average, 2–7 days). CHIKV infection causes high levels of viremia, which usually last for 4 to 6 days after the onset of symptoms. CHIKV infection is symptomatic in most children and adults who are infected, with less than 15% having asymptomatic sero-conversion.[53]

Symptoms

The symptoms (**Table 3**) are similar to those of other arboviruses, such as dengue and other common causes of febrile illnesses in the tropics; thus, accurate diagnosis is challenging.

During the acute phase of illness, the intensity of the clinical symptoms correlates with the viremia during the acute infection, usually lasting 1 week when anti-CHIKV IgM antibodies appear.[81] Following the onset of fever, intense myalgia and arthralgia occur. These symptoms can be severe and disabling, causing much morbidity.

Table 3 Clinical features of Chikungunya: symptoms and signs	
Stage	**Signs and Symptoms**

Acute stage	Common
	   Fever
	   Macular to maculopapular rash
	   edema of the face and extremities
	   Benign bleeding (gingival bleeding, epistaxis) in children
	   Pruritus
	   Myalgia
	   Arthralgia
	   Periorbital pain
	   Headache
	   Lymphadenopathy
	Less common
	   Diarrhea, vomiting, abdominal pain
	   Confusion
	   Optical neuritis
	   Oral or gingival ulceration
	   Conjunctivitis

Post-acute stage	Inflammatory arthralgia, joint stiffness Arthritis (synovitis with or without effusion) Tenosynovitis, bursitis Decompensation of pre-existing degenerative or traumatic arthropathy Osteoarthritis or sometimes-calcific tendinitis Entrapment syndromes Neuropathic pain Severe asthenia Neuropsychological disorders
Chronic stage	Joints: articular arthritis, synovitis, degenerative osteoarthritis, bursitis Tendons: tendinitis, enthesitis, tenosynovitis Edema Neuropathic pain Stiffness Loss of physical fitness Postural hypotension Mood disorders

Disabling polyarthralgia is a key symptom for differential diagnosis with a positive predictive value greater than 80%.[82] The joint pain is usually symmetric in both the arms and legs; the large joints are almost invariably symptomatic. Other common signs are nausea, fatigue, headache, back pain, and skin rash (50% of cases). The skin lesions are characterized by a macular or maculopapular transitory eruption often in the body extremities, palms, soles of the feed, torso, and face.[81,83] Gastrointestinal tract involvement can manifest as nausea, vomiting, and abdominal pain.[84] Ocular manifestations can occur during the acute phase with photophobia, retro-orbital pain, and conjunctivitis.[85]

The acute phase is usually followed by a post-acute stage, usually from the fourth week to the end of the third month.[86] This phase is characterized by persistence of the initial inflammatory events, including inflammatory arthralgia, arthritis (synovitis with or without effusion), tenosynovitis, bursitis, which slowly regress. It is often associated with decompensation of pre-existing degenerative or traumatic arthropathy (sometimes unknown) such as osteoarthritis or calcific tendinitis, and local events such as reactionary edema, entrapment syndromes, joint stiffness, or neuropathic pain.

The chronic stage (after the third month) is defined by the absence of return to pre-existing condition more than 3 months after the onset of CHIK. The chronic phase can last a few months to several years (more than 6 years for a small group of patients in Reunion Island). The observed clinical symptoms are the same as in the post-acute stage. It is common to observe painful rebounds on joints used too strongly considering their post-CHIK inflammatory condition. The diagnostic approach is to qualify the nosology of each patient according to the presence or absence of inflammatory symptoms (arthritis, enthesitis, tenosynovitis, inflammatory arthralgia) and the number of joints involved (polyarticular if ≥ 4 joints).

In infected newborns, symptoms generally develop on days 3 to 7 of life with fever, rash, and peripheral edema. Pathology typically reveals a bicytopenia, increased prothrombin time, and aspartate aminotransferase level. The presentation in infants is subsequently complicated by seizures, hemorrhagic syndrome, hemodynamic disorders, and myocardial dysfunction.[59,87] Neonatal symptoms range from mild presentation (43%) to severe infection with encephalitis (53%)[59] that requires intensive care. Fever and acute respiratory distress have also been reported.[88] Neurologic complications can have severe effects on postnatal neurologic development, such as lower development quotient at age of 2 years, and moderate to severe global neurodevelopmental delay.[89]

Atypical Features and Complications

Complications of the cardiovascular, renal, respiratory, hepatic gastrointestinal, and adrenal systems are associated with the infection and referred to as atypical features (**Table 4**). As reported during the Reunion Island outbreak in 2005, the proportion of atypical cases was 0.3%. Atypical cases were defined as patients with clinical presentation of fever, arthralgia, and other atypical signs. The median age of the cases was 70 years. Of the 610 atypical cases, 546 (89%) had underlying medical conditions, 479 (78%) were on medication before hospitalization. However, the involvement of the central nervous system is the most common complication of CHIK infection. Neurologic disease after CHIKV infection was first reported during an outbreak in 1964 in Madras, India.[90] In 2 studies investigating manifestations of CHIKV in patients requiring intensive care, a neurologic disorder was the primary issue in 61%[91] and 79%.[92] Given the large spectrum of neurologic disease and scarce epidemiologic data, estimating the incidence of neurologic disease among all systemically

Table 4
Clinical features of CHIKV: complications

Organ/System	Complication(s)
Nervous system	Frequent
	Encephalopathy and meningitis
	Myelopathy and myelitis
	Encephalomyelopathy
	Myeloneuropathy
	Encephalomyeloneuropathy
	Guillain-Barré syndrome
	Acute disseminated encephalomyelitis
	Neonatal hypotonia
	Optic neuritis
	Less frequent
	Seizures
	Sensorineural hearing loss
	Stroke
	Cerebellitis
	Third nerve palsy
	Encephalopathy
	Behavioral changes
	Carpal tunnel syndrome
	Bilateral ophthalmoplegia
Cardiovascular system	Heart failure
	Arrhythmias
	Myocarditis/pericarditis
	Blood pressure instability
	Acute myocardial infarction
Ocular	Conjunctivitis, episcleritis, nongranulomatous anterior uveitis, granulomatous anterior uveitis
	Keratitis, retinitis with vitritis, bilateral retinitis
	Multifocal choroiditis, optic neuritis, retrobulbar neuritis
	Exudative retinal detachment, pan-uveitis
Other organ involvement	Pre-renal failure
	Exacerbation of chronic renal failure
	Pneumonia and respiratory failure
	Hepatic insufficiency, subacute hepatitis
	Bullous dermatosis
	Pancreatitis
	Syndrome of inappropriate antidiuretic hormone secretion
	Hypoadrenalism

symptomatic CHIKV infections is difficult. In 1 study from the 2006 Indian outbreak, 18 (4.4%) of 405 suspected cases of CHIKV attending the recruiting hospital over 3 months developed neurologic complications.[90] An epidemiologic study of the 2005 to 2006 Reunion Island outbreak found approximately 0.3% of all CHIKV infections resulted in atypical cases,[93] of which 24.1% of the adults presented with abnormal neurology. Thus, approximately 0.1% (1 case per 1000) of all CHIKV infections developed neurologic disease. It has been observed that severe complications of CHIKV typically arise in patients with comorbidities. Studies from Reunion Island and from India show that underlying diseases play a role in neurologic disorders and other complication but are not an indispensable requisite. Age has been reported as a significant risk factor for severe manifestations in the elderly (>65 years)[90,93] and in infants.[94]

A recent systematic review[77] described the frequency of reported neurologic syndromes and diseases. The most frequent are encephalopathy and encephalitis, myelopathy and myelitis, Guillain-Barré syndrome, acute disseminated encephalomyelitis, neonatal hypotonia, and neuro-ocular disease. Other manifestations are described less frequently, such as behavioral changes, seizure with and without fever, stroke, cerebellitis, meningism, third nerve palsy, encephalopathy, and bilateral total ophthalmoplegia.

Mortality

Although morbidity is debilitating, CHIKV mortality rates are low. As with most viral illnesses, people at a higher risk for more severe disease include the newborn, the elderly, and those with comorbid illnesses such as diabetes, heart disease, chronic liver and kidney disease, and human immunodeficiency virus. An increase in mortality has been observed in the last epidemics, probably as a result of neurologic disorders mainly in neonates, immunocompromised patients, and the elderly.[55,63,95] In Europe, the case fatality rate was 2.5 per 1000 clinical cases,[30] lower than that reported in the 2007 outbreak in Italy (0.5%) but consistent with that reported from Reunion Island (1 death per 1000 clinical cases).[27,96]

LABORATORY DIAGNOSIS

Several laboratory tests are available for diagnosing CHIK using serum or plasma to detect the virus, viral nucleic acid, or virus-specific immunoglobulin (Ig) IgM, and neutralizing antibodies. Given the high viral load during viremia, CHIKV viral RNA can be detected during the first 5 to 8 days of illness using commercial tests with high sensitivity and specificity. The choice between the types of tests is dictated by the timing of the sampling with respect to the beginning of the symptoms and the volume of the samples available.

Serologic Tests

CHIKV IgM antibodies normally develop toward the end of the first week of illness, and to definitively rule out the diagnosis, convalescent-phase samples should be obtained from patients whose acute-phase samples test negative. Serologic diagnosis of CHIK is made by detecting CHIKV-specific IgM in serum samples for 5 to 7 days after symptom onset, or by demonstrating a 4-fold increase (or seroconversion) of CHIK-specific IgG antibody titers in a pair of serum samples at least 15 days apart (acute and convalescent phase of the disease). IgM antibodies specific for CHIKV may persist for up to 1 year, particularly in patients with long-term arthralgia, but typically persist for 3 to 4 months. The specific CHIKV IgG can be detected for many years after initial infection. Serologic cross-reactions and false-positive tests have been reported due to infection with closely related alphaviruses belonging to the Semliki forest virus. An enzyme-linked immunosorbent assay may confirm the presence of IgM and IgG anti-CHIKV antibodies. IgM antibody levels are highest 3 to 5 weeks after the onset of illness and persist for about 2 months. Samples collected during the first week after the onset of symptoms should be tested by both serologic and virologic methods (reverse transcriptase-polymerase chain reaction [RT-PCR]).

Molecular Diagnostic Tests

PCR detection of specific CHIKV RNA can be detected by RT-PCR in serum or plasma/EDTA samples obtained from patients during the acute phase of infection (typically ≤7 days after the onset of symptoms). CHIKV infection causes high levels of viremia, which usually last for 4 to 6 days after the onset of symptoms. This is a favorable situation for diagnosis. Real-time RT-PCR is the ideal test for the diagnosis of CHIKV infections in the acute phase of infection. RT-PCR can typically be performed within the first 7 days of symptom onset to confirm CHIKV infection. The virus may be isolated from the blood during the first few days of infection. Various RT-PCR methods are available but are of variable sensitivity. Some are suited to clinical diagnosis. RT-PCR products from clinical samples may also be used for genotyping of the virus, allowing comparisons with virus samples from various geographic sources.

Viral culture may detect the virus in the first 3 days of illness; however, CHIKV should be handled under biosafety level 3 conditions.

TREATMENT
Supportive Treatment

There is no effective antiviral treatment, and thus treatment of CHIK is supportive and symptomatic. It should be adapted to the clinical context and risk groups aimed at controlling fever and pain, treating dehydration, organ support, and preventing iatrogenic complications and functional impairment. Infection control procedures should be instituted to reduce the risk of iatrogenic infection to health care and laboratory workers.

Analgesics

Analgesia based on acetaminophen therapy is preferred. Using nonsteroidal anti-inflammatory drugs (NSAIDs) and salicylates is not recommended in the 14 days after onset of the disease because of the risk of bleeding complications related to dengue fever unless this diagnosis is ruled out, and Reye syndrome induced by aspirin. Using analgesics (weak opioids) is required if acetaminophen is not effective: tramadol alone or in combination with acetaminophen.

The treatment of the post-acute stage should be based primarily on analgesics (stages 1 and 2), neuropathic drugs, and NSAIDs.

Nonsteroidal Anti-Inflammatory Drugs

No NSAID class has demonstrated superiority of effectiveness on post-CHIK symptoms. A local anti-inflammatory therapy (topical or infiltration) should be prescribed in case of tenosynovitis, bursitis, tunnel syndrome, capsulitis, or synovitis inadequately controlled by oral treatment, to limit the therapeutic excess. The risk of drug toxicity by overdose (self-medication) or drug interaction is high for acetaminophen as well as for other analgesics, anti-inflammatory drugs, long-term treatments, and traditional medicines used for self-medication.[86]

Use of Steroids

The use of corticosteroids is not recommended. Steroids may also cause severe rebound of arthritis and tenosynovitis. Systemic corticosteroids should be used only for inflammatory polyarticular presentations, especially when associated with tenosynovitis, active synovitis, or in case of resistance or contraindication to NSAIDs.

Newer Therapies

Off-label use of other US Food and Drug Administration-approved drugs in a therapeutic manner has been proposed and is under consideration. In animal models of CHIKV infection, prophylaxis with CHIKV IgG or CHIKV-specific monoclonal antibodies was found to be protective,[97] suggesting that antibody-based therapies may be a promising disease prevention strategy for individuals who are at risk for severe

CHIKV infection. In cell-based screens of compounds against CHIKV infection, several drugs with antiviral activity have been identified, some of which target distinct steps in the CHIKV replication cycle. These include chloroquine[98] and chlorpromazine,[99] which affect virus entry. Harringtonine and homoharringtonine[100] have been found to affect viral protein translation. Others, including trigocherriolide A,[101] ribavirin,[102] interferon-alpha,[103] apigenin, and silybin[99] affect virus replication. More extensive preclinical evaluation of these and other identified drugs in animal models of CHIKV disease are necessary before they are proposed for use in humans.

PREVENTION

At present, there is no effective vaccine against CHIKV infection. The proximity of mosquito vector breeding sites to human habitation is a significant risk factor for CHIKV. Prevention and control rely on reducing the number of natural and artificial water-filled container habitats that support breeding of the mosquitoes. This requires mobilization of affected communities.

Vector Control and Breeding Reservoirs

Vector control depends on reducing the number of natural and artificial water-filled container habitats that support breeding of mosquitoes. Accumulation of stagnant water should be prevented. Water in vases should be changed once a week. Using saucers underneath flower pots should be avoided. Water containers should be tightly covered. Air-conditioner drip trays should be free of stagnant water. All used cans and bottles should be placed in covered dustbins. During outbreaks, insecticides may be sprayed to kill flying mosquitoes, applied to surfaces in and around containers where the mosquitoes land, and used to treat water in containers to kill the immature larvae.

Clothing and Insect Repellants

For protection during CHIK outbreaks, clothing that minimizes skin exposure to the day-biting vectors is advised. Repellents can be applied to exposed skin or to clothing in strict accordance with product label instructions. Repellents should contain DEET (N,N-diethyl-3-methylbenzamide), IR3535 (3-[N-acetyl-N-butyl]-aminopropionic acid ethyl ester), or icaridin (1-piperidinecarboxylic acid, 2-(2-hydroxyethyl)-1-methylpropylester). For those who sleep during the daytime, particularly young children, or sick or older people, insecticide-treated mosquito nets afford good protection. Mosquito coils or other insecticide vaporizers may also reduce indoor biting.

Miscellaneous Advice to Travelers

Basic precautions should be taken by people traveling to risk areas, and these include use of repellents, wearing long sleeves and pants, and ensuring rooms are fitted with screens to prevent mosquitoes from entering bedrooms. General measures on preventing mosquito-borne diseases include wearing loose, light-colored, long-sleeved tops and trousers, and use of insect repellent on exposed parts of the body and clothing. Use of fragrant cosmetics or skin care products should be avoided. Clothing, tents, and bed nets should be treated with permethrin (an insecticide). Travelers who return from affected areas and feel unwell, for example, have a fever, should be advised to seek medical advice promptly and provide travel details to the doctor.

Vaccines

After the reemergence of CHIKV in 2004 and its rapid expansion throughout the Indian Ocean and Southeast Asia, and unexpected autochthonous transmission in Europe in

2007 and later in 2017, there has been renewed interest in developing a vaccine against CHIKV. Several approaches have been used for the development of CHIKV vaccines, including noninfectious[104] and infectious DNA vaccines,[105] viruslike particles (VLP), and inactivated virus. Live attenuated vaccines under development include rationally attenuated alphavirus chimeras[106] and deletion mutants[107]; a vesicular stomatitis-vectored vaccine[108]; and an internal ribosome entry site-modified CHIKV strain.[109] To date, 3 CHIKV vaccines have progressed to clinical trials. The strain 181/clone25, developed by the US Army in the 1980s,[110] proved highly immunogenic

Table 5
CHIKV: addressing gaps in knowledge and strengthening public health preparedness

Knowledge Gaps/Needs	Actions Required
Understanding the epidemiology and pathogenesis of CHIKV across geographic settings	Appropriately funded, well-designed longitudinal and cross-sectional clinical, pathogenesis, and epidemiologic studies of sylvatic, rural, and urban cycles (animal and human studies)
The spectrum of the vertebrate intermediate hosts	Evaluate the possibility of endemic circulation of CHIKV by means of virus identification at the human-animal interface
Prevalent mosquito vectors and their behavior	Integrating entomologic and human surveillance
Improved diagnostic, treatment, prognostic, prevention, and surveillance tools	More investments into development and evaluation of: a. Newer, affordable, field-friendly rapid diagnostic tests and sequencing platforms b. New biomarkers of disease progression c. Newer treatments (antivirals, immunotherapies, and host-directed therapies) d. New vaccines
Defining the animal and environmental host reservoirs	Cross-sectional and longitudinal studies at the human-animal interface
Customization of vector control measures adapted to local culture and norms in the context of the population behavior	Close collaboration between medical and social science/anthropologists/animal-human-environmental sectors and local communities
Establish the cocirculation of other arboviruses	Appropriate use of serology and metagenomics analysis during outbreaks
Lack of understanding of factors underlying the pathogenesis of organ involvement and complications; eg, acute and persisting synovial pathology and arthritis; and of maternal-infant transmission and infection rate of newborns	Longitudinal cohort studies during outbreaks
New surveillance tools, early warning systems, and real-time data management	The integration of different surveillance tools and the combination with entomologic surveillance in a One Health dedicated surveillance system should facilitate the detection, response, and control of arboviruses spreading, including CHIKV

but mildly reactogenic in phase 2 trials.[111] A VLP vaccine produced by expression of the CHIKV structural proteins in vertebrate cells demonstrated efficacy in preclinical studies in mice or Rhesus macaques.[112] Phase 1 clinical studies showed strong immunogenicity after 2 to 3 doses. Currently, this vaccine is not licensed to a commercial partner. A CHIKF vaccine in advanced stages of clinical development uses an attenuated measles virus strain as a vector to express the CHIKV structural proteins.[113] In a phase 1 trial, this vaccine was well tolerated and induced neutralizing antibodies in 44% of volunteers receiving a single low dose, 92% receiving a medium dose, and 90% receiving a high dose. A booster raised seroconversion to 100%, and immunogenicity was not affected by pre-existing anti-measles immunity. This vaccine is now in a phase 2 trial.[114]

SUMMARY

Several challenges are involved in the development of tools and strategies for prevention of zoonotic and re-emerging infections with epidemic potential, including CHIK (**Table 5**): early identification of human cases, developing rapid point of care diagnostics, and effective treatments and vaccines. The establishment of more effective collaborative research networks involving different disciplines, such as medical entomologists, virologists, veterinarians, infectious diseases clinicians, social science experts, anthropologists, community leaders, and policymakers, is required to enable more effective definition of host reservoirs, improving outbreak response and control activities. Given the unpredictability and paucity of CHIK and other zoonotic outbreaks, public health response and preparedness should be ready to perform research immediately during an outbreak, allowing for evaluation of existing and newer diagnostics, treatments, and vaccines. These are being addressed through increasing research capacity during interepidemic periods with an integrated One Health (human-environmental-animal health) approach[115,116] to assist in rapid investigations of zoonotic outbreaks and development of local capacity to improve national public health institutions.

DISCLOSURE

All authors have an interest in global public health and emerging and re-emerging infections. All authors are part of the PANDORA-ID-NET Consortium (EDCTP reg/grant RIA2016E-1609) funded by the European and Developing Countries Clinical Trials Partnership (EDCTP2) program, which is supported under Horizon 2020, the European Union's Framework Programme for Research and Innovation. A. Zumla is in receipt of a National Institutes of Health Research (NIHR) senior investigator award. F. Ntoumi and A. Zumla acknowledge support from EDCTP (CANTAM2). F. Vairo and G. Ippolito acknowledge financial support from the Italian Ministry of Health, grants to Ricerca Corrente linea 1 to National Institute for Infectious Diseases, Lazzaro Spallanzani, IRCCS.

REFERENCES

1. Diallo M, Thonnon J, Traore-Lamizana M, et al. Vectors of Chikungunya virus in Senegal: current data and transmission cycles. Am J Trop Med Hyg 1999;60: 281–6.
2. Mason PJ, Haddow AJ. An epidemic of virus disease in Southern Province, Tanganyika Territory, in 1952-53; an additional note on Chikungunya virus isolations and serum antibodies. Trans R Soc Trop Med Hyg 1957;51:238–40.

3. Ross RW. The Newala epidemic. III. The virus: isolation, pathogenic properties and relationship to the epidemic. J Hyg (Lond) 1956;54:177–91.

4. Weaver SC, Forrester NL. Chikungunya: evolutionary history and recent epidemic spread. Antiviral Res 2015;120:32–9.

5. Weinbren MP. The occurrence of Chikungunya virus in Uganda. II. In man on the Entebbe peninsula. Trans R Soc Trop Med Hyg 1958;52:258–9.

6. Powers AM, Brault AC, Tesh RB, et al. Re-emergence of Chikungunya and O'nyong-nyong viruses: evidence for distinct geographical lineages and distant evolutionary relationships. J Gen Virol 2000;81:471–9.

7. Volk SM, Chen R, Tsetsarkin KA, et al. Genome-scale phylogenetic analyses of chikungunya virus reveal independent emergences of recent epidemics and various evolutionary rates. J Virol 2010;84:6497–504.

8. Tsetsarkin KA, Chen R, Leal G, et al. Chikungunya virus emergence is constrained in Asia by lineage-specific adaptive landscapes. Proc Natl Acad Sci U S A 2011;108:7872–7.

9. Nunes MR, Faria NR, de Vasconcelos JM, et al. Emergence and potential for spread of Chikungunya virus in Brazil. BMC Med 2015;13:102.

10. Mourya DT, Thakare JR, Gokhale MD, et al. Isolation of chikungunya virus from *Aedes aegypti* mosquitoes collected in the town of Yawat, Pune District, Maharashtra State, India. Acta Virol 2001;45:305–9.

11. Rausalu K, Utt A, Quirin T, et al. Chikungunya virus infectivity, RNA replication and non-structural polyprotein processing depend on the nsP2 protease's active site cysteine residue. Sci Rep 2016;6:37124.

12. Metz SW, Pijlman GP. Production of Chikungunya virus-like particles and subunit vaccines in insect cells. Methods Mol Biol 2016;1426:297–309.

13. Khan AH, Morita K, Parquet MD, et al. Complete nucleotide sequence of chikungunya virus and evidence for an internal polyadenylation site. J Gen Virol 2002; 83:3075–84.

14. Voss JE, Vaney MC, Duquerroy S, et al. Glycoprotein organization of Chikungunya virus particles revealed by X-ray crystallography. Nature 2010;468:709–12.

15. Snyder AJ, Sokoloski KJ, Mukhopadhyay S. Mutating conserved cysteines in the alphavirus e2 glycoprotein causes virus-specific assembly defects. J Virol 2012; 86:3100–11.

16. Melton JV, Ewart GD, Weir RC, et al. Alphavirus 6K proteins form ion channels. J Biol Chem 2002;277:46923–31.

17. Snyder JE, Kulcsar KA, Schultz KL, et al. Functional characterization of the alphavirus TF protein. J Virol 2013;87:8511–23.

18. Solignat M, Gay B, Higgs S, et al. Replication cycle of chikungunya: a re-emerging arbovirus. Virology 2009;393:183–97.

19. Lum FM, Ng LF. Cellular and molecular mechanisms of chikungunya pathogenesis. Antiviral Res 2015;120:165–74.

20. Rupp JC, Sokoloski KJ, Gebhart NN, et al. Alphavirus RNA synthesis and non-structural protein functions. J Gen Virol 2015;96:2483–500.

21. Powers AM. Vaccine and therapeutic options to control Chikungunya virus. Clin Microbiol Rev 2017;31 [pii:e00104-16].

22. Fortuna C, Remoli ME, Rizzo C, et al. Imported arboviral infections in Italy, July 2014-October 2015: a National Reference Laboratory report. BMC Infect Dis 2017;17:216.

23. Wahid B, Ali A, Rafique S, et al. Global expansion of chikungunya virus: mapping the 64-year history. Int J Infect Dis 2017;58:69–76.

24. Sergon K, Yahaya AA, Brown J, et al. Seroprevalence of Chikungunya virus infection on Grande Comore Island, union of the Comoros, 2005. Am J Trop Med Hyg 2007;76:1189–93.
25. Josseran L, Paquet C, Zehgnoun A, et al. Chikungunya disease outbreak, Reunion Island. Emerg Infect Dis 2006;12:1994–5.
26. Grandadam M, Caro V, Plumet S, et al. Chikungunya virus, southeastern France. Emerg Infect Dis 2011;17:910–3.
27. Rezza G, Nicoletti L, Angelini R, et al. Infection with chikungunya virus in Italy: an outbreak in a temperate region. Lancet 2007;370:1840–6.
28. Delisle E, Rousseau C, Broche B, et al. Chikungunya outbreak in Montpellier, France, September to October 2014. Euro Surveill 2015;20. https://doi.org/10.2807/1560-7917.es2015.20.17.21108.
29. Calba C, Guerbois-Galla M, Franke F, et al. Preliminary report of an autochtonous chikungunya outbreak in France, July to September 2017. Euro Surveill 2017;22(39). https://doi.org/10.2807/1560-7917.ES.2017.22.39.17-00647.
30. Vairo F, Mammone A, Lanini S, et al. Local transmission of chikungunya in Rome and the Lazio region, Italy. PLoS One 2018;13:e0208896.
31. Bordi L, Carletti F, Lalle E, et al. Molecular characterization of autochthonous Chikungunya cluster in Latium region, Italy. Emerg Infect Dis 2018;24(1). https://doi.org/10.3201/eid2401.171605.
32. Diallo D, Sall AA, Buenemann M, et al. Landscape ecology of sylvatic chikungunya virus and mosquito vectors in southeastern Senegal. PLoS Negl Trop Dis 2012;6:e1649.
33. Jupp PG, McIntosh BM. Aedes furcifer and other mosquitoes as vectors of chikungunya virus at Mica, northeastern Transvaal, South Africa. J Am Mosq Control Assoc 1990;6:415–20.
34. Coffey LL, Failloux AB, Weaver SC. Chikungunya virus-vector interactions. Viruses 2014;6:4628–63.
35. Gubler DJ. The global emergence/resurgence of arboviral diseases as public health problems. Arch Med Res 2002;33:330–42.
36. Lounibos LP. Invasions by insect vectors of human disease. Annu Rev Entomol 2002;47:233–66.
37. Powers AM, Logue CH. Changing patterns of chikungunya virus: re-emergence of a zoonotic arbovirus. J Gen Virol 2007;88:2363–77.
38. Schuffenecker I, Iteman I, Michault A, et al. Genome microevolution of chikungunya viruses causing the Indian Ocean outbreak. PLoS Med 2006;3:e263.
39. Tsetsarkin KA, Vanlandingham DL, McGee CE, et al. A single mutation in chikungunya virus affects vector specificity and epidemic potential. PLoS Pathog 2007;3:e201.
40. Vashishtha M, Phalen T, Marquardt MT, et al. A single point mutation controls the cholesterol dependence of Semliki Forest virus entry and exit. J Cell Biol 1998;140:91–9.
41. Venturi G, Di Luca M, Fortuna C, et al. Detection of a chikungunya outbreak in Central Italy, August to September 2017. Euro Surveill 2017;22(39). https://doi.org/10.2807/1560-7917.ES.2017.22.39.17-00646.
42. Bordi L, Carletti F, Castilletti C, et al. Presence of the A226V mutation in autochtonous and imported Italian chikungunya virus strains. Clin Infect Dis 2008;47:428–9.
43. Tsetsarkin KA, Chen R, Yun R, et al. Multi-peaked adaptive landscape for chikungunya virus evolution predicts continued fitness optimization in *Aedes albopictus* mosquitoes. Nat Commun 2014;5:4084.

44. Tsetsarkin KA, McGee CE, Volk SM, et al. Epistatic roles of E2 glycoprotein mutations in adaption of chikungunya virus to *Aedes albopictus* and *Ae. aegypti* mosquitoes. PLoS One 2009;4:e6835.
45. Horwood PF, Buchy P. Chikungunya. (Special Issue: New developments in major vector-borne diseases. Part II: important diseases for veterinarians.). Sci Tech Rev Off Int Epiz 2015;34:479–89.
46. Mavale M, Parashar D, Sudeep A, et al. Venereal transmission of chikungunya virus by *Aedes aegypti* mosquitoes (Diptera: Culicidae). Am J Trop Med Hyg 2010;83:1242–4.
47. Agarwal A, Dash PK, Singh AK, et al. Evidence of experimental vertical transmission of emerging novel ECSA genotype of Chikungunya Virus in *Aedes aegypti*. PLoS Negl Trop Dis 2014;8:e2990.
48. Chompoosri J, Thavara U, Tawatsin A, et al. Vertical transmission of Indian Ocean Lineage of chikungunya virus in *Aedes aegypti* and *Aedes albopictus* mosquitoes. Parasit Vectors 2016;9:227.
49. Jain J, Kushwah RBS, Singh SS, et al. Evidence for natural vertical transmission of chikungunya viruses in field populations of *Aedes aegypti* in Delhi and Haryana states in India-a preliminary report. Acta Trop 2016;162:46–55.
50. Furuya-Kanamori L, Liang S, Milinovich G, et al. Co-distribution and co-infection of chikungunya and dengue viruses. BMC Infect Dis 2016;16:84.
51. Boga JA, Alvarez-Arguelles ME, Rojo-Alba S, et al. Simultaneous detection of Dengue virus, Chikungunya virus, Zika virus, Yellow fever virus and West Nile virus. J Virol Methods 2019;268:53–5.
52. Appassakij H, Khuntikij P, Kemapunmanus M, et al. Viremic profiles in asymptomatic and symptomatic chikungunya fever: a blood transfusion threat? Transfusion 2013;53:2567–74.
53. Brouard C, Bernillon P, Quatresous I, et al. Estimated risk of Chikungunya viremic blood donation during an epidemic on Reunion Island in the Indian Ocean, 2005 to 2007. Transfusion 2008;48:1333–41.
54. Liumbruno GM, Calteri D, Petropulacos K, et al. The Chikungunya epidemic in Italy and its repercussion on the blood system. Blood Transfus 2008;6:199–210.
55. Kee AC, Yang S, Tambyah P. Atypical chikungunya virus infections in immunocompromised patients. Emerg Infect Dis 2010;16:1038–40.
56. Dalla Gasperina D, Balsamo ML, Garavaglia SD, et al. Chikungunya infection in a human immunodeficiency virus-infected kidney transplant recipient returning to Italy from the Dominican Republic. Transpl Infect Dis 2015;17:876–9.
57. Girão ES, Rodrigues Dos Santos BG, do Amaral ES, et al. Chikungunya infection in solid organ transplant recipients. Transpl Proc 2017;49:2076–81.
58. Couderc T, Gangneux N, Chrétien F, et al. Chikungunya virus infection of corneal grafts. J Infect Dis 2012;206:851–9.
59. Gérardin P, Barau G, Michault A, et al. Multidisciplinary prospective study of mother-to-child chikungunya virus infections on the island of La Réunion. PLoS Med 2008;5:e60.
60. Couderc T, Chrétien F, Schilte C, et al. A mouse model for Chikungunya: young age and inefficient type-I interferon signaling are risk factors for severe disease. PLoS Pathog 2008;4:e29.
61. Contopoulos-Ioannidis D, Newman-Lindsay S, Chow C, et al. Mother-to-child transmission of Chikungunya virus: a systematic review and meta-analysis. PLoS Negl Trop Dis 2018;12:e0006510.
62. Patterson J, Sammon M, Garg M. Dengue, Zika and Chikungunya: emerging arboviruses in the new world. West J Emerg Med 2016;17:671–9.

63. Bandeira AC, Campos GS, Rocha VF, et al. Prolonged shedding of Chikungunya virus in semen and urine: a new perspective for diagnosis and implications for transmission. IDCases 2016;6:100–3.

64. Matusali G, Colavita F, Bordi L, et al. Tropism of the Chikungunya Virus. Viruses 2019;11 [pii:E175].

65. Sourisseau M, Schilte C, Casartelli N, et al. Characterization of reemerging chikungunya virus. PLoS Pathog 2007;3:e89.

66. Kam YW, Ong EK, Rénia L, et al. Immuno-biology of Chikungunya and implications for disease intervention. Microbes Infect 2009;11:1186–96.

67. Lohachanakul J, Phuklia W, Thannagith M, et al. Differences in response of primary human myoblasts to infection with recent epidemic strains of Chikungunya virus isolated from patients with and without myalgia. J Med Virol 2015;87:733–9.

68. Hoarau JJ, Jaffar Bandjee MC, Krejbich Trotot P, et al. Persistent chronic inflammation and infection by Chikungunya arthritogenic alphavirus in spite of a robust host immune response. J Immunol 2010;184:5914–27.

69. Zhang X, Huang Y, Wang M, et al. Differences in genome characters and cell tropisms between two chikungunya isolates of Asian lineage and Indian Ocean lineage. Virol J 2018;15:130.

70. Lokireddy S, Vemula S, Vadde R. Connective tissue metabolism in chikungunya patients. Virol J 2008;5:31.

71. Chow A, Her Z, Ong EK, et al. Persistent arthralgia induced by Chikungunya virus infection is associated with interleukin-6 and granulocyte macrophage colony-stimulating factor. J Infect Dis 2011;203:149–57.

72. Goupil BA, McNulty MA, Martin MJ, et al. Novel lesions of bones and joints associated with Chikungunya virus infection in two mouse models of disease: new insights into disease pathogenesis. PLoS One 2016;11:e0155243.

73. Yoon IK, Alera MT, Lago CB, et al. High rate of subclinical chikungunya virus infection and association of neutralizing antibody with protection in a prospective cohort in the Philippines. PLoS Negl Trop Dis 2015;9:e0003764.

74. Burt FJ, Chen W, Miner JJ, et al. Chikungunya virus: an update on the biology and pathogenesis of this emerging pathogen. Lancet Infect Dis 2017;17:e107–17.

75. Morrison TE. Reemergence of chikungunya virus. J Virol 2014;88:11644–7.

76. Colavita F, Vita S, Lalle E, et al. Overproduction of IL-6 and type-I IFN in a lethal case of Chikungunya virus infection in an elderly man during the 2017 Italian outbreak. Open Forum Infect Dis 2018;5:ofy276.

77. Mehta R, Gerardin P, de Brito CAA, et al. The neurological complications of chikungunya virus: a systematic review. Rev Med Virol 2018;28:e1978.

78. Dhanwani R, Khan M, Bhaskar AS, et al. Characterization of Chikungunya virus infection in human neuroblastoma SH-SY5Y cells: role of apoptosis in neuronal cell death. Virus Res 2012;163:563–72.

79. Abere B, Wikan N, Ubol S, et al. Proteomic analysis of chikungunya virus infected microglial cells. PLoS One 2012;7:e34800.

80. Abraham R, Mudaliar P, Padmanabhan A, et al. Induction of cytopathogenicity in human glioblastoma cells by chikungunya virus. PLoS One 2013;8:e75854.

81. Thiberville SD, Moyen N, Dupuis-Maguiraga L, et al. Chikungunya fever: epidemiology, clinical syndrome, pathogenesis and therapy. Antiviral Res 2013;99:345–70.

82. Capeding MR, Chua MN, Hadinegoro SR, et al. Dengue and other common causes of acute febrile illness in Asia: an active surveillance study in children. PLoS Negl Trop Dis 2013;7:e2331.

83. Simon F, Javelle E, Oliver M, et al. Chikungunya virus infection. Curr Infect Dis Rep 2011;13:218–28.

84. Rahman M, Yamagishi J, Rahim R, et al. East/Central/South African Genotype in a Chikungunya Outbreak, Dhaka, Bangladesh, 2017. Emerg Infect Dis 2019;25: 370–2.

85. de Andrade GC, Ventura CV, Mello Filho PA, et al. Arboviruses and the eye. Int J Retina Vitreous 2017;3:4.

86. Simon F, Javelle E, Cabie A, et al. French guidelines for the management of chikungunya (acute and persistent presentations). November 2014. Med Mal Infect 2015;45:243–63.

87. Ramful D, Carbonnier M, Pasquet M, et al. Mother-to-child transmission of Chikungunya virus infection. Pediatr Infect Dis J 2007;26:811–5.

88. Torres JR, Falleiros-Arlant LH, Dueñas L, et al. Congenital and perinatal complications of chikungunya fever: a Latin American experience. Int J Infect Dis 2016; 51:85–8.

89. Gérardin P, Sampériz S, Ramful D, et al. Neurocognitive outcome of children exposed to perinatal mother-to-child Chikungunya virus infection: the CHIMERE cohort study on Reunion Island. PLoS Negl Trop Dis 2014;8:e2996.

90. Tandale BV, Sathe PS, Arankalle VA, et al. Systemic involvements and fatalities during Chikungunya epidemic in India, 2006. J Clin Virol 2009;46:145–9.

91. Crosby L, Perreau C, Madeux B, et al. Severe manifestations of chikungunya virus in critically ill patients during the 2013-2014 Caribbean outbreak. Int J Infect Dis 2016;48:78–80.

92. Lemant J, Boisson V, Winer A, et al. Serious acute chikungunya virus infection requiring intensive care during the Reunion Island outbreak in 2005-2006. Crit Care Med 2008;36:2536–41.

93. Economopoulou A, Dominguez M, Helynck B, et al. Atypical Chikungunya virus infections: clinical manifestations, mortality and risk factors for severe disease during the 2005-2006 outbreak on Réunion. Epidemiol Infect 2009;137:534.

94. Gérardin P, Couderc T, Bintner M, et al. Chikungunya virus-associated encephalitis: a cohort study on La Réunion Island, 2005-2009. Neurology 2016;86: 94–102.

95. Chusri S, Siripaitoon P, Hirunpat S, et al. Case reports of neuro-Chikungunya in southern Thailand. Am J Trop Med Hyg 2011;85:386–9.

96. Charrel RN, de Lamballerie X, Raoult D. Chikungunya outbreaks—the globalization of vectorborne diseases. N Engl J Med 2007;356:769–71.

97. Couderc T, Khandoudi N, Grandadam M, et al. Prophylaxis and therapy for Chikungunya virus infection. J Infect Dis 2009;200:516–23.

98. Khan M, Santhosh SR, Tiwari M, et al. Assessment of in vitro prophylactic and therapeutic efficacy of chloroquine against Chikungunya virus in vero cells. J Med Virol 2010;82:817–24.

99. Pohjala L, Utt A, Varjak M, et al. Inhibitors of alphavirus entry and replication identified with a stable Chikungunya replicon cell line and virus-based assays. PLoS One 2011;6:e28923.

100. Kaur P, Thiruchelvan M, Lee RC, et al. Inhibition of chikungunya virus replication by harringtonine, a novel antiviral that suppresses viral protein expression. Antimicrob Agents Chemother 2013;57:155–67.

101. Bourjot M, Leyssen P, Neyts J, et al. Trigocherrierin A, a potent inhibitor of chikungunya virus replication. Molecules 2014;19:3617–27.
102. Albulescu IC, Tas A, Scholte FE, et al. An in vitro assay to study chikungunya virus RNA synthesis and the mode of action of inhibitors. J Gen Virol 2014;95: 2683–92.
103. Schilte C, Couderc T, Chretien F, et al. Type I IFN controls chikungunya virus via its action on nonhematopoietic cells. J Exp Med 2010;207:429–42.
104. Mallilankaraman K, Shedlock DJ, Bao H, et al. A DNA vaccine against chikungunya virus is protective in mice and induces neutralizing antibodies in mice and nonhuman primates. PLoS Negl Trop Dis 2011;5:e928.
105. Tretyakova I, Hearn J, Wang E, et al. DNA vaccine initiates replication of live attenuated chikungunya virus in vitro and elicits protective immune response in mice. J Infect Dis 2014;209:1882–90.
106. Wang E, Volkova E, Adams AP, et al. Chimeric alphavirus vaccine candidates for chikungunya. Vaccine 2008;26:5030–9.
107. Hallengärd D, Kakoulidou M, Lulla A, et al. Novel attenuated Chikungunya vaccine candidates elicit protective immunity in C57BL/6 mice. J Virol 2014;88: 2858–66.
108. Chattopadhyay A, Wang E, Seymour, et al. A chimeric vesiculo/alphavirus is an effective alphavirus vaccine. J Virol 2013;87:395–402.
109. Plante K, Wang E, Partidos CD, et al. Novel chikungunya vaccine candidate with an IRES-based attenuation and host range alteration mechanism. PLoS Pathog 2011;7:e1002142.
110. Levitt NH, Ramsburg HH, Hasty SE, et al. Development of an attenuated strain of chikungunya virus for use in vaccine production. Vaccine 1986;4:157–62.
111. Edelman R, Tacket CO, Wasserman SS, et al. Phase II safety and immunogenicity study of live chikungunya virus vaccine TSI-GSD-218. Am J Trop Med Hyg 2000;62:681–5.
112. Chang LJ, Dowd KA, Mendoza FH, et al. Safety and tolerability of chikungunya virus-like particle vaccine in healthy adults: a phase 1 dose-escalation trial. Lancet 2014;384:2046–52.
113. Ramsauer K, Schwameis M, Firbas C, et al. Immunogenicity, safety, and tolerability of a recombinant measles-virus-based chikungunya vaccine: a randomised, double-blind, placebo-controlled, active-comparator, first-in-man trial. Lancet Infect Dis 2015;15:519–27.
114. Reisinger EC, Tschismarov R, Beubler E, et al. Immunogenicity, safety, and tolerability of the measles-vectored chikungunya virus vaccine MV-CHIK: a double-blind, randomised, placebo-controlled and active-controlled phase 2 trial. Lancet 2019;392:2718–27.
115. Zumla A, Dar O, Kock R, et al. Taking forward a 'One Health' approach for turning the tide against the Middle East respiratory syndrome coronavirus and other zoonotic pathogens with epidemic potential. Int J Infect Dis 2016;47:5–9.
116. McCloskey B, Dar O, Zumla A, et al. Emerging infectious diseases and pandemic potential: status quo and reducing risk of global spread. Lancet Infect Dis 2014;14(10):1001–10.

Human Monkeypox
Epidemiologic and Clinical Characteristics, Diagnosis, and Prevention

Eskild Petersen, MD, DMSc, DTMH[a,b,c,*], Anu Kantele, MD, PhD[d],
Marion Koopmans, DVM, PhD[e], Danny Asogun, MBBS, FWACP[f,g],
Adesola Yinka-Ogunleye, BDS, MPH[h],
Chikwe Ihekweazu, MBBS, MPH, FFPH[h],
Alimuddin Zumla, MBChB, MSc, PhD, MD, FRCP(Lond), FRCP(Edin), FRCPath(UK), FAAS[i]

KEYWORDS

• Monkeypox • Smallpox • West Africa • Epidemic

KEY POINTS

• Human monkeypox is a zoonosis caused by the monkeypox virus (MPXV), a double-stranded DNA virus of the family Poxviridae.

• The frequency and geographic distribution of human monkeypox cases across West and Central Africa have increased in recent years.

Continued

All authors contributed equally.
A. Zumla, D. Asogun, and C. Ihekweazu are members of the PANDORA-ID-NET Consortium. PANDORA-ID-NET (EDCTP Reg/Grant RIA2016E-1609) is funded by the European and Developing Countries Clinical Trials Partnership (EDCTP2) programme, which is supported under Horizon 2020, the European Union's Framework Programme for Research and Innovation. A. Zumla is in receipt of a National Institutes of Health Research senior investigator award.
Conflicts of Interest: All authors have an interest in global public health and emerging and re-emerging infections. All authors have no other conflict of interest to declare.
[a] Institute of Clinical Medicine, University of Aarhus, Palle Juul-Jensens Boulevard 82, Aarhus N DK-8200, Denmark; [b] The Royal Hospital, Muscat, Oman; [c] European Society for Clinical Microbiology and Infectious Diseases, Task Force for Emerging Infections, Basel, Switzerland; [d] Inflammation Center, Helsinki University Hospital and Helsinki University, Stenbäckinkatu 9, PO BOX 100, Helsinki FI-00029 HUS, Finland; [e] Viroscience Department, Erasmus Medical Centre, Postbus 2040, Rotterdam 3000 CA, the Netherlands; [f] Department of Public Health, College of Medicine, Ambrose Alli University, Ekpoma, Nigeria; [g] Department of Public Health, and Institute of Lassa Fever Research and Control, Irrua Specialist Teaching Hospital, Irrua, Nigeria; [h] Nigeria Centre for Disease Control, Plot 801, Ebitu Ukiwe Street, Jabi, Abuja, Nigeria; [i] Division of Infection and Immunity, Center for Clinical Microbiology, University College London, The National Institute of Health Research Biomedical Research Centre at UCL Hospitals, Gower Street, London WC1E 6BT, UK
* Corresponding author. Directorate General for Communicable Disease Surveillance and Control, Ministry of Health, 18th November Street, 101 Muscat, Sultanate of Oman.
E-mail address: eskild.petersen@gmail.com

Continued

- The clinical presentation of monkeypox is similar to that of smallpox, in terms of symptom onset, timing of rash occurrence, and rash distribution, but generally less severe than smallpox with lower fatality rate and scarification.
- Most confirmed Monkeypox cases are younger than 40 years with a median age of 31 years, a population born only after discontinuation of the smallpox vaccination campaign, and thus may reflect a lack of cross-protective immunity.

INTRODUCTION

Human monkeypox virus (MPXV) is a double-stranded DNA virus of the Orthopoxvirus genus of the family Poxviridae.[1-4] Two genetic clades of the monkeypox virus have been characterized: West African and Central African. MPXV is one of the 4 orthopoxvirus species pathogenic for humans, the other 3 being (1) variola major virus (VARV), the causative agent of smallpox, now eradicated, (2) variola minor virus, and (3) cowpox virus (CPXV). There is a range of animal poxviruses, several of which have zoonotic potential. Infections in humans have been described for vaccinia virus, cowpox virus, buffalopox virus, and sporadic cases of camelpox.[5,6] Monkeypox infects a wide range of mammalian species, but its natural host reservoir remains unknown.

PUBLIC HEALTH IMPORTANCE

Thought to be a rare and self-limiting disease,[7] monkeypox has not attracted much attention since its discovery 70 years ago. The frequency and geographic distribution of human monkeypox cases have increased in recent years in a specific region of Africa (**Fig. 1**),[8] and monkeypox has been recognized as an increasing public health threat, particularly in regions in West Africa where there is close interaction between humans and wild animal reservoirs and in particular where there is evidence that the infection attack rate is increasing. The clinical presentation of monkeypox is similar to that of smallpox[2] in terms of symptom onset, timing of rash occurrence, and rash distribution,[7] but generally less severe than smallpox in terms of complication rate, case fatality rate, and levels of scarification.

Recently, concern has been raised about the emergence of MPXV as well as the resemblance of its clinical presentation to that of smallpox, a deadly disease globally eradicated by vaccination 40 years ago.[9] During outbreaks, it has been challenging to clinically distinguish monkeypox from chickenpox, an unrelated herpesvirus infection. However, sporadic zoonotic infections with other orthopoxviruses also call for vigilance. Outbreaks of buffalopox have occurred with multiple human cases in India.[10] Similarly, during outbreaks of vaccinia virus infection in cattle in Brazil, there is documented evidence of human infections.[11]

Cross-Immunity and Protection

Various orthopoxvirus species share genetic and antigenic features,[12-14] and an infection by any of these species may confer substantial protection against infection by the others.[15] Vaccination with vaccinia virus protects against disease caused by VARV, MPXV, or CPXV.[16] The immunologic mechanisms underlying cross-protection by immunization with vaccinia virus seem to be diverse, with neutralizing antibodies among the principal components.[17] Consistent with the ability of smallpox vaccine to provide

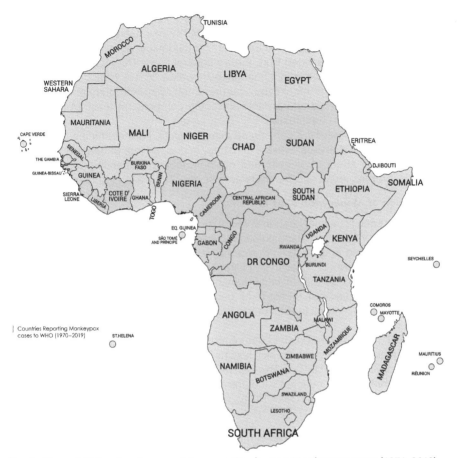

Fig. 1. Map of Africa showing countries reporting human Monkeypox cases (1971–2019).

cross-protection for humans against monkeypox, monkeys can be protected against monkeypox by immunization with the human smallpox vaccine.[18,19]

Ever since smallpox vaccinations were discontinued in 1978, cross-protective immunity to various orthopoxviruses has waned, particularly in younger individuals lacking vaccinia-induced immunity, and the number of unvaccinated, susceptible individuals has grown worldwide. Indeed, these changes have been accompanied by an increased frequency and geographic distribution of human monkeypox cases in recent years.

EPIDEMIOLOGY
Discovery and Animal Reservoirs

MPXV was first detected in 1958 in an outbreak of a vesicular disease among captive monkeys transported to Copenhagen, Denmark from Africa for research purposes. Hence the name "monkeypox."[20] The term is inappropriate because the largest animal reservoirs of the virus have been found in rodents, including squirrels and giant pouched rats, both of which are hunted for food.[21] Rodents are the largest group of mammals with more than 1500 species. The extent of the wild animal reservoir, the natural history, and pathogenesis of monkeypox in both animals and humans remains unknown, requiring characterization through ecologic and epidemiologic studies. Thus far, MPXV has been detected in diverse animal species: squirrels (rope and tree), rats, striped mice, dormice, and monkeys. In 1985, the virus was isolated from a rope squirrel in the Democratic Republic of Congo (DRC) and a dead infant mangabey monkey in Tai National Park, Cote d'Ivoire.[22] During a large monkeypox outbreak following introduction of the virus through animals imported into an animal trading company, at least 14 species of rodents were found to be infected.[23]

Like humans, monkeys are considered disease hosts. Further studies are needed to understand how the virus persists in nature, and to explore pathogen-host associations and the effect of climatic and ecologic factors influencing the shifts between geographic areas and the virus as a cause of disease in humans.[24]

Transmission of Monkeypox Virus to Humans

Not only the specific animal host reservoir of monkeypox but also the mode of transmission of MPXV from animals to humans remain unknown. Aerosol transmission has been demonstrated in animals,[25,26] and may explain a nosocomial outbreak in the Central African Republic.[27] However, indirect or direct contact with live or dead animals is assumed to be the driver of human monkeypox infections in humans.[28,29] Poverty and continued civil unrest force people to hunt small mammals (bushmeat) to obtain protein-rich food, thus increasing exposure to wild rodents, which may carry monkeypox.[30]

In August 1970 the first human case of monkeypox was identified in a 9-year-old child with smallpox-like vesicular skin lesions in the village of Bukenda in the Equatorial region of Zaire (now DRC).[31] This patient was found during a period of intensified smallpox surveillance conducted 9 months after the World Health Organization (WHO) the eradication of smallpox in the DRC had certified the eradication of smallpox in the DRC.

Geographic Endemicity and Increase in Number of Cases

Ever since its discovery, the disease has been endemic to Central and West Africa with intermittent, sporadic cases of monkeypox transmitted from local wildlife reported among humans. Retrospective studies indicated that similar cases had occurred in 1970 to 1971 in the Ivory Coast, Liberia, Nigeria, and Sierra Leone.[32–35] Subsequent enhanced surveillance observed a steady increase in the rate of human monkeypox cases. The number of cases of human monkeypox has increased exponentially over the past 20 years, and has already exceeded that accumulated during the first 45 years since its first discovery.[28,29,36–45]

A comprehensive enhanced surveillance study in the DRC in 2004 to 2005 showed a steep increase in incidence compared with data from a WHO enhanced surveillance program carried out from 1970 to 1986 reporting 404 cases.[46] The incidence was highest in forested regions, and in lower age groups not vaccinated as part of the smallpox eradication program.[42] To date, human monkeypox cases have been reported from 10 African countries: DRC, Republic of the Congo, Cameroon, Central African Republic, Nigeria, Ivory Coast, Liberia, Sierra Leone, Gabon, and South Sudan.[1,36,47] The growing incidence of human monkeypox cases in Central and West Africa is considered a consequence of waning cross-protective immunity among the population after smallpox vaccination was discontinued in the early 1980s, following the eradication of smallpox.[28,42] The deteriorating immunologic status is not only related to waning vaccine-induced protection among those initially vaccinated, but probably—and even more—to the increasing proportion of those never given the vaccine, that is, nonvaccinated younger age groups. Both mechanisms lead to a growing percentage of susceptible individuals in the endemic areas in Central and West Africa. Another central factor considered to contribute to the incidence of monkeypox is related to increasing contact between humans and small mammals potentially carrying MPXV. Humans invade jungles and forests, the natural environment of the reservoir species. Civil wars, refugee displacement, farming, deforestation, climate change, demographic changes, and population movement may have led to a spread of monkeypox-infected animals and increased their interaction with humans across West and Central Africa.

Monkeypox Cases in the United States

Monkeypox remained an ignored global public health threat and was only given international attention when the first cases outside Africa were detected in the United States in 2003.[48] After several Midwesterners developed fever, rash, respiratory symptoms, and lymphadenopathy, outbreak investigation linked the symptoms to exposure to pet prairie dogs (*Cynomys* species), and monkeypox virus was identified as a causative agent.[48] It spread rapidly. Monkeypox cases were reported from 6 states—Illinois, Indiana, Kansas, Missouri, Ohio, and Wisconsin—during the outbreak.[49] Molecular investigations identified a monkeypox virus of the West African genetic group (clade). Epidemiologic studies concluded that the virus had been imported into the United States, more specifically to Texas, from Ghana on April 9, 2003, with a shipment of small mammals of 9 different species, including 6 genera of African rodents.[50] These comprised rope squirrels (*Funiscuirus* sp.), tree squirrels (*Heliosciurus* sp.), African giant pouched rats (*Cricetomys* sp.), brush-tailed porcupines (*Atherurus* sp.), dormice (*Graphiurus* sp.), and striped mice (*Lemniscomys* sp.). Some of the infected animals were housed in close proximity to prairie dogs later sold as pets.

Monkeypox Cases in the United Kingdom and Israel

In September 2018, monkeypox again drew the attention of global media, politicians, and scientists when 3 individual patients in the United Kingdom were diagnosed with monkeypox.[51] The first 2 had recently traveled in Nigeria, a country with an ongoing outbreak of the disease,[52] and both were symptomatic during their flight home. The third case of monkeypox in the United Kingdom was diagnosed in a health care worker caring for 1 of these first 2 patients. As the clinical picture of the 3 patients' disease raised a concern over an exotic disease, special infection control measures were taken well before monkeypox was suspected. One of the primary cases reported contact with a person with suspected rash at a family gathering, and the consumption of bushmeat.[52] Secondary and tertiary human-to-human transmission of monkeypox does occur in endemic areas.[53,54] Of note, definitive confirmation of human-to-human transmission in endemic areas is somewhat problematic, because even the secondary and tertiary cases may have been exposed to infected animals. The disease contracted by the British health care worker provides indisputable evidence of human-to-human transmission from an infected patient.

In October 2018, Israel reported a monkeypox case imported from Nigeria.[55] It is well known that travelers can act as sentinels of infectious disease epidemics in the region visited. Not consistent with the reports of low levels of transmission in Nigeria, 3 cases imported to other countries from there within a couple of months should raise the concern of health authorities.[56]

Ongoing Monkeypox Outbreak in West Africa

On September 22, 2017, the Nigeria Center for Disease Control (NCDC) commenced an outbreak investigation following the identification of a suspected case of monkeypox in an 11-year-old child.[57] The data available indicate that the current outbreak is either a multisource outbreak or one stemming from previously undetected endemic transmission, because the cases were not epidemiologically linked.[28,58–60] The exact zoonotic origin and role of environmental and ecologic factors in the Nigerian outbreak are not yet known. New cases of monkeypox continue to be detected in the country. Since the beginning of the outbreak on September 22, 2018, as of January 1, 2019 there have been 311 suspected cases reported from 26 states (132 confirmed cases affecting children and adults of all ages) and 7 deaths reported.[60] Most of the confirmed monkeypox patients are aged between 21 and 40 years, with a median age of 31 years, similar to the observed age range in DRC.[42] It is noteworthy that all were born after 1978, when the global vaccination programs for smallpox were discontinued.

MODES OF TRANSMISSION OF MONKEYPOX VIRUS TO HUMANS

The exact mode of MPXV transmission to humans remains unknown. Primary animal-to-human infection is assumed to occur when handling monkeypox-infected animals, through direct (touch, bite, or scratch) or indirect contact, although the exact mechanism(s) remains to be defined. The virus is assumed to enter the body through broken skin, respiratory tract, or the mucous membranes (eyes, nose, or mouth). Secondary human-to-human transmission is considered common,[37,53,61] presumably through large respiratory droplets or direct or indirect contact with body fluids, lesion material, and contaminated surfaces or other material, such as clothing or linens. Prolonged contact with patients renders hospital staff and family members at greater risk of infection. Nosocomial transmission has been described.[38] There is no evidence to date that human-to-human transmission alone can sustain monkeypox infections in the human population.

There have only been a few genomic studies of the origins of monkeypox outbreaks. Human-to-human transmission has been described from primary human cases and secondary cases,[53,62,63] and serial transmission across 4 cases has been observed.[64] In the current monkeypox outbreak in Nigeria, genomic studies of monkeypox virus isolates from humans[60] indicate that the index case was not imported into Nigeria. Thus, the outbreak is considered to be a spillover from multiple sources of introduction into the human population. The zoonotic source(s) of the outbreak are being investigated at present, and it is unclear what, if any, environmental or ecologic changes might have facilitated the sudden re-emergence of monkeypox in Nigeria. Case clustering has been identified within the various states, but no epidemiologic linkages between them have been detected thus far. Three family clusters have been identified, suggesting human-to-human transmission.[58–60] In one family the secondary attack rate was 71%. However, most patients had no obvious epidemiologic linkage or person-to-person contact, indicating a probable multiple-source outbreak or, possibly, an endemic disease previously unrecognized.

CLINICAL FEATURES

The incubation period has been estimated at 5 to 21 days, and duration of symptoms and signs at 2 to 5 weeks. The illness begins with nonspecific symptoms and signs that include fever, chills, headaches, lethargy, asthenia, lymph node swellings, back pain, and myalgia (muscle ache) and begins with a fever before rashes appear. Within 1 to 5 days after the onset of fever, rashes of varying sizes appear, first on the face (**Fig. 2**), then across the body (**Fig. 3**), hands (**Fig. 4A**), and legs and feet (**Fig. 4B**). The rash undergoes several stages of evolution from macules, papules, vesicles (fluid-filled blisters) (see **Fig. 2**), and pustules (see **Fig. 3B, D**), followed by resolution over time with crusts and scabs (**Fig. 5**), which drop off on recovery. Various stages of the rash may show at the same time (see **Figs. 3B and 5**). Areas of erythema (see **Fig. 2A**) and/or skin hyperpigmentation (see **Fig. 5**) are often seen around discrete lesions. Detached scabs may be considerably smaller than the original lesion. Inflammation of the pharyngeal, conjunctival, and genital mucosae may also be seen.

The clinical presentation of monkeypox includes symptoms and lesions that are difficult to distinguish from smallpox.[37,60,65,66] Although the clinical manifestations of monkeypox are milder than smallpox, the disease can prove fatal, death rates ranging from 1% to 10%. Mortality is higher among children and young adults and the course is more severe in immunocompromised individuals.[67] A range of complications has been reported, such as secondary bacterial infections, respiratory distress, broncho-pneumonia, encephalitis, corneal infection with ensuing loss of vision, gastrointestinal

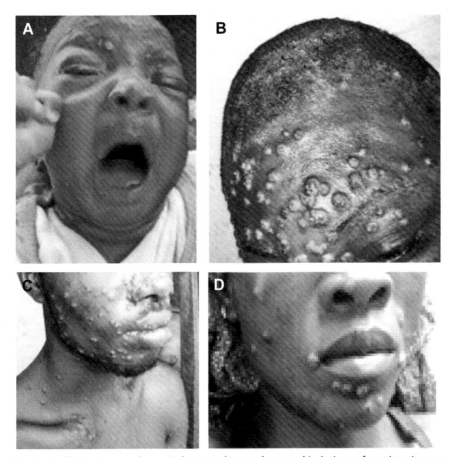

Fig. 2. (*A–D*) Maculo-papular-vesicular-pustular monkeypox skin lesions of varying sizes on the face. (*Courtesy of* Nigeria Centre for Disease Control, Abuja, Nigeria.)

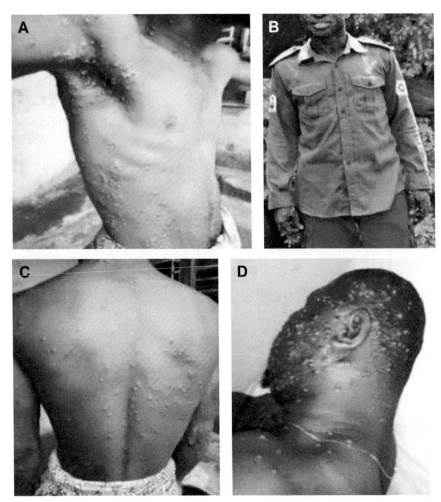

Fig. 3. (*A–D*) Papular-vesicular-pustular monkeypox skin lesions of varying sizes across the body. (*Courtesy of* Nigeria Centre for Disease Control, Abuja, Nigeria.)

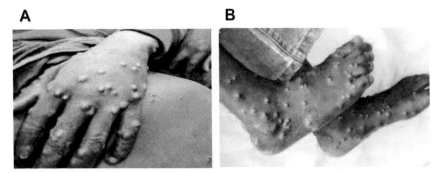

Fig. 4. (*A, B*) Papular-pustular monkeypox skin lesions on the hands, legs, and feet. (*Courtesy of* Nigeria Centre for Disease Control, Abuja, Nigeria.)

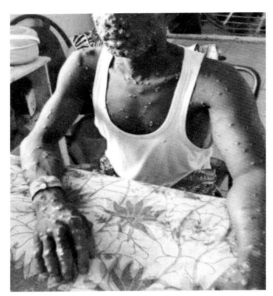

Fig. 5. Extensive papulo-pustular monkeypox rashes with crust and scar formation. (*Courtesy of* Nigeria Centre for Disease Control, Abuja, Nigeria.)

involvement, vomiting, and diarrhea with dehydration. Case fatality rates have varied between 1% and 10% in outbreaks, deaths occurring mostly among young adults and children. Particularly those with immunosuppression are at risk of severe disease. Lymphadenopathy is seen in up to 90% of patients and appears to be a clinical feature distinguishing human monkeypox from smallpox.

Previous smallpox vaccination confers some cross-protection against monkeypox and modifies the clinical picture toward a milder disease. Between 1980 and 1990, the clinical presentation of human monkeypox seems to have changed: primary human cases have increasingly been seen among those never vaccinated against smallpox. Compared with those vaccinated, the clinical picture described for the unvaccinated was more severe, with more vigorous and pleomorphic rashes and higher mortality.[62,66,68–70]

The primary differential diagnosis is severe chickenpox with lesions in palms and soles.[7,65] The lesions in chickenpox are more superficial and occur in clusters of the same stage, with denser manifestations on the trunk than on the face and extremities. Because of the nonspecific nature of the symptoms and signs of monkeypox, a wide variety of differential diagnoses should be considered, ranging from chickenpox, molluscum contagiosum, measles, rickettsial infections, bacterial skin infections (such as those caused by *Staphylococcus aureus*), anthrax, scabies, syphilis, and drug reactions to other noninfectious causes of rash. A clinical sign differentiating monkeypox from smallpox and chickenpox is the presence of enlarged lymph nodes, particularly submental, submandibular, cervical, and inguinal nodes.[71]

SMALLPOX VACCINATION, MONKEYPOX PREVALENCE, AND CHANGING CLINICAL PRESENTATIONS

In 1980, the Global Commission for the Certification of Smallpox Eradication (GCCSE) continued to designate monkeypox as a public health threat, recommending that the epidemiologic, ecologic, and surveillance program on monkeypox be continued.[35,72]

In response, the WHO supported an active surveillance program for human monkeypox from 1970 to 1986.[46] It was assumed to be endemic to DRC, but other Central and West African countries also reported cases of monkeypox in humans or circulation in wildlife. At the end of the smallpox eradication campaign, the GCCSE stated that smallpox vaccination to prevent monkeypox was no longer justified, even if cross-protective immunity could not be relied on for long because of the vaccinations being discontinued. In retrospect, this resolution may have been an error.

Experimental studies of monkeys have shown immunization with smallpox vaccine to give cross-protection against monkeypox.[19]

Several reviews have summarized human monkeypox outbreaks over the past 38 years.[28,29,42] Between November 2005 and November 2007, population-based surveillance studies conducted in 9 health zones in central DRC identified 760 laboratory-confirmed human monkeypox cases. The average annual cumulative incidence across the zones was 5.53 per 10,000 (2.18–14.42). Factors associated with increased risk of infection included living in forested areas, male sex, age less than 15 years, and absence of smallpox vaccination scar. Among those vaccinated, the risk of monkeypox was found to be 5.2-fold lower than among those unvaccinated (0.78 versus 4.05 per 10,000). Compared with surveillance data from the same region recorded in the 1980s, a 20-fold increase in human monkeypox incidence was observed. Between January 2001 and December 2004, the DRC Ministry of Health surveillance program reported 2734 cases of suspected human monkeypox in 11 provinces, showing an annual upward trend: 380 cases in 2001, 545 in 2002, 783 in 2003, and 1026 in 2004. Most cases (94%) were observed in children and adults younger than 25 years.[41] These patients had not been vaccinated against smallpox. Surveillance activities have been halted since 2005 because of the civil war.

DIAGNOSIS: LABORATORY, VIROLOGIC, AND HISTOLOGIC FEATURES

Optimal clinical specimens for laboratory analyses include specimens from skin lesions such as swabs of vesicular lesions, exudate, or crusts stored in a dry, sterile tube (no viral transport media) and kept cold. A viral culture should be obtained by an oropharyngeal or nasopharyngeal swab. Skin biopsies of vesiculopustular rash or a sample of the roof of an intact skin vesicular lesion are valuable for analyses. Reference laboratories with high containment facilities are required to make a definitive diagnosis using electron microscopy, culture and molecular analysis identification by polymerase chain reaction, and sequencing. Serologic testing requires paired acute and convalescent sera for MPXV-specific immunoglobulin M detection within 5 days of presentation, or immunoglobulin G detection after 8 days.

Histology and immunohistochemistry of papular lesions may show acanthosis, individual keratinocyte necrosis, and basal vacuolization, along with a superficial and deep perivascular lymphohistiocytic infiltrate in the dermis. Vesicular lesions show spongiosis with reticular and ballooning degeneration, multinucleated epithelial giant cells with epidermal necrosis with numerous eosinophils and neutrophils, and features of vasculitis and viral inclusions in keratinocytes. Intracytoplasmic, round-to-oval inclusions with sausage-shaped structures centrally, measuring 200 to 300 μm, may be seen on electron microscopic observation.

TREATMENT

There is no specific treatment for monkeypox. Supportive care, symptomatic management, and treatment of secondary bacterial infections remain the main recommendations.

PREVENTION

Prevention of MPXV spread in endemic areas is highly challenging, and consists of avoiding any contact with rodents and primates as well as limiting direct exposure to blood and inadequately cooked meat. Efforts to halt bushmeat trade and consumption of wild animals are extremely difficult both culturally and economically because this meat may be the only protein source available for the poorest people. Massive health education campaigns are needed to increase general awareness and to advise on proper handling of potential animal reservoir species (gloves, protective clothing, surgical mask) as well as avoiding close contact with anyone infected.

Infection control measures are vital to prevention of human-to-human transmission in health care. Improved nursing (gloves, protective clothing, surgical masks) and isolation practices require education as well as adequate facilities and staffing.

National health authorities should consider arranging immunization against smallpox for health care workers and those treating or exposed to patients with monkeypox or their samples. Smallpox vaccination has been estimated to provide 85% cross-protection against monkeypox infection.[32] The Centers for Disease Control and Prevention (CDC) recommended smallpox vaccination within 2 weeks, ideally before 4 days, after significant, unprotected exposure to a diseased animal or a confirmed human case.

During an outbreak, the spread of monkeypox virus may be controlled by quarantining (at least for 6 weeks from the date of last exposure) the infected animals and tracing their contacts. Adherence to specific instructions from the local and global public health authorities is mandatory. Increasing awareness and action (adequate decisions, medical staff, sampling, surveillance, education) both by local and international authorities are of central importance.

At hospitals in developed countries, when suspecting a case of monkeypox (eg, a patient with fever, skin lesions, and history of visiting endemic area or contact with patients), the patient should immediately be placed in a negative air pressure isolation room, or a private room if such facilities are unavailable. Standard, contact, and droplet precautions should all be taken. Infection control personnel should be contacted without delay. In developed countries, likewise, increasing awareness among health care personnel about the disease and its endemic areas is an important precaution.

VACCINES AGAINST MONKEYPOX

Although new vaccines are being developed for monkeypox, there is a need for conducting controlled clinical trials to evaluate the impact of the use of smallpox vaccines for prevention of monkeypox or modifying disease severity. Studies should focus on the cost/benefit of population-level vaccination and investigation of alternative vaccination strategies such as targeting vaccination to affected areas, contacts, and health care workers, and wider geographic areas. Currently the CDC recommends pre-exposure smallpox vaccination for field investigators, veterinarians, animal control personnel, contacts of monkeypox patients, researchers, and health care workers caring for such patients and their contacts.[3]

Can the Smallpox Vaccine Available Be Used to Protect Against Monkeypox?

Percutaneous inoculation with vaccinia virus elicits a broad and heterogeneous serum antibody response targeting a large number of antigenic determinants of vaccinia virus.[73,74] The viral inhibitory activity of serum from immune subjects with cross-neutralizing activity to vaccinia virus, MPXV, and VARV is presumably composed of antibodies with diverse specificities.[75–77]

Production of first-generation live attenuated vaccine has been reviewed by the WHO in 1988.[9] A considerable proportion of the population may have contraindications for the vaccine candidates: 15.2% to 15.8% of the United States population has been estimated to have potential contraindications for taking the live attenuated smallpox vaccine.[78]

The rates of side effects associated with the live attenuated vaccinia virus in the United States in 1968 were 74 complications and 1 death per 1 million primary vaccinations. Morbidity and mortality rates were highest for infants, with 112 complications and 5 deaths per million primary vaccinations.[79] In 2002, the US Department of Defense resumed a program for widespread smallpox vaccinations because of a perceived threat of biological warfare. A total of 540,824 military personnel were vaccinated with a New York City Board of Health (NYCBH) strain of vaccinia, "DryVax," from December 2002 through December 2003. Dryvax was produced by infecting the skin of calves using the NYCBH strain as seed virus. Of these, 67 (1 in 8000) developed myopericarditis.[80,81]

The highest rate of postvaccine encephalitis (pvE) was found with the Bern strain (44.9 expected cases per million vaccines), followed by the Copenhagen strain (33.3 per million vaccines), the Lister strain (26.2 per million vaccines), and the NYCBH strain with the lowest rate (2.9 per million vaccinations).[82]

ADDRESSING GAPS IN KNOWLEDGE AND STRENGTHENING PUBLIC HEALTH PREPAREDNESS

Most data available on monkeypox are obtained from individual case or outbreak reports, and from passive intermittent surveillance, none of which convey an accurate overall picture. The current major gaps in monkeypox knowledge, the changing epidemiologic and clinical presentations, and the multifarious factors involved in monkeypox transmission argue the need to strengthen outbreak preparedness efforts. There remains an urgent need for developing public health and surveillance capacities in Central and West Africa to guide appropriate surveillance, data collection, prevention, preparedness, and response activities to monkeypox and other emerging and reemerging infections with epidemic potential. Advancing public health preparedness and aligning proactive surveillance activities to priority research will require coordinated, locally led, multidisciplinary efforts adjusted closely to capacity development and training.

SUMMARY

The spread of monkeypox across West Africa over the past decade and the ongoing outbreak in Nigeria indicates that it is no longer "a rare viral zoonotic disease that occurs primarily in remote parts of Central and West Africa, near tropical rainforests." Its potential for further spread both regionally and internationally remains a major concern.[28,29] The ecologic, zoonotic, epidemiologic, clinical, and public health aspects of monkeypox remain inadequately characterized.[33,36,44,45] The first-generation live attenuated vaccinia virus vaccines stored for emergency purposes in many countries cannot be used because of severe adverse reactions. Discontinuing the smallpox vaccination program has created an ecologic gap whereby an increasing proportion of the population has either waning or nonexistent immunity to MPXV. This development will further increase the risk of both the animal-to-human and human-to-human spread of the virus. Therefore, priority research and surveillance should urgently be conducted through a joint "One-Human-Animal-Environmental Health" effort across Central and West Africa.[83–85]

ACKNOWLEDGMENTS

The authors thank the NCDC staff for providing the clinical photographs from the ongoing 2019 monkeypox outbreak in Nigeria, and the patients who gave permission to have the photos taken.

REFERENCES

1. WHO. Human monkeypox 2019. Available at: https://www.who.int/emergencies/diseases/monkeypox/en/. Accessed February 22, 2019.
2. WHO. Smallpox 2019. Available at: https://www.who.int/biologicals/vaccines/smallpox/en/. Accessed February 20, 2019.
3. CDC. Monkeypox. MMWR Morb Mortal Wkly Rep 2018;67:306–10.
4. Shchelkunov SN, Totmenin AV, Babkin IV, et al. Human monkeypox and smallpox viruses: genomic comparison. FEBS Lett 2001;509:66–70.
5. Pauli G, Blümel J, Burger R, et al. Orthopox viruses: infections in humans. Transfus Med Hemother 2010;37:351–64.
6. Bera BC, Shanmugasundaram K, Barua S, et al. Zoonotic cases of camelpox infection in India. Vet Microbiol 2011;152:29–38.
7. Cook GC, Zumla A. Chapter 47. Cutaneous viral diseases. Monkeypox. In: Cook GC, Zumla A, editors. Manson's tropical diseases. 22nd edition. London: Harcourt Brace Saunders, Publishing Group; 2009. p. 839–40.
8. Petersen E, Abubakar I, Ihekweazu C, et al. Monkeypox—Enhancing public health preparedness for an emerging lethal human zoonotic epidemic threat in the wake of the smallpox post-eradication era. Int J Infect Dis 2019;78:78–84.
9. Fenner F, Henderson DA, Arita I, et al. Smallpox and its eradication. Geneva (Switzerland): World Health Organisation; 1988.
10. Singh RK, Hosamani M, Balamurugan V, et al. Buffalopox: an emerging and re-emerging zoonosis. Anim Health Res Rev 2007;8:105–14.
11. Oliveira JS, Figueiredo PO, Costa GB, et al. Vaccinia virus natural infections in Brazil: the good, the bad, and the ugly. Viruses 2017;9(11) [pii:E340].
12. Hughes AL, Irausquin S, Friedman R. The evolutionary biology of poxviruses. Infect Genet Evol 2010;10:50–9.
13. Ichihashi Y, Oie M. Epitope mosaic on the surface proteins of orthopoxviruses. Virology 1988;163:133–44.
14. Stanford MM, McFadden G, Karupiah G, et al. Immunopathogenesis of poxvirus infections: forecasting the impending storm. Immunol Cell Biol 2007;85:93–102.
15. McConnell S, Herman YF, Mattson DE, et al. Protection of rhesus monkeys against monkeypox by vaccinia virus immunization. Am J Vet Res 1964;25:192–5.
16. Hammarlund E, Lewis MW, Carter SV, et al. Multiple diagnostic techniques identify previously vaccinated individuals with protective immunity against monkeypox. Nat Med 2005;11:1005–11.
17. Moss B. Smallpox vaccines: targets of protective immunity. Immunol Rev 2011; 239:8–26.
18. Gispen R, Verlinde JD, Zwart P. Histopathological and virological studies on monkeypox. Arch Gesamte Virusforsch 1967;21:205–16.
19. McConnell S, Hickman RL, Wooding WL Jr, et al. Monkeypox: experimental infection in chimpanzee (*Pan satyrus*) and immunization with vaccinia virus. Am J Vet Res 1968;29:1675–80.

20. von Magnus P, Anderson EK, Petersen KB, et al. A pox-like disease in cynomolgus monkeys. Acta Pathol Microbiol Scand 1959;46:156–76.
21. Doty JB, Malekani JM, Kalemba LN, et al. Assessing monkeypox virus prevalence in small mammals at the human-animal interface in the democratic Republic of the Congo. Viruses 2017;9(10) [pii:E283].
22. Radonić A, Metzger S, Dabrowski PW, et al. Fatal monkeypox in wild-living sooty mangabey, Côte d'Ivoire, 2012. Emerg Infect Dis 2014;20:1009–11.
23. Hutson CL, Lee KN, Abel J, et al. Monkeypox zoonotic associations: insights from laboratory evaluation of animals associated with the multi-state US outbreak. Am J Trop Med Hyg 2007;76:757–68.
24. Thomassen HA, Fuller T, Asefi-Najafabady S, et al. Pathogen-host associations and predicted range shifts of human monkeypox in response to climate change in central Africa. PLoS One 2013;8:e66071.
25. Prier JE, Sauer RM. A pox disease of monkeys. Ann N Y Acad Sci 1960;85:951–9.
26. Wenner HA, Macasaet D, Kamitsuka PS, et al. Monkeypox I. Clinical, virologic and immunologic studies. Am J Epidemiol 1968;87:551–66.
27. Nakoune E, Lampaert E, Ndjapou SG, et al. A nosocomial outbreak of human monkeypox in the Central African Republic. Open Forum Infect Dis 2017;4: ofx168.
28. Durski KN, McCollum AM, Nakazawa Y, et al. Emergence of monkeypox—West and Central Africa, 1970-2017. MMWR Morb Mortal Wkly Rep 2018;67:306–10.
29. Sklenovská N, Van Ranst M. Emergence of monkeypox as the most important orthopoxvirus infection in humans. Front Public Health 2018;6:241.
30. Quiner CA, Moses C, Monroe BP, et al. Presumptive risk factors for monkeypox in rural communities in the Democratic Republic of the Congo. PLoS One 2017;12: e0168664.
31. Marennikova SS, Seluhina EM, Malceva NN, et al. Isolation and properties of the causal agent of a new variola-like disease (monkeypox) in man. Bull World Health Organ 1972;46:599–611.
32. Fine PE, Jezek Z, Grab B, et al. The transmission potential of monkeypox virus in human populations. Int J Epidemiol 1988;17:643–50.
33. Heymann DL, Szczeniowski M, Esteves K. Reemergence of monkeypox in Africa: a review of the past six years. Br Med Bull 1998;54:693–702.
34. Breman JG, Kalisa R, Steniowski MV, et al. Human monkeypox, 1970-79. Bull World Health Organ 1980;58:165–82.
35. WHO. 1980 the global eradication of smallpox: final report of the Global Commission for the Certification of Smallpox Eradication. Geneva (Switzerland): World Health Organization; 1980.
36. WHO. Human monkeypox (MPX) 2018. Available at: http://www.who.int/emergencies/diseases/monkeypox/en/. Accessed February 22, 2019.
37. Hutin YJ, Williams RJ, Malfait P, et al. Outbreak of human monkeypox, Democratic Republic of Congo, 1996 to 1997. Emerg Infect Dis 2001;7:434.
38. Learned LA, Reynolds MG, Wassa DW, et al. Extended interhuman transmission of monkeypox in a hospital community in the Republic of the Congo, 2003. Am J Trop Med Hyg 2005;73:428–34.
39. Reynolds MG, Emerson GL, Pukuta E, et al. Detection of human monkeypox in the Republic of the Congo following intensive community education. Am J Trop Med Hyg 2013;88:982–5.
40. Khodakevich L, Widy-Wirski R, Arita I, et al. Monkey pox virus infection in humans in the Central African Republic. Bull Soc Pathol Exot Filiales 1985;78: 311–20.

41. Rimoin AW, Kisalu N, Kebela-Ilunga B, et al. Endemic human monkeypox, Democratic Republic of Congo, 2001-2004. Emerg Infect Dis 2007;13:934–7.

42. Rimoin AW, Mulembakani PM, Johnston SC, et al. Major increase in human monkeypox incidence 30 years after smallpox vaccination campaigns cease in the Democratic Republic of Congo. Proc Natl Acad Sci U S A 2010;107: 16262–7.

43. Kantele A, Chickering K, Vapalahti O, et al. Emerging diseases—the monkeypox epidemic in the Democratic Republic of the Congo. Clin Microbiol Infect 2016;22: 658–9.

44. Hoff NA, Doshi RH, Colwell B, et al. Evolution of a disease surveillance system: an increase in reporting of human monkeypox disease in the Democratic Republic of the Congo, 2001-2013. Int J Trop Dis Health 2017;25 [pii:IJTDH.35885].

45. Yinka-Ogunleye A, Aruna O, Ogoina D, et al. Reemergence of human Monkeypox in Nigeria, 2017. Emerg Infect Dis 2018;24:1149–51.

46. Jezek Z, Fenner F. Human monkeypox. Monographs in virology, vol. 17. Basel (Switzerland): Karger; 1988. p. 49. Tabel 7.

47. Formenty P, Muntasir MO, Damon I, et al. Human monkeypox outbreak cause by novel virus belonging to Congo Basin clade, Sudan, 2005. Emerg Infect Dis 2010; 16:1539–45.

48. Centers for Disease Control and Prevention (CDC). Update: multistate outbreak of monkeypox–Illinois, Indiana, Kansas, Missouri, Ohio, and Wisconsin, 2003. MMWR Morb Mortal Wkly Rep 2003;52(27):642–6.

49. Centers for Disease Control and Prevention (CDC). Update: multistate outbreak of monkeypox–Illinois, Indiana, Kansas, Missouri, Ohio, and Wisconsin, 2003. MMWR Morb Mortal Wkly Rep 2003;52(25):589–90.

50. CDC, Centers for Disease Control and Prevention. Monkeypox in the United States. 2003 Outbreak. Available at: https://www.cdc.gov/poxvirus/monkeypox/outbreak.html. Accessed February 22, 2019.

51. Public Health England. Cases of monkeypox confirmed in England. Available at: https://www.gov.uk/government/news/monkeypox-case-in-england. Accessed March 28, 2019.

52. Vaughan A, Aarons E, Astbury J, et al. Two cases of monkeypox imported to the United Kingdom, September 2018. Euro Surveill 2018;23(38). https://doi.org/10.2807/1560-7917.

53. Jezek Z, Arita I, Mutombo M, et al. Four generations of probable person-to-person transmission of human monkeypox. Am J Epidemiol 1986;123:1004–12.

54. Kalthan E, Tenguere J, Ndjapou SG, et al. Investigation of an outbreak of monkeypox in an area occupied by armed groups, Central African Republic. Med Mal Infect 2018;48:263–8.

55. Ministry of Health, State of Israel. Monkeypox patient diagnosed. Available at: https://www.health.gov.il/English/News_and_Events/Spokespersons_Messages/Pages/12102018_1.aspx. Accessed February 19, 2019.

56. WHO. Human monkeypox in Nigeria 2018. Available at: https://www.who.int/csr/don/05-october-2018-monkeypox-nigeria/en/. Accessed February 22, 2019.

57. Eteng WE, Mandra A, Doty J, et al. Notes from the field: responding to an outbreak of monkeypox using the one health approach—Nigeria, 2017-2018. MMWR Morb Mortal Wkly Rep 2018;67:1040–1.

58. Nigeria CDC. An update of monkeypox outbreak in Nigeria 2018. Available at: https://ncdc.gov.ng/diseases/sitreps/?cat=8&name=An%20Update%20of%20Monkeypox%20Outbreak%20in%20Nigeria. Accessed February 22, 2019.

59. Nigeria CDC. Monkeypox 2019. Available at: https://ncdc.gov.ng/diseases/sitreps/?cat=8&name=An%20Update%20of%20Monkeypox%20Outbreak%20in%20Nigeria. Accessed February 22, 2019.

60. Faye O, Pratt CB, Faye M, et al. Genomic characterisation of human monkeypox virus in Nigeria. Lancet Infect Dis 2018;18:246.

61. Jezek Z, Grab B, Szczeniowski MV, et al. Human monkeypox: secondary attack rates. Bull World Health Organ 1988;66:465–70.

62. Jezek Z, Grab B, Dixon H. Stochastic model for interhuman spread of monkeypox. Am J Epidemiol 1987;126:1082–92.

63. Jezek Z, Szczeniowski M, Paluku KM, et al. Human monkeypox: clinical features of 282 patients. J Infect Dis 1987;156:293–8.

64. Nolen LD, Osadebe L, Katomba J, et al. Extended human-to-human transmission during a monkeypox outbreak in the Democratic Republic of the Congo. Emerg Infect Dis 2016;22:1014–21.

65. Jezek Z, Szczeniowski M, Paluku KM, et al. Human monkeypox: confusion with chickenpox. Acta Trop 1988;45:297–307.

66. Di Giulio DB, Eckburg PB. Human monkeypox: an emerging zoonosis. Lancet 2004;4:15–25.

67. Gordon SN, Cecchinato V, Andresen V, et al. Smallpox vaccine safety is dependent on T cells and not B cells. J Infect Dis 2011;203:1043–53.

68. Huhn GD, Bauer AM, Yorita K, et al. Clinical characteristics of human monkeypox, and risk factors for severe disease. Clin Infect Dis 2005;41:1742–51.

69. Damon IK. Status of human monkeypox: clinical disease, epidemiology and research. Vaccine 2011;29(Suppl 4):D54–9.

70. McCollum AM, Damon IK. Human monkeypox. Clin Infect Dis 2014;58:260–7.

71. Osadebe L, Hughes CM, Shongo Lushima R, et al. Enhancing case definitions for surveillance of human monkeypox in the Democratic Republic of Congo. PLoS Negl Trop Dis 2017;11:e0005857.

72. WHO. The current status of human monkeypox: memorandum from a WHO Meeting. Bull World Health Organ 1984;62:703–13.

73. Davies DH, Liang X, Hernandez JE al. Profiling the humoral immune response to infection by using proteome microarrays: high-throughput vaccine and diagnostic antigen discovery. Proc Natl Acad Sci U S A 2005;102:547–52.

74. Davies DH, Molina DM, Wrammert, et al. Proteome-wide analysis of the serological response to vaccinia and smallpox. Proteomics 2007;7:1678–86.

75. Hughes CM, Newman FK, Davidson WB, et al. Analysis of variola and vaccinia virus neutralization assays for smallpox vaccines. Clin Vaccine Immunol 2012; 19:1116–8.

76. Kennedy JS, Gurwith M, Dekker CL, et al. Safety and immunogenicity of LC16m8, an attenuated smallpox vaccine in vaccinia-naive adults. J Infect Dis 2011;204: 1395–402.

77. Gilchuk I, Gilchuk P, Sapparapu G, et al. Cross-neutralizing and protective human antibody specificities to poxvirus infections. Cell 2016;167:684–94.

78. Carlin EP, Giller N, Katz R. Estimating the size of the U.S. population at risk of severe adverse events from replicating smallpox vaccine. Public Health Nurs 2017; 34:200–9.

79. Lane JM, Ruben FL, Neff JM, et al. Complications of smallpox vaccination, 1968. N Engl J Med 1969;281:1201–8.

80. Eckart RE, Love SS, Atwood JE, et al, Department of Defense Smallpox Vaccination Clinical Evaluation Team. Incidence and follow-up of inflammatory

cardiac complications after smallpox vaccination. J Am Coll Cardiol 2004;44: 201–5.

81. Neff J, Modlin J, Birkhead GS, et al, and the Advisory Committee on Immunization. Practices; Armed Forces Epidemiological Board. Monitoring the safety of a smallpox vaccination program in the United States: report of the joint Smallpox Vaccine Safety Working Group of the advisory committee on immunization practices and the Armed Forces Epidemiological Board. Clin Infect Dis 2008; 46(Suppl 3):258–70.

82. Kretzschmar M, Walinga J, Teunis P, et al. Frequency of adverse events after vaccination with different vaccinia strains. PLoS Med 2006;3(8):e272.

83. Bass J, Tack DM, McCollum AM, et al. Enhancing health care worker ability to detect and care for patients with monkeypox in the Democratic Republic of the Congo. Int Health 2013;5:237–43.

84. Zumla A, Dar O, Kock R, et al. Taking forward a 'One Health' approach for turning the tide against the Middle East respiratory syndrome coronavirus and other zoonotic pathogens with epidemic potential. Int J Infect Dis 2016;47:5–9.

85. Doshi RH, Guagliardo SAJ, Dzabatou-Babeaux A, et al. Strengthening of surveillance during monkeypox outbreak, Republic of the Congo, 2017. Emerg Infect Dis 2018;24:1158–60.

Viral Hepatitis
Etiology, Epidemiology, Transmission, Diagnostics, Treatment, and Prevention

Simone Lanini, MD, MSc[a],[*],[1], Andrew Ustianowski, MD, PhD, FRCP[b],[1],
Raffaella Pisapia, MD[a],
Alimuddin Zumla, MBChB, MSc, PhD, MD, FRCP(Lond), FRCP(Edin), FRCPath(UK), FAAS[c],
Giuseppe Ippolito, MD, FRCP, FRCPath[d]

KEYWORDS

- Acute viral hepatitis • Chronic viral hepatitis • HAV • HBV • HCV • HDV • HEV

KEY POINTS

- Viral hepatitis owing to hepatitis A virus, hepatitis B virus, hepatitis C virus, hepatitis D virus, and hepatitis E viruses affects hundreds of millions of people globally.
- Hepatitis may present with a range of clinical features from asymptomatic, or acute with relatively rapid onset, or chronically.
- A large proportion of infected people are asymptomatic and are unaware of having an infection that can result in liver cirrhosis and liver cancer.
- Although hepatitis is associated with significant morbidity, most deaths from viral hepatitis are due to hepatitis B and hepatitis C.
- The development of new diagnostics and highly effective, pangenotypic direct-acting antivirals provide opportunities to cure and eradicate chronic hepatitis C virus infection globally.

INTRODUCTION

Viral hepatitis is a major global public health problem (**Fig. 1**) affecting hundreds of millions of people and is associated with significant morbidity and mortality (**Fig. 2**). Five biologically unrelated hepatotropic viruses cause most of the global burden

Conflicts of Interest: All authors have an interest in global public health and emerging and re-emerging infections. All authors have no other conflict of interest to declare.
[a] National Institute for Infectious Diseases, Lazzaro Spallanzani, IRCCS via Portuense 292, Rome 00149, Italy; [b] North Manchester General Hospital, Delaunays Road, Crumpsall, Manchester M8 5RB, UK; [c] Center for Clinical Microbiology, University College London, Royal Free Campus 2nd Floor, Rowland Hill Street, London NW3 2PF, UK; [d] National Institute for Infectious Diseases, Lazzaro Spallanzani, IRCCS via Portuense 292, Rome 00149, Italy
[1] Authors contributed equally.
* Corresponding author. Epidemiology and Preclinical Research Department, INMI Lazzaro Spallanzani, Via Portuense 292, Rome 00149, Italy.
E-mail address: simone.lanini@inmi.it

Infect Dis Clin N Am 33 (2019) 1045–1062
https://doi.org/10.1016/j.idc.2019.08.004
0891-5520/19/© 2019 Elsevier Inc. All rights reserved.
id.theclinics.com

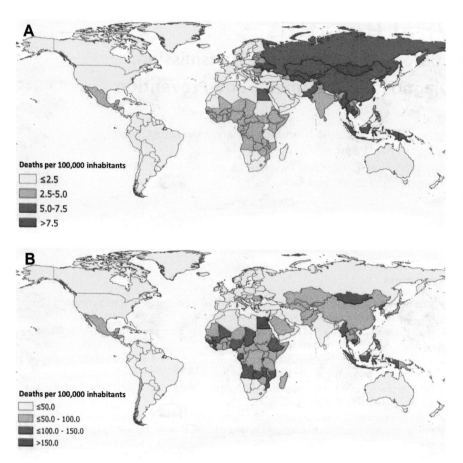

Fig. 1. Global distribution of deaths owing to viral hepatitis. The Global Burden of Disease Study estimates that in 2017 viral hepatitis has caused about 1.4 million deaths (range, 1.2–1.6; see **Fig. 2**). This analysis reports the number of deaths per 100,000 inhabitants owing to viral hepatitis in 196 territories worldwide for 2017 (fatality rate) for (*A*) people aged less than 50 years and (*B*) people aged 50 years or more. The burden of viral hepatitis is the heaviest among older adults as the consequence of late sequalae of chronic infections and severe presentation of acute viral hepatitis. Asia, Egypt, and Sub-Saharan Africa are the geographic areas where viral hepatitis took most life in 2017. Fatalities for viral hepatitis in Italy and Japan were still relatively high among older people owing historical issues. In contrast, Russia and Eastern European countries experienced a relatively high number of fatalities among young people; this phenomenon is alarming and potentially associated with the surging number of new infections reported in these areas since the early 1990s. (*Data from*: Estimates: Global Burden of Disease Collaborative Network. Global Burden of Disease Study 2017 (GBD 2017) Results. Seattle, United States: Institute for Health Metrics and Evaluation (IHME), 2018. Available from http://ghdx.healthdata.org/gbd-results-tool. Maps: Esri, HERE, Garmin, Intermap, increment P Corp., GEBCO, USGS, FAO, NPS, NRCAN, GeoBase, IGN, Kadaster NL, Ordnance Survey, Esri Japan, METI, Esri China (Hong Kong), swisstopo, © OpenStreetMap contributors, and the GIS User Community.)

of viral hepatitis: hepatitis A virus (HAV), hepatitis B virus (HBV), hepatitis C viruses (HCV), hepatitis D (delta) virus (HDV), and hepatitis E viruses (HEV). HBV, HCV, HDV, and occasionally HEV can also produce chronic infections, whereas HAV does not. HBV and HCV are associated with significant chronic morbidity. Most

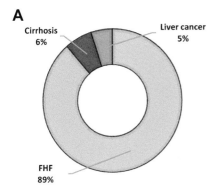

A

Cirrhosis 6% Liver cancer 5% FHF 89%

Clinical condition	GBD estimates (2017)		
	Deaths	Range	
HAV FHF	9,323	6,139	12,841
HEV FHF	1,427	893	2,094
HBV FHF	7,188	4,250	10,358
HBV cirrhosis	1,052	786	1,385
HBV liver cancer	1,085	973	1,217
HCV FHF	2,162	1,095	3,788
HCV cirrhosis	401	291	542
HCV liver cancer	38	28	49
Overall deaths	22,676	14,455	32,274

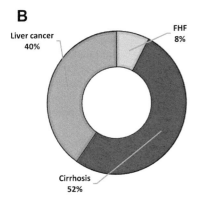

B

Liver cancer 40% FHF 8% Cirrhosis 52%

Clinical condition	GBD estimates (2017)		
	Deaths	Range	
HAV FHF	9,319	5,933	13,400
HEV FHF	13,259	8257	19,855
HBV FHF	82,402	60,576	95,638
HBV cirrhosis	382,919	333888	447,536
HBV liver cancer	324,362	298743	353,462
HCV FHF	1,311	504	2,889
HCV cirrhosis	341842	298785	394852
HCV liver cancer	234298	213763	255745
Overall deaths	1,389,712	1,220,449	1,583,377

Fig. 2. Global number of deaths associated with viral hepatitis according to clinical conditions. (*A*) people aged less than 50 years and (*B*) people aged 50 years or more. (*Data from* Global Burden of Disease Collaborative Network. Global Burden of Disease Study 2017 (GBD 2017) Results. Seattle, United States: Institute for Health Metrics and Evaluation (IHME), 2018. Available from http://ghdx.healthdata.org/gbd-results-tool.)

deaths from viral hepatitis are due to hepatitis B and hepatitis C. Globally, an estimated 257 million people were living with HBV and 71 million people were living with HCV. The first global hepatitis report[1,2] published in 2017 indicated that 1.4 million persons died in 2015 from the consequences of viral hepatitis infection. More than 90% of this burden was due to cirrhosis and hepatocellular carcinoma (HCC), which are consequences of chronic hepatitis B (CHB) and chronic hepatitis C (CHC) infection. In 2015, the United Nations adopted a resolution calling for specific action to combat viral hepatitis as part of the Agenda for Achieving Sustainable Development Goals 2030, followed with the World Health Organization's first global elimination strategy for viral hepatitis in 2016.[3]

We review the epidemiology, biology, clinical features, treatment, and prevention of viral hepatitis. We also review new agents for treatment of hepatitis C allowing the conceptual framework permitting the development of elimination programs, and the rich pipeline of potential new therapies for HBV and HDV that may allow cure in future years. Recent outbreaks of HAV and HEV and the increasing recognition of atypical presentations are highlighted.

VIRAL HEPATITIS A
Virology and Pathogenesis

HAV is single strain positive sense RNA virus belonging to *Hepatovirus* genus[4] and consists of 6 genotypes. Genotypes I to III infect humans.[5] HAV is present in the host in 2 forms: naked virions (shed in the feces) and quasi-enveloped virions (that circulate in the blood). Both forms are infectious and the synthetic genome length RNA is infectious itself.[5] HAV does not have a significant direct cytopathic effect and most liver damage is due to the host immune response. Cellular immunity seems to be responsible for viral clearance after primary infection, whereas humoral response has a direct role in the prevention of infection. Deficits of cellular immune response, such as human immunodeficiency virus (HIV) infection, can produce longer shedding (and infectivity) but without an apparent increase of symptom severity.[6,7]

Natural History

HAV causes an acute self-limiting hepatitis that normally resolves spontaneously. The average incubation period is between 2 and 4 weeks (but can be up $\leq$8 weeks).[8] Clinical manifestations are characterized by the appearance of dark urine and sometimes clay-colored stool, often accompanied or followed by jaundice.[9] The proportion of asymptomatic infections range between 30% in adults up to 90% in children under the age of 5 years.[5,8] Fulminant hepatic failure (FHF) is rare, and occurs more frequently among people older than 50 years and those with liver comorbidities. FHF is due to an excessive host response, associated with a reduction in viral load but a marked increase in the international normalized ratio, bilirubin, and alanine aminotransferase.[5,6] Several studies suggested that HAV superinfection may lead to clearance of HBV and HCV chronic hepatitis.[5] Relapse of acute hepatitis A occurs in 3% to 20% of cases and prolonged or persistent cholestasis after infection, although HAV is not associated with chronic infection. Rarely, HAV has extrahepatic manifestations such as pancreatitis, rash, acute kidney injury with interstitial nephritis or glomerular nephritis, pneumonitis, pericarditis, hemolysis, acute cholecystitis, mononeuritis, Guillain-Barre syndrome, encephalitis, and central myelitis. HAV infection can precipitate autoimmune hepatitis.

Global Epidemiology and Transmission Route

HAV infects between 1 and 2 million people annually.[10] Mortality rates are low at 0.3%.[5,6,11] HAV is a human infection transmitted by the feco-oral route via contaminated food and water and oro-anal sex.[12,13] In high endemic areas with poor sanitation, HAV is mainly a waterborne infection. In these settings 90% or more of the population have anti-HAV IgG by the age of 10 years; thus, large epidemics are paradoxically infrequent because most people contract Acute hepatitis A (AHA) during childhood as asymptomatic infection or have mild infection.[14] In intermediate endemic areas, HAV is mainly transmitted through contaminated food and water. These areas include countries with transitional economies or geographic settings. In these areas the prevalence of anti-HAV IgG is 50% or greater by age 30 but less than 50% at the age of 15 years. The wide circulation of HAV causes large-scale outbreaks.[14-16] In low endemic areas, HAV infections are associated with travel to high endemic areas and with oro-anal sex. Infection rates are very low and fewer than 50% of people older than 30 are immune to HAV.[14] Owing to the heterogeneity of transmission modes,[14] AHA may occur as sporadic cases in travelers,[17] small epidemic clusters,[8,16] and large epidemics associated with special alimentary habits,[18] sexual behaviors,[19] or special populations.[20] HAV vaccination in low and intermediate endemic settings is shifting the age to a disease of adults rather than early childhood.[21] Foodborne outbreaks are becoming more frequent in high-income countries and among the HIV-infected population, men who have sex with men,[22] the homeless, and intravenous drug users.[23]

Diagnosis

Serology remains the gold standard for diagnosis of AHA. Anti-HAV IgM is recommended for new infection and can be detected at the same time as symptom onset. Anti-HAV IgG represent past infection and generally persists for life. Detection of HAV RNA, and analysis of clinical viral variant, may be useful for the molecular investigation of epidemic clusters.[5,8] HAV RNA is present in blood and feces soon after infection (while an individual is asymptomatic) until 1 to 2 weeks after the onset of symptoms. Longer shedding in feces can occur in children and those infected with HIV. HAV is also shed in saliva and urine, but no assays are available to detect this.[24]

Treatment and Prevention

There is no specific therapy for hepatitis A. The majority of cases require no specific treatment.[11] Liver transplantation is an option in the rare cases of FHF. Pre-exposure prophylaxis can prevent HAV infection. Two types of HAV vaccines are currently available: formaldehyde-inactivated vaccines and live attenuated vaccines (available only in China and India).[14,25] Traditionally, a 2-dose schedule is recommended but, in healthy individuals, a high level of immunity can be also achieved with a single dose.[14,22,23] Inactivated HAV vaccine is also available in combination with typhoid vaccine or HBV vaccine (3 doses). Serologic response to the inactivated vaccine may be diminished in those infected with HIV[26] and in older adults.[27] Targeted vaccination might be the most cost-effective intervention in low endemic areas,[14,28] universal vaccination campaigns are most helpful in intermediate endemic areas.[29] In high HAV endemic settings, universal vaccine campaigns should be implemented along with improving sanitation and provision of safe drinking water. Suboptimal vaccine campaigns can lead to an increment of the age of exposure with an increased incidence of severe clinical presentations.[5,8,14,16,18] Postexposure prophylaxis with either inactivated vaccine or specific anti-HAV IgG is effective when administered within 2 weeks of exposure. The inactivated vaccine is noninferior to specific anti-HAV IgG, and confers long-lasting immunity.[30]

VIRAL HEPATITIS B
Virology

HBV is an enveloped, partially double-stranded DNA virus belonging to *Orthohepadnavirus* genus. It is classified in into 10 genotypes (A–J).[31] The genome consists of 3020 to 3320 nucleotides (for the full-length strand) and 1700 to 2800 nucleotides (for the short length strand). It contains 4 genes that encode for 5 main proteins, including the polymerase (gene P); hepatitis B core protein on gene C, hepatitis B envelope antigen created by a different splicing of gene C (HBeAg); hepatitis B surface antigen on gene S (HBeAg), and a replication cofactor on gene X.[32] The HBV genome exists in different forms in infected individuals. The Dane particles are the infective enveloped visions. The covalently closed circular DNA episomial nucleic acid moieties in the nucleus (5–50 molecules per infected cell) serve as an intranuclear transcriptional template for the synthesis of viral RNAs. Finally, HBV may also exist as proviral DNA integrated in the nucleus (which has roles in the pathogenesis of chronic infection and oncogenesis).[33]

Natural History

Acute hepatitis B occurs 45 to 180 days after exposure to HBV. The rate of symptomatic infection is associated with age, being less than 10% in children and about 50% in adults. FHF is rare, occurring in up to 1% to 4% of cases depending of patient's clinical background.[34] HBV may persist after acute infection and produce CHB infection, which is inversely associated with age, that is, more than 90% in infants and less than 10% in those who develop acute hepatitis B in adulthood. The natural history of CHB is schematically divided into 5 phases.[35]

1. HBeAg-positive chronic infection is a long period of asymptomatic infection that is frequent among young patients and especially those perinatally infected. This phase is characterized by high viral replication (HBeAg and HBsAg positivity with high HBV DNA levels) and minimal (if any) liver damage.
2. HBeAg positive chronic hepatitis may immediately follow an acute infection or may start after several decades of chronic infection. This phase is characterized by sustained viral replication (HBeAg and HBsAg positivity with high HBV DNA levels) and significant liver damage.
3. HBeAg-negative chronic infection follows the loss of HBeAg and is characterized by suppression of viral replication with minimal on-going liver inflammation (HBV DNA levels of <2000 U/L and normal plasma transaminases). This phase is associated with a low risk of liver disease progression.
4. HBeAg-negative chronic hepatitis may directly follow an acute hepatitis or start after decades of chronic HBeAg positive infection. This phase is characterized by the absence of HBeAg and persistent viral replication and liver damage (HBV DNA levels of >2000 U/L and increased plasma transaminase levels).
5. HBsAg-negative phase is characterized by negative serum HBsAg and positive antibodies to hepatitis B core antigen, with or without detectable antibodies to HBsAg. If HBsAg loss has occurred before the onset of cirrhosis, a minimal risk of liver disease progression occurs. However, this phase can be associated with positive viremia, known as occult HBV infection. HBV DNA can integrate into the hepatocyte genome, and all patients with CHB are at risk of HCC, regardless the level of liver damage.

Global Epidemiology and Transmission Route

HBV only causes disease in humans. It is transmitted through sexual contact, via blood, and vertically from mother to child. HBV infectivity is very high. HBV genotypes are congruent with distinct geographic distribution and mode of transmission. Genotype A is frequent in Africa, North America, and western European countries. It is more common among those with sexually acquired infection and it is associated with high rates of HCC. Genotypes B and C are common in Asia, where they are associated with perinatal infection. Genotype D predominates in the Mediterranean basin, Middle East, and Central Asia; it has been historically associated with HBeAg-negative cirrhosis and HCC. Genotype E is an African genotype and has been correlated with high rates of HBeAg positivity and perinatal transmission. Genotype F is associated with high rates of HCC in South America and the Arctic Circle. Genotype H has not been well-studied, and genotype G is usually found in a recombinant form, mostly with genotype A. Genotype I has recently been reported in Vietnam and Laos. The latest HBV genotype J has been identified in the Ryukyu Islands in Japan.[36]

Diagnosis

HBsAg is the primary marker of active disease. Hepatitis B core antigen antibodies reflect virus exposure with either active or resolved natural infection. HBeAg reflects active viral replication. Antibodies to HBsAg represent the marker of immunity in vaccinated people and or resolved infection after natural exposure. Quantification of HBV DNA in blood is recommended for monitoring therapy and for diagnosis of occult hepatitis. Increased alanine transaminase levels indicate active liver inflammation.

Treatment and Prevention

A rich pipeline of novel therapies are shown in **Table 1**. These range from therapeutic vaccinations and other strategies to adapt the immune response (eg, check-point inhibitors), to agents that directly target steps in the virus life cycle (for instance, entry inhibitors, capsid inhibitors), therapies to decrease surface antigen production and release, and therapies that target the HBV nucleic acid (such as small interfering RNA). It is probable that a combination of such new therapies will be needed to induce long-term off-treatment viral control, HBsAg loss, or loss of covalently closed circular DNA.

The main goals of antiviral therapy are sustained suppression of HBV replication and hepatic inflammation, thereby decreasing progression to cirrhosis and HCC. Severe acute hepatitis B, characterized by coagulopathy or a protracted course, can be treated with nucleos(t)ide analogues. Patients should be considered for liver transplantation in the case of FHF. Long-term administration of nucleos(t)ide analogues with high barrier to resistance (ie, entecavir, tenofovir disoproxil, or tenofovir alafenamide) represents the treatment of choice for patients with CHB.[37] Pegylated interferon-alfa treatment can also be considered in mild to moderate CHB. Therapy is indicated if there is evidence of significant HBV replication and elevated plasma transaminases, or significant hepatic fibrosis (all cirrhotic patients with detectable HBV DNA should be treated). Other indications for HBV therapy include the prevention of mother to child transmission in pregnant women with high viremia and the prevention of HBV reactivation and flares in patients requiring immunosuppression and chemotherapy.[36]

Universal vaccination of children (using the recombinant anti-HBV vaccine) is the most effective intervention to control HBV globally. Perinatal vaccination of infants born to mothers with HBV, catch-up vaccination programs, sterile medical and other equipment, safe sexual practice and mitigation measures for persons who inject drugs should be included in hepatitis control programs.[38] Pharmacologic treatment of HBV infection with nucleos(t)ide analogues or interferon may be indicated but has only a low impact as a public health intervention (with rates of clearance of <3%).[37]

Hepatitis D Virus Coinfection

HDV is a defective virus (virusoid) that can replicate only in persons with HBV infection. HDV can be transmitted either via simultaneous infection with HBV (coinfection) or via infection superimposed on CHB (superinfection). It is estimated that globally about 5% to 10% of patients with CHB are coinfected with HDV with higher prevalence in persons who inject drugs populations[39] High-prevalence areas include the Mediterranean basin, Middle East, Indian Subcontinent, Japan, Taiwan, Greenland, the Horn of Africa, West Africa, the Amazon Basin, and certain areas of the Pacific. HDV epidemiology and potential intervention for control are the same of HBV.[40]

Table 1
Current clinical pipeline and therapies for HBV and HDV

	Phase 1	Phase 2	Phase 3	Licensed in US/Europe
Hepatitis B pipeline and current therapies				
Life-cycle target				
Nucleos(t)ide analogues		CMX 157		Adefovir Entecavir Lamivudine Telbivudine Tenofovir Disoproxil Fumarate Tenofovir Alafenamide
Small interfering RNA based	AB-729 DCR-HBVS	ARB-1467 ARO-HBV RG6004 Vir-2218		
Entry inhibitor		Myrcludex B		
Capsid inhibitor	AB-423 AB-506 ABI-H2158 QL-007 RG7907	ABI-H0731 JNJ 56136379 Morphothiadin		
HBsAg inhibitors		REP 2139 REP 2165		
Antisense molecules		GSK3228836 GSK33389404		
Immune system targeting				
Interferons				Interferon alfa-2a Interferon alfa-2b
Therapeutic vaccines	AIC 649 HB-110 HepTcell INO-1800 TG1050			
Innate immune activators	GS9688 RG7854 S9688	Inarigivir RG7795		
Apoptosis inducers	APG-1387			
Anti-sAg antibodies		GC1102		
Farnesoid X receptor agonist	EYP001			
HDV pipeline and current therapies				
Varied		Ezetimibe Myrcludex B Lonafarnib REP 2139 REP 2165	Interferon-lambda	Interferon alfa-2a Interferon alfa-2b

VIRAL HEPATITIS C
Virology

HCV is an enveloped positive sense single-stranded RNA virus belonging to *Flaviviridae*. It is currently classified in into 8 genotypes (1–8).[37,41,42] The genome consists of 9600 nucleotides within a unique open reading frame (ORF) encoding for a unique polyprotein. This large preprotein is cleaved by cellular and viral proteases into the 10 viral mature proteins. Structural proteins are assembled into mature viral particles and include the core protein (C) and the 2 envelope proteins (E1 and E2) that are important for cell entry. Nonstructural (NS) proteins are essential for viral replication within the host but are not assembled into mature viral particles. The p7 protein is in the endoplasmic reticulum and plays a role in virus morphogenesis. NS2 integrates with the cellular membrane and has protease activity for viral particle maturation. NS3 is located within the endoplasmic reticulum and forms a heterodimeric complex with NS4A. NS3/NS4A complex has serine protease activity (NS3 N-terminal domain) and helicase activity (NS3 C-terminal domain). NS4B is located within the endoplasmic reticulum where it contributes to a structure known as the membranous web that plays an important role in viral particle assembly. NS5A binds to endoplasmic reticulum and plays a role in viral replication through modulation of cell signaling pathways and the interferon response. NS5B is the RNA-dependent RNA polymerase.

Natural History

Humans are the only natural host of HCV. The incubation period of HCV infection is 14 to 180 days. Only less than 15% of infected people develop acute disease. Viral clearance occurs naturally in about 15% of these, whereas the remainder develop CHC. About one-third of patients with CHC develop cirrhosis over the subsequent 30 years, especially males with coinfections and certain comorbidities[43,44] such as HBV, *Schistosomiases*, HIV, alcoholics, obesity, and insulin resistance.[45] Once cirrhosis occurs, there is a 1% to 5% annual risk of developing HCC and a 3% to 6% risk of hepatic decompensation. The development of ascites is associated with a 1-year survival of 50%, spontaneous bacterial peritonitis,[46] variceal hemorrhage,[47] hepatic encephalopathy, and the hepatorenal syndrome. CHC also induces extrahepatic metabolic and immunologic disorders.[48] HCV may have a direct role in the pathogenesis of insulin resistance and affects lipid metabolism pathways. HCV circulates in blood associated with lipoproteins forming "lipoviroparticles" and uses low-density lipoprotein receptors for hepatic cell entry. HCV affects lipid metabolism in 3 ways: (a) enhancement of lipogenesis, (b) reduction of lipoprotein degradation, and (c) impairment of lipoprotein export (liver steatosis).[49] Chronic stimulation of B cells by HCV may lead to type 2 or 3 mixed cryoglobulinemia, ischemia, kidney injury, and vasculitic syndromes. Persistent antigenic stimulation may induce malignant transformation of B cells resulting in lymphoma. HCV is epidemiologically associated with autoimmune conditions[50] such as porphyria cutanea tarda, Sjögren's syndrome, lichen planus, and inflammatory arthritis.

Epidemiology and Routes of Transmission

Hepatitis C is transmitted from person to person mainly through the bloodborne route. Modes of transmission include the use of contaminated needles in persons who inject drugs. Perinatal transmission occurs in about 3% to 10% of children born to HCV-infected mothers.[51] An increased risk of HCV through sex has been reported only for HIV-positive men who have sex with men.[3] Different genotypes have different geographic distributions.[52] Genotype in Europe and North America accounts for more than 60% of HCV infections. Genotype 2 is locally endemic to west Africa and Latin America.[53] Genotype 3 in India and Pakistan, and genotype 6 in Thailand,[54] Myanmar, Laos, and Vietnam.[55] Genotype 4 is predominant in North Africa and the Middle East and has been associated with an iatrogenic epidemic in Egypt.[56] Genotype 5 in Southern Africa occurs in up to 40% of HCV infections.[57] Genotype 7 was isolated in the Democratic Republic of Congo in 2014.[46] Genotype 8 was reported in 2018 among the Punjabi people living in Canada.[47]

Diagnostics

The diagnosis of HCV infection is carried out by a combination of serology (anti-HCV IgG) and detection of HCV RNA in blood. Anti-HCV IgG are the biomarker for lifelong contact with infection whereas HCV RNA in essential for the diagnosis of active infection. Nonprotective anti-HCV IgG may indeterminately persist after resolution of infection. HCV RNA is also crucial for monitoring response to anti-HCV therapy. Recently, HCV-Ag has been proposed as substitute of HCV RNA testing in settings with low diagnostic capability. Laboratory tests for distinguishing between acute and chronic infection require validation.[58]

Treatment and Prevention

Multiple direct-acting antivirals (DAAs) target specific steps within the HCV replication cycle, targeting specific NS proteins. Four classes of DAAs, which are defined by their mechanism of action and therapeutic target are NS proteins 3/4A (NS3/4A) protease inhibitors, NS5B nucleoside polymerase inhibitors, NS5B non-nucleoside polymerase inhibitors, and NS5A inhibitors. European[59] and North American guidelines[60] recommend therapy for CHC using combination therapy comprising 2 or 3 DAAs. Treatment duration and DAA combination may change according to stage of liver diseases, genotype, and previous failure with interferon. Infection clearance may be obtained in almost all naïve patients within 8 to 12 weeks, whereas patients with cirrhosis may require longer therapy. All HCV RNA-positive patients should be initiated as soon as possible, especially in patients with decompensated liver diseases who are not eligible for liver transplantation and those eligible for liver transplantation and a Model for End-stage Liver Disease score of less than 18. **Table 2** shows recommended interferon and ribavirin free treatment for patients with CHC. Patients with a Model for End-stage Liver Disease score of greater than 18 who are eligible for liver transplant might best be treated after transplantation.

HIV and HBV coinfected patients should be treated similarly to HCV monoinfected patients, but modification of antiretroviral therapy may be required before starting DAA treatment, and clinicians need to be alert to HBV flares associated with successful HCV treatment in HBV/HCV-coinfected individuals.[61,62] All DAAs are contraindicated in patients receiving cytochrome P450–inducing agents owing to the risk of significantly reduced concentrations of DAA. NS3/4A inhibitors are contraindicated in those with decompensated liver disease.

Resolution of CHC is associated with remission of HCV extrahepatic manifestations[54,63] and clearance of HCV may arrest progression of liver disease, and possibly revert fibrosis and hepatic decompensation.[64,65] Because clearance of chronic infection stops further transmission, anti-HCV therapy is considered to be useful in preventing further transmission.

VIRAL HEPATITIS E
Virology and Pathogenesis

HEV is a single-stranded, positive-sense RNA virus belonging to *Orthohepevirus* genus. There are 8 HEV genotypes within a unique serotype. HEV-1 and HEV-2 are human viruses, and other HEV genotypes are enzootic viruses mainly found in swine (HEV-3 to HEV-6), rodents (HEV-3 and HEV-4), and camels (HEV-7 and HEV-8). The RNA is made of 7.2 kb and contains 3 or 4 ORFs. ORF1 polyprotein contains the replication machinery of the virus, including methyltransferase, RNA helicase, and RNA-dependent RNA polymerase. ORF2 contains the capsid protein and ORF3 encodes a functional ion channel that mediates the release of infectious viral particles. HEV-1 expresses an additional ORF (ORF4) that produces a NS protein that has a role in viral replication in human cells.[61] HEV is shed in faces as a nonenveloped virus, but exists in a lipid-enveloped form in blood. The lipid envelopment is essential for immune escape and viral dissemination to different body compartments.[62] HEV is a noncytopathic virus and clinical presentations of the infection, including hepatic and extrahepatic manifestation, are determined by the host immune response.[66]

Natural History

HEV1 and HEV2 are transmitted person to person, and are generally associated with acute, self-limiting hepatitis. However, HEV1 can cause severe infection in pregnancy, where it is associated with FHF and stillbirth.[67] HEV3, HEV4, and HEV7 are associated with self-limiting hepatitis in immunocompetent hosts, although rarely this infection can progress to FHF in the elderly.[68] Infection in immunocompromised hosts results in persistent infection associated with rapid progression toward cirrhosis and liver decompensation.[61] The clinical relevance of HEV5, HEV6, and HEV8 is unclear. HEV1 and HEV3 cause a wide range of extrahepatic manifestations, including acute neurologic diseases, myositis, renal diseases, acute pancreatitis, arthritis, autoimmune thyroiditis, and myocarditis. HEV has been isolated in the cerebrospinal fluid, suggesting a potential causal link between HEV infection and neurologic diseases, including Guillain–Barré syndrome, neuralgic amyotrophy, encephalitis, and acute myelitis.[69] The immunopathologic mechanisms associated with the increased HEV virulence during pregnancy, the persistence of infection in immunocompromised hosts, and the extrahepatic manifestation are unclear. Whether humoral immunity mediated by anti-HEV IgG can protect from reinfection remains to be defined.[70,71]

Global Epidemiology and Transmission Route

HEV has received increased attention recent as an emerging infection.[72] The distribution of HEV genotypes is congruent with specific geographic areas and different modes of transmission.[73] HEV1 and HEV2 are human pathogens transmitted largely through the waterborne route causing outbreaks in poor setting in Asia,[74] Africa,[75,76] and Latin America.[77] HEV1 and HEV2 cause about 20.1 million new infections annually and 70,000 deaths.[78] HEV3, HEV4, and HEV7[79] are enzootic viruses associated with small clusters of infection among people with close contact with animals or after consumption of animal products. HEV4 can infect humans and swine and is associated with zoonotic infections in high-income Asian countries.[80] Apart from rare cases of iatrogenic transmission there is no strong evidence of direct person-to-person transmission of HEV other than genotype 1 and 2.[81]

Table 2
Recommended interferon and ribavirin treatment for patients with CHC

HCV Genotype	Type of Patient	SOF/VEL 1QD	GLE/PIB 3QD	SOF/LDV 1QD	GZR/EBR 1QD	3D[e] 2QD + 1BID
1a	Naive without cirrhosis	12	8	8[a,c]	12[b]	
	Naive with cirrhosis	12	12	12	12[b]	
	Experienced without cirrhosis	12	8		12[b]	
	Experienced with cirrhosis	12	12		12[b]	
1b	Naive without cirrhosis	12	8	8[a,c]	8[a]	8[a]
	Naive with cirrhosis	12	12	12	12	12
	Experienced without cirrhosis	12	8	12	12	12
	Experienced with cirrhosis	12	12	12	12	12
2	Naive without cirrhosis	12	8			
	Naive with cirrhosis	12	12			
	Experienced without cirrhosis	12	8			
	Experienced with cirrhosis	12	12			
3	Naive without cirrhosis	12	8			
	Naive with cirrhosis	12[d]	12			
	Experienced without cirrhosis	12	12			
	Experienced with cirrhosis	12[d]	16			
4	Naive without cirrhosis	12	8	12	12[b]	
	Naive with cirrhosis	12	12	12	12[b]	
	Experienced without cirrhosis	12	8			
	Experienced with cirrhosis	12	12			
5	Naive without cirrhosis	12	8	12		
	Naive with cirrhosis	12	12	12		
	Experienced without cirrhosis	12	8			
	Experienced with cirrhosis	12	12			
6	Naive without cirrhosis	12	8	12		
	Naive with cirrhosis	12	12	12		
	Experienced without cirrhosis	12	8			
	Experienced with cirrhosis	12	12			

Figures indicate the duration of treatment in weeks; Black square indicates that the treatment is not recommended.

Abbreviations: 1BID, 1 tablet 2 times daily; 1QD, 1 tablet 1 time daily; 2QD, 2 tablets 1 time daily; 3D, ombitasvir/paritaprevir/ritonavir/dasabuvir; GLE/PIB, glecaprevir/pibrentasvir; GZR/EBR, grazoprevir/elbasvir; SOF/LDV 1QD, sofosbuvir/ledipasvir; SOF/VEL, sofosbuvir/velpatasvir.

[a] A 12-week treatment required if patients has Metavir F3 fibrosis.

[b] Recommended only for patients with an HCV RNA of ≤800,00 IU/mL.

[c] A 12-week treatment is needed for those who are Afro-Caribbean in origin, HIV infected, or those who have an HCV RNA level of <6 million IU/mL.

[d] Only recommended for patients who tested negative for Y93H RAS at baseline, all other patients need addition of voxilaprevir or ribavirin if it is unavailable.

[e] Ombitasvir/paritaprevir/ritonavir/dasabuvir is not available in fixed doses combination; it requires ombitasvir/paritaprevir/ritonavir 2 tablets once daily and 1 tablet of dasabuvir twice daily.

Diagnostics

Serologic and molecular tests for detecting acute and past HEV infection have been developed for both epidemiologic and diagnostic purposes. The detection of HEV RNA in blood or plasma represents the gold standard for diagnosis of acute hepatitis E (AHE). Serologic tests detecting anti-HEV IgM and HEV antigen. Anti-HEV IgG antibodies can last more than 10 years after infection and recognize past infection. There are 9 different serology assays for the detection of anti-HEV IgG.[82] Interassay concordance is suboptimal and a recent meta-analysis suggested that results from population studies performed with different assays cannot be compared directly.[83] Molecular testing for direct assessment of the viral load is the more appropriate modality in immunocompromised patients.[70] Neurologic involvement seems to be directly associated with recent HEV infection and cerebrospinal fluid abnormalities may be found in patients with mild (anicteric) HEV infection.[84,85]

Therapy and Prevention

AHE does not require treatment. However, pregnant women with acute infection should be strictly monitored because they may develop FHF. HEV3 and HEV4 have been associated with persistent infection in immunocompromised patients, including organ transplant recipients, patients with AIDS, and those with hematologic malignancies. The mainstay of management is to ensure optimal antiretroviral therapy for HIV-infected patients and a decrease in immunosuppression in transplant recipients. In patients with persisting HEV replication for more than 3 months, ribavirin treatment for 12 weeks is recommended. Twelve additional weeks of therapy can be given to nonresponders. Nonresponse to ribavirin may be associated with single nucleotide variants in the virus, which may be present as a baseline minor variant.[86] Therapy with pegylated interferon alpha may be considered in liver transplant recipients who did not respond to ribavirin.[70] Prevention of human HEV genotypes (HEV1 and HEV2) involves providing better sanitation standards in low-income countries. Zoonotic genotype spread (HEV3, 4, and 7) in more affluent settings can be prevented by avoiding the consumption of raw or undercooked meat products, or attempts to decrease the prevalence of this infection via animal husbandry. In the Democratic Republic of China, a recombinant vaccine (Hecolin) is available based on a 239 amino acid peptide derived from the Chinese HEV1 strain. The protective efficacy of this vaccine for symptomatic disease has been demonstrated in areas with known circulation of HEV1 and HEV4, but its efficacy against other HEV genotypes is unknown.[87]

SUMMARY: TOWARD GLOBAL CONTROL OF VIRAL HEPATITIS

Viral hepatitis owing to HAV, HBV, HCV, HDV, and HEV affects hundreds of millions of people globally. Most deaths from viral hepatitis are due to hepatitis B and hepatitis C. The World Health Organization has set the ambitious target to eliminate viral hepatitis by achieving a 90% reduction of new HBV and HCV infections by 2030. A shift in emphasis from the current focus on individuals to a coordinated public health to interrupt transmission is required to achieve this. Endemic infections may be eradicated by immunizing susceptible patients or depleting the reservoir of chronically infected patients by mass treatment. In HBV the former is possible, and the pipeline of future therapies may allow us to explore the potential of the latter in future years. A major challenge for the elimination of HBV and HCV globally is the lack of guaranteed access to diagnostics, vaccine, and drugs.

ACKNOWLEDGMENTS

Authors Professor G. Ippolito and Sir A. Zumla are members of the PANDORA-ID-NET consortium and acknowledge support from the European and Developing Countries Clinical Trials Partnership (EDCTP2) programme (Grant Agreement RIA2016E-1609) which is supported under Horizon 2020, the European Union's Framework Programme for Research and Innovation. Sir A. Zumla is in receipt of a UK NIHR Senior Investigator Award. Authors acknowledge support from theg Italian Ministry of Health research programme -*Ricerca Corrente*.

REFERENCES

1. Global hepatitis report 2017. Geneva (Switzerland): World Health Organization; 2017. Licence: CC BY-NC-SA 3.0 IGO. Available at: https://www.who.int/hepatitis/publications/global-hepatitis-report2017/en/. Accessed March 3, 2019.
2. Global health sector strategy on viral hepatitis, 2016–2021. Geneva (Switzerland): WHO; 2016. WHO/HIV/2016.06. Available at: http://apps.who.int/iris/bitstream/10665/246177/1/WHO-HIV-2016.06-eng.pdf?ua=1. Accessed March 3, 2019.
3. Lanini S, Easterbrook PJ, Zumla A, et al. Hepatitis C: global epidemiology and strategies for control. Clin Microbiol Infect 2016;22:833–8.
4. Najarian R, Caput D, Gee W, et al. Primary structure and gene organization of human hepatitis A virus. Proc Natl Acad Sci U S A 1985;82:2627–31.
5. Lemon SM, Ott JJ, Van Damme P, et al. Type A viral hepatitis: a summary and update on the molecular virology, epidemiology, pathogenesis and prevention. J Hepatol 2018;68:167–84.
6. Shin EC, Jeong SH. Natural history, clinical manifestations, and pathogenesis of hepatitis A. Cold Spring Harb Perspect Med 2018;8:a031708.
7. Hirai-Yuki A, Hensley L, McGivern DR, et al. MAVS-dependent host species range and pathogenicity of human hepatitis A virus. Science 2016;353:1541–5.
8. McFarland N, Dryden M, Ramsay M, et al. An outbreak of hepatitis A affecting a nursery school and a primary school. Epidemiol Infect 2011;139:336–43.
9. Matheny SC, Kingery JE. Hepatitis A. Am Fam Physician 2012;86:1027–34.
10. WHO. WHO position paper on Hepatitis A vaccines. Wkly Epidiol Rec 2012; 87:15.
11. GBD 2016 Causes of Death Collaborators. Global, regional, and national age-sex specific mortality for 264 causes of death, 1980-2016: a systematic analysis for the Global Burden of Disease Study 2016. Lancet 2017;390:1151–210.
12. Lanini S, Pisapia R, Capobianchi MR, et al. Global epidemiology of viral hepatitis and national needs for complete control. Expert Rev Anti Infect Ther 2018;16: 625–39.
13. World Health Organization Hepatitis 2018. Available at: https://www.who.int/newsroom/fact-sheets/detail/hepatitis-a. Accessed September 14, 2019.
14. Alventosa Mateu C, Urquijo Ponce JJ, Diago Madrid M. An outbreak of acute hepatitis due to the hepatitis A virus in 2017: are we witnessing a change in contagion risk factors? Rev Esp Enferm Dig 2018;110:675–6.
15. Wang H, Gao P, Chen W, et al. Changing epidemiological characteristics of Hepatitis A and warning of Anti-HAV immunity in Beijing, China: a comparison of prevalence from 1990 to 2017. Hum Vaccin Immunother 2019;15(2):420–5.
16. Croker C, Hathaway S, Marutani A, et al. Outbreak of hepatitis A virus infection among adult patients of a mental hospital - Los Angeles County, 2017. Infect Control Hosp Epidemiol 2018;39:881.

17. Gassowski M, Michaelis K, Wenzel JJ, et al. Two concurrent outbreaks of hepatitis A highlight the risk of infection for non-immune travellers to Morocco, January to June 2018. Euro Surveill 2018;23(27). pii=1800329.
18. Viray MA, Hofmeister MG, Johnston DI, et al. Public health investigation and response to a hepatitis A outbreak from imported scallops consumed raw-Hawaii, 2016. Epidemiol Infect 2018;17:1–8.
19. Lanini S, Minosse C, Vairo F, et al. A large ongoing outbreak of hepatitis A predominantly affecting young males in Lazio, Italy; August 2016 - March 2017. PLoS One 2017;12:e0185428.
20. Foster M, Ramachandran S, Myatt K, et al. Hepatitis A virus outbreaks associated with drug use and homelessness - California, Kentucky, Michigan, and Utah, 2017. MMWR Morb Mortal Wkly Rep 2018;67:1208–10.
21. Lemon SM, Walker CM. Enterically transmitted non-A, non-B Hepatitis and the discovery of hepatitis E virus. Cold Spring Harb Perspect Med 2019;9(8) [pii: a033449].
22. Ott JJ, Wiersma ST. Single-dose administration of inactivated hepatitis A vaccination in the context of hepatitis A vaccine recommendations. Int J Infect Dis 2013; 17:e939–44.
23. Souto FJD, de Brito WI, Fontes CJF. Impact of the single-dose universal mass vaccination strategy against hepatitis A in Brazil. Vaccine 2019;37:771–5.
24. Joshi MS, Bhalla S, Kalrao VR, et al. Exploring the concurrent presence of hepatitis A virus genome in serum, stool, saliva, and urine samples of hepatitis A patients. Diagn Microbiol Infect Dis 2014;78:379–82.
25. Nelson NP, Link-Gelles R, Hofmeister MG, et al. Update: recommendations of the Advisory Committee on Immunization Practices for use of hepatitis A vaccine for postexposure prophylaxis and for preexposure prophylaxis for international travel. MMWR Morb Mortal Wkly Rep 2018;67:1216–20.
26. Lin KY, Chen GJ, Lee YL, et al. Hepatitis A virus infection and hepatitis A vaccination in human immunodeficiency virus-positive patients: a review. World J Gastroenterol 2017;23:3589–606.
27. Link-Gelles R, Hofmeister MG, Nelson NP. Use of hepatitis A vaccine for postexposure prophylaxis in individuals over 40 years of age: a systematic review of published studies and recommendations for vaccine use. Vaccine 2018; 36(20):2745–50.
28. Castillo EM, Chan TC, Tolia VM, et al. Effect of a computerized alert on emergency department hepatitis a vaccination in homeless patients during a large regional outbreak. J Emerg Med 2018;55:764–8.
29. Stuurman AL, Marano C, Bunge EM, et al. Impact of universal mass vaccination with monovalent inactivated hepatitis A vaccines – A systematic review. Hum Vaccin Immunother 2017;13:724–36.
30. Victor JC, Monto AS, Surdina TY, et al. Hepatitis A vaccine versus immune globulin for postexposure prophylaxis. N Engl J Med 2007;357:1685–94.
31. Lin CL, Kao JH. Natural history of acute and chronic hepatitis B: the role of HBV genotypes and mutants. Best Pract Res Clin Gastroenterol 2017;31:249–55.
32. Nguyen DH, Ludgate L, Hu J. Hepatitis B virus-cell interactions and pathogenesis. J Cell Physiol 2008;216:289–94.
33. Tu T, Budzinska MA, Shackel NA, et al. HBV DNA integration: molecular mechanisms and clinical implications. Viruses 2017;9:E75.
34. Xiong QF, Xiong T, Huang P, et al. Early predictors of acute hepatitis B progression to liver failure. PLoS One 2018;13:e0201049.

35. European Association for the Study of the Liver. EASL 2017 Clinical Practice Guidelines on the management of hepatitis B virus infection. J Hepatol 2017; 67:370–98.

36. Mikulska M, Lanini S, Gudiol C, et al. ESCMID Study Group for Infections in Compromised Hosts (ESGICH) Consensus Document on the safety of targeted and biological therapies: an infectious diseases perspective (Agents targeting lymphoid cells surface antigens [I]: CD19, CD20 and CD52). Clin Microbiol Infect 2018;24(Suppl 2):S71–82.

37. Smith DB, Bukh J, Kuiken C, et al. Expanded classification of hepatitis C virus into 7 genotypes and 67 subtypes: updated criteria and genotype assignment web resource. Hepatology 2014;59:318–27.

38. World Health Organization. Hepatitis B vaccines: WHO position paper, July 2017 - recommendations. Vaccine 2019;37(2):223–5.

39. Chen HY, Shen DT, Ji DZ, et al. Prevalence and burden of hepatitis D virus infection in the global population: a systematic review and meta-analysis. Gut 2019; 68:512–21.

40. Botelho-Souza LF, Vasconcelos MPA, Dos Santos AO, et al. Hepatitis delta: virological and clinical aspects. Virol J 2017;14:177.

41. Murphy DG, Sablon E, Chamberland J, et al. Hepatitis C virus genotype 7, a new genotype originating from central Africa. J Clin Microbiol 2015;53:967–72.

42. Borgia SM, Hedskog C, Parhy B, et al. Identification of a novel hepatitis C virus genotype from Punjab, India: expanding classification of hepatitis C virus into 8 genotypes. J Infect Dis 2018;218:1722–9.

43. Gasim GI, Bella A, Adam I. Schistosomiasis, hepatitis B and hepatitis C co-infection. Virol J 2015;12:19.

44. Antonucci G, Goletti D, Lanini S, et al. HIV/HCV co-infection: putting the pieces of the puzzle together. Cell Death Differ 2003;10(Suppl 1):S25–6.

45. Lingala S, Ghany MG. Natural history of Hepatitis C. Gastroenterol Clin North Am 2015;44:717–34.

46. Sheer TA, Runyon BA. Spontaneous bacterial peritonitis. Dig Dis 2005;23:39–46.

47. D'Amico G, De Franchis R. Upper digestive bleeding in cirrhosis. Post-therapeutic outcome and prognostic indicators. Hepatology 2003;38:599–612.

48. Westbrook RH, Dusheiko G. Natural history of hepatitis C. J Hepatol 2014;61: S58–68.

49. Lanini S, Scognamiglio P, Pisapia R, et al. Recovery of metabolic impairment of patients who cleared HCV infections after direct-acting antiviral therapy. Int J Antimicrob Agents 2018;53(5):559–63.

50. Younossi Z, Park H, Henry L, et al. M. Extrahepatic manifestations of hepatitis C: a meta-analysis of prevalence, quality of life, and economic burden. Gastroenterology 2016;150:1599–608.

51. Yeung CY, Lee HC, Chan WT, et al. Vertical transmission of hepatitis C virus: current knowledge and perspectives. World J Hepatol 2014;6:643–51.

52. Messina JP, Humphreys I, Flaxman A, et al. Global distribution and prevalence of hepatitis C virus genotypes. Hepatology 2015;61:77–87.

53. Markov PV, van de Laar TJ, Thomas XV, et al. Colonial history and contemporary transmission shape the genetic diversity of hepatitis C virus genotype 2 in Amsterdam. J Virol 2012;86:7677–87.

54. Wasitthankasem R, Vongpunsawad S, Siripon N, et al. Genotypic distribution of hepatitis C virus in Thailand and Southeast Asia. PLoS One 2015;10:e0126764.

55. Li C, Barnes E, Newton PN, et al. An expanded taxonomy of hepatitis C virus genotype 6: characterization of 22 new full-length viral genomes. Virology 2015;476: 355–63.

56. Strickland GT. Liver disease in Egypt: hepatitis C superseded schistosomiasis as a result of iatrogenic and biological factors. Hepatology 2006;43:915–22.

57. Al Naamani K, Al Sinani S, Deschênes M. Epidemiology and treatment of hepatitis C genotypes 5 and 6. Can J Gastroenterol 2013;27:e8–12.

58. Araujo AC, Astrakhantseva IV, Fields HA, et al. Distinguishing acute from chronic hepatitis C virus (HCV) infection based on antibody reactivities to specific HCV structural and nonstructural proteins. J Clin Microbiol 2011;49:54–7.

59. European Association for the Study of the Liver. EASL recommendations on treatment of hepatitis C 2018. J Hepatol 2018;69:461–511.

60. The American Association for the Study of Liver Diseases and the Infectious Diseases Society of America Present HCV Guidance: recommendations for testing, managing, and treating hepatitis C. Available at: https://www.hcvguidelines.org/. Accessed September 14, 2019.

61. Nair VP, Anang S, Subramani C, et al. Endoplasmic reticulum stress induced synthesis of a novel viral factor mediates efficient replication of genotype-1 hepatitis E virus. PLoS Pathog 2016;12:e1005521.

62. Yin X, Li X, Feng Z. Role of Envelopment in the HEV Life Cycle. Viruses 2016;8: E229.

63. Cacoub P, Desbois AC, Comarmond C, et al. Impact of sustained virological response on the extrahepatic manifestations of chronic hepatitis C: a meta-analysis. Gut 2018;67:2025–34.

64. Gentile I, Scotto R, Coppola C, et al. Treatment with direct-acting antivirals improves the clinical outcome in patients with HCV-related decompensated cirrhosis: results from an Italian real-life cohort (Liver Network Activity-LINA cohort). Hepatol Int 2019;13:66–74.

65. Stournaras E, Neokosmidis G, Stogiannou D, et al. Effects of antiviral treatment on the risk of hepatocellular cancer in patients with chronic viral hepatitis. Eur J Gastroenterol Hepatol 2018;30:1277–82.

66. Kamar N, Izopet J, Pavio N, et al. Hepatitis E virus infection. Nat Rev Dis Primers 2017;3:17086.

67. Chaudhry SA, Verma N, Koren G. Hepatitis E infection during pregnancy. Can Fam Physician 2015;61:607–8.

68. Haffar S, Shalimar, Kaur RJ, et al. Acute liver failure caused by hepatitis E virus genotype 3 and 4: a systematic review and pooled analysis. Liver Int 2018;38: 1965–73.

69. Mclean BN, Gulliver J, Dalton HR. Hepatitis E virus and neurological disorders. Pract Neurol 2017;17:282–8.

70. European Association for the Study of the Liver. EASL clinical practice guidelines on hepatitis E virus infection. J Hepatol 2018;68:1256–71.

71. Su YY, Huang SJ, Guo M, et al. Persistence of antibodies acquired by natural hepatitis E virus infection and effects of vaccination. Clin Microbiol Infect 2017; 23:336.e1-4.

72. Sooryanarain H, Meng XJ. Hepatitis E virus: reasons for emergence in humans. Curr Opin Virol 2018;34:10–7.

73. Nan Y, Wu C, Zhao Q, et al. Vaccine development against zoonotic hepatitis E virus: open questions and remaining challenges. Front Microbiol 2018;9:266.

74. Gurley ES, Hossain MJ, Paul RC, et al. Outbreak of hepatitis E in urban Bangladesh resulting in maternal and perinatal mortality. Clin Infect Dis 2014; 59:658–65.

75. Browne LB, Menkir Z, Kahi V, et al. Notes from the field: hepatitis E outbreak among refugees from South Sudan - Gambella, Ethiopia, April 2014-January 2015. MMWR Morb Mortal Wkly Rep 2015;64:537.

76. Wang B, Akanbi OA, Harms D, et al. A new hepatitis E virus genotype 2 strain identified from an outbreak in Nigeria, 2017. Virol J 2018;15:163.

77. Spina A, Lenglet A, Beversluis D, et al. A large outbreak of Hepatitis E virus genotype 1 infection in an urban setting in Chad likely linked to household level transmission factors, 2016-2017. PLoS One 2017;12:e0188240.

78. Hepatitis E vaccine: WHO position paper, May 2015. Wkly Epidemiol Rec 2015; 90:185–200.

79. Sridhar S, Teng JLL, Chiu TH, et al. Hepatitis E virus genotypes and evolution: emergence of camel hepatitis E variants. Int J Mol Sci 2017;18:E869.

80. Nimgaonkar I, Ding Q, Schwartz RE, et al. Hepatitis E virus: advances and challenges. Nat Rev Gastroenterol Hepatol 2018;15:96–110.

81. Izopet J, Lhomme S, Chapuy-Regaud S, et al. HEV and transfusion-recipient risk. Transfus Clin Biol 2017;24:176–81.

82. Al-Sadeq DW, Majdalawieh AF, Mesleh AG, et al. Laboratory challenges in the diagnosis of hepatitis E virus. J Med Microbiol 2018;67:466–80.

83. Hartl J, Otto B, Madden RG, et al. Hepatitis E Seroprevalence in Europe: a meta-analysis. Viruses 2016;8:E211.

84. van Eijk JJJ, Dalton HR, Ripellino P, et al. Clinical phenotype and outcome of hepatitis E virus-associated neuralgic amyotrophy. Neurology 2017;89:909–17.

85. Fritz M, Berger B, Schemmerer M, et al. Pathological cerebrospinal fluid findings in patients with neuralgic amyotrophy and acute hepatitis E virus infection. J Infect Dis 2018;217:1897–901.

86. Todt D, Meister TL, Steinmann E. Hepatitis E virus treatment and ribavirin therapy: viral mechanisms of nonresponse. Curr Opin Virol 2018;32:80–7.

87. WHO. Hepatitis E vaccine: WHO position paper, May 2015–Recommendations. Vaccine 2016;34:304–5.

Multidrug and Extensively Drug-resistant Tuberculosis
Epidemiology, Clinical Features, Management and Treatment

Simon Tiberi, MD[a],*,
Alimuddin Zumla, MBChB, MSc, PhD, MD, FRCP(Lond), FRCP(Edin), FRCPath(UK), FAAS[b],
Giovanni Battista Migliori, FRCP, FERS[c]

KEYWORDS

- Drug-resistant tuberculosis • Multidrug-resistant TB (MDR-TB)
- GeneXpert MTB/RIF Assay • Treatment guidelines • Surgery • Rehabilitation
- Workplace safety

KEY POINTS

- Drug-resistant tuberculosis (TB) currently is a threat to global health security, with an estimated 558,000 new multidrug-resistant (MDR)/rifampicin-resistant TB infections in 2017 (160,684 notified cases) and 230,000 deaths.
- MDR-TB is a lethal form of TB caused by *Mycobacterium tuberculosis* strains, which are resistant to rifampicin and isoniazid. It should be suspected in patients living in high MDR-TB endemic areas or those who have had previous TB treatment. New rapid molecular-based diagnostic tests, such as the GeneXpert MTB/RIF assay, can provide results operationally within a day.
- MDR-TB requires treatment with second-line drugs, usually 4 or more anti-TB drugs for a period extending between 18 months and 24 months. Under ideal program conditions, MDR-TB cure rates can be above 70%. An all-oral treatment regimen has been recently approved by the World Health Organization (WHO).
- Surgery for drug-resistant TB remains an option when there is a lesion that is resectable together with poor response, lack of drugs, and intolerance to medications.
- Pulmonary rehabilitation is useful for patients with reduced exercise performance and impaired quality of life.

Disclosure Statement: The authors have nothing to disclose.
[a] Department of Infection, Royal London Hospital, Blizard Institute, Barts and The London School of Medicine and Dentistry, Queen Mary, Barts Health NHS Trust, 80 Newark Street, London E1 2ES, UK; [b] Center for Clinical Microbiology, University College London, Royal Free Campus 2nd Floor, Rowland Hill Street, London NW3 2PF, United Kingdom; [c] Respiratory Diseases Clinical Epidemiology Unit, Istituti Clinici Scientifici Maugeri (Istituto di Ricovero e Cura a Carattere Scientifico), Crotto Roncaccio Street, 16 - 21049 Tradate (Varese), Italy
* Corresponding author.
E-mail address: Simon.Tiberi@nhs.net

Infect Dis Clin N Am 33 (2019) 1063–1085
https://doi.org/10.1016/j.idc.2019.09.002
0891-5520/19/© 2019 Elsevier Inc. All rights reserved.
id.theclinics.com

DEFINITIONS

Drug-sensitive (susceptible) tuberculosis (TB) is defined as TB caused by *Mycobacterium tuberculosis* sensitive to all first-line TB drugs.

Rifampicin-resistant TB (RR-TB) is now managed as multidrug-resistant (MDR)-TB, since the World Health Organization (WHO) 2016 MDR-TB guidelines update.[1]

Isoniazid-monoresistant TB has been recently reviewed[2] and guidance updated.[3]

Polyresistant TB is defined as multiple resistances but not fulfilling the MDR-TB definition, that is, resistance to isoniazid, streptomycin, ethambutol, and pyrazinamide.

MDR-TB is defined as TB resistance to rifampicin and isoniazid.

Extensively drug-resistant TB (XDR-TB) is defined as MDR-TB with additional resistance to a fluoroquinolone and a second-line injectable (capreomycin, amikacin, or kanamycin).

Acquired drug-resistant TB. Acquired drug resistance is the selection of mutant-resistant *M tuberculosis* strains due to inadequate, incomplete, or poor-quality treatment or suboptimal patient compliance with quadruple therapy. Simultaneous natural mutations in *M tuberculosis* resulting in resistance to more than 1 TB drug occur but are rare.

Primary drug-resistant TB. Patients are infected with a drug-resistant strain of *M tuberculosis*. The natural history of infection is similar to that of drug-susceptible TB. Drug-resistant TB was noted after the first clinical trial using streptomycin in monotherapy.[4] The most common cause of drug resistance is through acquired drug resistance and predominantly by adding a single active drug to a failing regimen.[5]

Latent *M tuberculosis* infection (LTBI): LTBI is defined by the WHO as "a state of persistent immune response to *M tuberculosis* antigens with no evidence of clinically active TB disease."

INTRODUCTION, BACKGROUND, AND EPIDEMIOLOGY

TB is an infectious disease caused by *M tuberculosis*. TB has plagued humankind for millennia. Today TB it is the most common cause of death from an infectious disease and the ninth cause of death globally.[6] The WHO annual TB report (2018) estimated that 10 million people (3.2 million women and 1 million children) developed TB. TB caused 1.3 million deaths in non–human immunodeficiency virus (HIV)-infected and an additional 300,000 HIV-positive people.[6] TB caused by *M tuberculosis* strains resistant to TB drugs is harder to treat than those infected with drug-susceptible strains.

TB frequently affects adults in the prime of their productive life and makes an enormous impact on the poor and socially disadvantaged, costing the global economy $617 billion from 2000 to 2015, with this number set to rise to $983 billion from 2015 to 2030. These figures are even more significant when taking into account that a majority of highest incidence countries are developing economies.[7]

Drug-resistant TB is a new threat; globally, 3.8% of all new cases have MDR-TB and it is now estimated that there were 558,000 new MDR/RR-TB infections (160,684 notified cases) and 230,000 deaths. Europe has the highest proportion of drug-resistant cases, with 17% of all new cases of TB MDR/RR-TB. Of concern, the number of MDR-TB cases increases year on year.[6] A recent model calculation has estimated that a third of TB cases in Russia will be drug resistant by 2040.[6–8] Drug-resistant cases threaten to replace susceptible cases and delay/hamper TB elimination; hence, it constitutes a considerable challenge to health programs. **Fig. 1** illustrates 3 defined

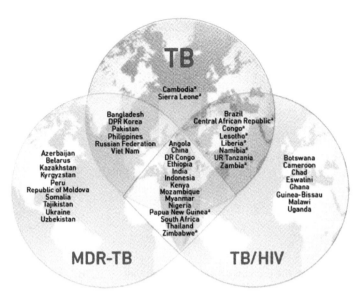

Fig. 1. In 2015, WHO defined 3 high-burden country (HBC) lists for the period 2016 to 2020: 1 for TB, 1 for MDR-TB, and 1 for TB/HIV ;the figure demonstrates overlap of these lists. [a] Indicates countries that are included in the list of 30 high TB burden countries on the basis of the severity of their burden (i.e., TB incident cases per 100 000 population per year), as opposed to the top 20, which are included on the basis of their absolute number of incident cases per year(see also Table 2.4). (*From* Falzon D, Schünemann HJ, Harausz E, et al. World Health Organization treatment guidelines for drug-resistant tuberculosis, 2016 update. European Respiratory Journal Mar 2017, 49 (3) 1602308; DOI: 10.1183/13993003.02308-2016; with permission.)

high-burden country lists for TB, MDR-TB, and TB/HIV. **Fig. 2** shows estimated WHO global MDR-TB incidence for 2017.

CLINICAL PRESENTATION

Drug-resistant TB presents in the same way as drug-susceptible TB (**Figs. 3–5**) and currently is less likely to occur through primary transmission because of the low prevalence of drug-resistant cases.

Pulmonary TB is the most common presentation of drug-resistant TB cases and, in cases of HIV or other causes of immunosuppression, features of extrapulmonary TB may be present. There are factors that make resistance more probable. Prior TB treatment increases the risk of drug-resistant TB; alcoholism and homelessness increase the likelihood of resistance, as does being in contact with a patient with active drug-resistant TB. Drug-resistant TB should be suspected in patients who are not responding to treatment and are not smear and culture converting after 2 months of adhering to standard quadruple TB drugs.

Patients give a history of chronic cough and nonspecific constitutional symptoms of anorexia, lethargy, and fever. Over time, the cough becomes productive, with purulent sputum and sometimes blood stained (hemoptysis), pleuritic chest pain, and breathlessness. As the disease progresses, there are worsening breathlessness, night sweats, weight loss, and general wasting, such that patients feel tired, sleepy, and unable to perform a day's work.

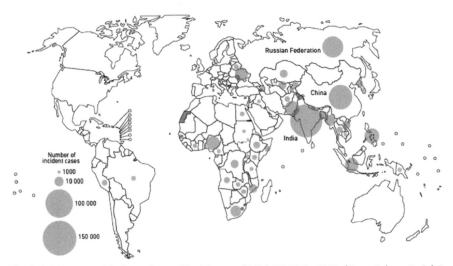

Fig. 2. WHO map with the estimated incidence of MDR/RR-TB in 2017. (*From* Falzon D, Schü-nemann HJ, Harausz E, et al. World Health Organization treatment guidelines for drug-resistant tuberculosis, 2016 update. European Respiratory Journal Mar 2017, 49 (3) 1602308; DOI: 10.1183/13993003.02308-2016; with permission.)

DIAGNOSIS OF DRUG-RESISTANT TUBERCULOSIS

Early and accurate diagnosis of TB and MDR-TB is important for successful treatment outcomes. The gold standard for making a specific diagnosis of TB is identifying the presence of *M tuberculosis* from a clinical sample (which can be sputum, pleural fluid, urine, pus, cerebrospinal fluid, bone marrow, biopsies, or excised tissue). Imaging can help localize sites of disease and associated pathology and allows for imaging-guided aspiration of lesion, abscess, or biopsy of tissue for microbiological and molecular examination. The choice of the optimal microbiological or molecular diagnostic method for TB diagnosis is dependent on clinical context, available laboratory capacity, and resources.[1]

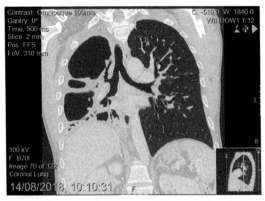

Fig. 3. Computer tomography scan of a 35-year-old man with a destroyed right lung from TB.

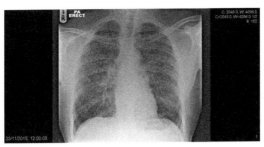

Fig. 4. Chest radiograph of a 20-year-old man living with HIV presenting with miliary changes; mycobacterial blood cultures isolated *M tuberculosis*.

Culture-based Methods

Culture of clinical specimens for *Mtb* is a laboratory method for diagnosis of active TB, with sensitivity of 65% and specificity of 100%. Traditionally solid Löwenstein-Jensen culture medium has been replaced by automated liquid culture systems using the limit of detection of approximately 10 organisms per milliliter based on modified Middlebrook 7H9 Broth with an oxygen-sensitive fluorescent detection technology; the system scans for increased fluorescence (reflecting presence of viable mycobacteria) every 60 minutes. Liquid culture is now recommended by the WHO as the gold standard confirmatory test for TB[9,10]; however, although it is more sensitive than solid media culture, it is more expensive and complex, with contamination a technical challenge. Once TB is isolated, phenotypic drug susceptibility tests (DSTs) and genotyping for further molecular epidemiology studies can be performed.[11] The disadvantage of culture methods is the time needed for the growth of mycobacteria. Liquid cultures require at least 9 days to 10 days for positive results and 6 weeks for being considered negative.[9,10]

Molecular-based Methods

The WHO guidelines[1] have simplified diagnosing MDR-TB by the programmatic rollout of TB–polymerase chain reaction testing, mainly with the GeneXpert MTB/RIF assay (Cepheid, Sunnyvale, California)[12,13] and to a lesser extent by Hain Lifescience Nehren, line probe assay and other molecular methods.[14] Culture-based methods remain the gold standard to determine drug resistance; however, these may be replaced in the future by whole genome sequencing.[15]

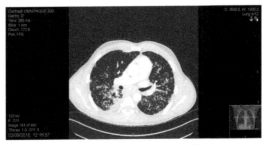

Fig. 5. Computer tomography scan of chest of a 40-year-old man with multinodular–tree-in-bud appearance in both lung fields; the patient was positive for AFB on sputum smear microscopy examination.

The GeneXpert MTB/RIF Assay

The WHO has recommended the GeneXpert MTB/RIF assay as a rapid, near-point-of-care test for detecting *Mtb* and also rifampicin resistance simultaneously for patients with pulmonary TB.[16] This test is a nested polymerase chain reaction assay for amplifying *Mtb* DNA and part of the *rpoB* gene encoding rifampicin resistance.[13] This assay now updated with the RIF/Ultra cartridge can give a result in under 2 hours and operationally in hospitals and TB clinics within 24 hours. The GeneXpert MTB/RIF assay and acid-fast bacilli (AFB) sputum smear microscopy have the same specificity, but sensitivity of GeneXpert is much higher than AFB smear microscopy on sputum. A single GeneXpert MTB/RIF test directly on sputum detects 99% of smear-positive patients and 80% of patients with smear-negative disease. Mean time to detection is less than 1 day for GeneXpert MTB/RIF, 1 day for microscopy, 17 days for liquid culture, and more than 30 days for solid culture.[16] In HIV-infected individuals, the GeneXpert increases case detection of TB by 45% compared with microscopy in HIV-infected individuals. It facilitates earlier diagnosis and reduces time to initiation of TB treatment. The timeliness of detection of rifampicin resistance in adults and children living with HIV using GeneXpert MTB/RIF may facilitate timely initiation of MDR-TB treatment. **Fig. 6**) shows how a diagnostic algorithm can incorporate the GeneXpert (**Figs. 7** and **8**).

MANAGEMENT OF DRUG-RESISTANT TUBERCULOSIS

The management of drug-resistant TB requires the use of several drugs in combination; the currently available new and repurposed drugs are shown in **Table 1**,[17] and discussed separately elsewhere.[18,19] This section focuses on the WHO guidelines for the management of MDR-TB, which have been based on a recent individual patient data metanalysis of 12,030 patients, which demonstrated better outcomes with line-zolid, fluoroquinolones, bedaquiline, clofazimine, and the β-lactamase inhibitor/carbapenems and worse tolerability and outcomes with prothionamide and second-line injectables.[20]

WORLD HEALTH ORGANIZATION GUIDELINES FOR MULTIDRUG-RESISTANT TUBERCULOSIS MANAGEMENT

The current guidance on the management of MDR-TB is embodied in the following WHO publications in 2011, with an update in 2016 and a recent one in 2019.[1,16,17]

The 2011 World Health Organization Multidrug-resistant Tuberculosis Guidelines

In 2011 anti-TB drugs were classified into 5 groups: group 1 drugs included the first-line oral drugs (rifampicin, isoniazid, ethambutol, and pyrazinamide); group 2, the injectable second-line drugs (amikacin, kanamycin, and capreomycin plus streptomycin, with the latter considered first line but also an injectable and grouped accordingly); group 3, the fluoroquinolones; group 4, the second-line old bacteriostatic drugs (ethionamide/prothionamide, para-aminosalicylic acid [PAS], and cycloserine/terizidone); and group 5 the new or repurposed drugs at the time considered of unclear efficacy.[16] Group 5 comprised several drugs like linezolid, carbapenems, and clofazimine, which were promoted to a higher rank in future adaptations of the WHO guidelines.[17]

The WHO 2011 guidelines were focusing on culture and DST as well as on rapid molecular diagnostic methods.[16] The recommended regimen included pyrazinamide, 1 fluoroquinolone, a second-line injectable drug (to be administered for the duration

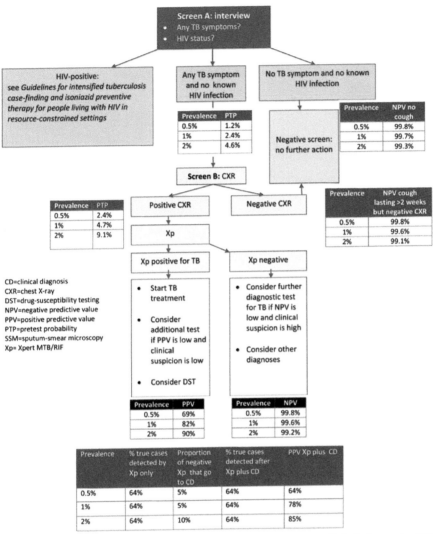

Fig. 6. Diagnostic algorithm incorporating use of GeneXpert. CD, clinical diagnosis; CXR, chest X-ray; NPV, negative predictive value; PPV, positive predictive value; PTP, pretest probability; SSM, sputum-smear microscopy; Xp, Xpert MTB/RIF. (*From* Falzon D, Jaramillo E, Schünemann HJ, et al. WHO guidelines for the programmatic management of drug-resistant tuberculosis: 2011 update. Eur Respir J 2011;38:516-28. 10.1183/09031936.00073611; with permission.)

of the intensive phase), ethionamide or prothionamide ,and either cycloserine or PAS. The total duration was 20 months or more, with an intensive phase of 8 months. They also recommended early initiation of antiretroviral treatment in HIV-positive individuals.[16]

The 2016 World Health Organization Multidrug-resistant Tuberculosis Guidelines

The 2016 WHO guidelines,[1] reorganized the classification of anti-TB drugs in groups A, B, C, and D, based on their safety and efficacy. Group A drugs included the

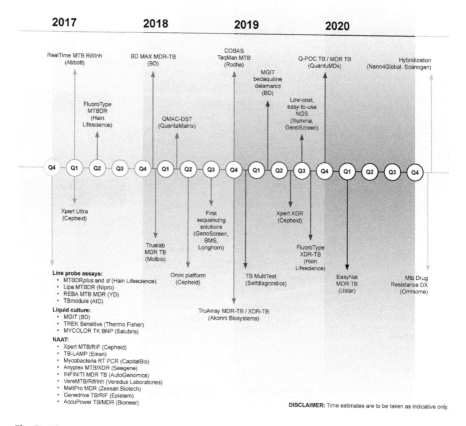

Fig. 7. Diagnostic landscape for sputum-based testing methods for *M tuberculosis* detection and susceptibility determination. *Courtesy of* the Foundation for Innovative New Diagnostics (FIND), Geneva, Switzerland; with permission.

fluoroquinolones, group B the second-line injectables, and the group C the other core second-line agents (ethionamide/prothionamide; cycloserine/terizidone plus linezolid and clofazimine). Group D (the add-on agents) was subdivided in 3 subgroups: group D1 included pyrazinamide, ethambutol, and high-dose isoniazid (High dose isoniazid

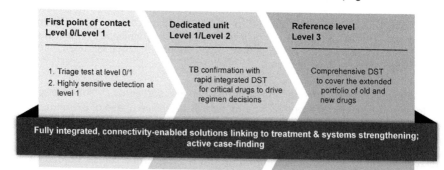

Fig. 8. Vision for a diagnostic cascade for *M tuberculosis* detection and susceptibility determination. *Courtesy of* the Foundation for Innovative New Diagnostics (FIND), Geneva, Switzerland; with permission.

Table 1
New World Health Organization drug classification for multidrug-resistant tuberculosis regimens

Groups and Steps	Medicine	
Group A: include all 3 medicines	Levofloxacin OR moxifloxacin	Lfx Mfx
	Bedaquiline[2,3]	Bdq
	Linezolid[4]	Lzd
Group B: add 1 or both medicines	Clofazimine	Cfz
	Cycloserine OR terizidone	Cs Trd

Group C:
  add to complete the
  regimen and when
  medicines from
  groups A and B
  cannot be used
	Ethambutol	E

	Delamanid[3,5]	Dlm
	Pyrazinamide[6]	Z
	Imipenem-cilastatin OR meropenem[7]	Ipm-Cln Mpm
	Amikacin (OR streptomycin)[8]	Am (S)
	Ethionamide OR prothionamide[9]	Eto Pto
	Para-aminosalicylic acid[9]	PAS

From Annex III, Flow charts of algorithms for screening and diagnosing tuberculosis (TB) in adults, with modelled yields and predictive values Systematic Screening for Active Tuberculosis: Principles and Recommendations. Geneva: World Health Organization; 2013. Accessed April 5, 2019; with permission.

is very important in the shorter regimen); group D2, bedaquiline and delamanid; and group D3, PAS and the carbapenems (imipenem and meropenem to be used with clavulanic acid to protect from β-lactamase action).

The new recommendations of these guidelines, in addition to the reclassification of the anti-TB drugs, included the following: the introduction of the WHO shorter regimen, a new recommendation for treatment in children based on pediatric individual meta-analytic data, and a new recommendation on partial lung resection surgery.

A regimen was recommended to include at least 5 effective medicines during the intensive phase of treatment, including pyrazinamide and 4 core second-line TB drugs, 1 from group A, 1 from group D2 and, if necessary, 1 or more agents from group D3 to reach a total of 5.

The World Health Organization Shorter Regimen

The World Health Organization Shorter Regimen was known previously as the Bangladesh regimen. The original Bangladesh study[21] achieved a relapse-free cure of 87.9% among 206 patients with infrequent and manageable adverse events. The regimen recommended by WHO was the same, the only difference being the use of moxifloxacin to replace gatifloxacin.[1]

The 9 months to 12 months standardized WHO shorter regimen is composed of 4 months to 6 months of kanamycin or amikacin, moxifloxacin, prothionamide or ethionamide, clofazimine, pyrazinamide, high-dose isoniazid, and ethambutol followed by 5 months of moxifloxacin, clofazimine, pyrazinamide, and ethambutol.

Importantly, no modifications were considered possible out of the drugs, discussed previously, due to lack of evidence. The recommendation applied to adults, children, and people living with HIV.

The indication was for patients with RR TB or MDR-TB, who have not been previously treated with second-line drugs, and in whom resistance to fluoroquinolones and second-line injectable agents has been excluded or considered highly unlikely.

The guidelines suggested the following checklist to define eligibility. If any answer yes to following the questions, the case was not considered eligible for the WHO shorter regimen:

- Confirmed resistance or suspected ineffectiveness to a medicine in the shorter MDR-TB regimen (except isoniazid resistance)?
- Exposure to greater than 1 second-line medicine in the shorter MDR-TB regimen for greater than 1 month?
- Intolerance to greater than 1 medicine in the shorter MDR-TB regimen or risk of toxicity (eg, drug-drug interactions)?
- Pregnancy?
- Extrapulmonary disease?
- At least 1 medicine in the shorter MDR-TB regimen unavailable?

The clear advantages of the WHO shorter regimen included lower costs (<$1000 in drug costs per patient) and improved adherence due to the shorter duration.

The WHO strongly recommended monitoring for effectiveness, relapse, and harms through the active TB drug safety monitoring and management project.

Although initial observational studies achieved better outcomes in patients treated with the shorter regimen in comparison with the longer regimen (eg, the regimen designed as per WHO guidelines in force) and treatment success rates exceeding 90% in Bangladesh, Cameroon, and Niger,[22] a controlled clinical trial (STREAM [Standard Treatment Regimen of Anti-Tuberculosis drugs for patients with MDR-TB]) was conducted to assess comparatively efficacy and safety of the 2 regimens.

The preliminary and final results of the STREAM trial,[23,24] showed a success rate of 78.1% with the shorter regimen and 80.6% with the longer one. Moreover, the short regimen used in STREAM was noninferior to the WHO long regimen at primary efficacy outcome and similar to the long regimen in terms of safety, even though the shorter regimen yielded more severe adverse events (grades 3–5), mortality (particularly among HIV-coinfected patients), and QT prolongation exceeding 500 milliseconds.[24]

Considerations on the World Health Organization Shorter Regimen

Using rapid molecular-line probe tests, it is possible to identify, as discussed previously in a specific paragraph of this review, the genes usually associated with resistance to isoniazid. In the presence of *inhA* alone, isoniazid is considered effective at normal doses, but resistance to ethionamide and prothionamide is usually present. In the presence of *katG* alone, high-dose isoniazid usually is effective against the majority of *M tuberculosis* strains (2 out of 99 strains had intermediate resistance to isoniazid).[25] In cases of both *inhA* and *katG* are present, high-dose isoniazid is considered ineffective.[26,27] Because resistance to ethionamide and protionamide also is present, the shorter regimen cannot be used.[26,27]

A scientific debate took place on the interpretation of the WHO recommendations, the more controversial points being the eligibility (or not) in settings where MDR-TB is common and the eligibility of the cases harboring strains of *M tuberculosis* resistant to ethambutol (and pyrazinamide), considering the unreliability of DST for these drugs. In Europe, where DST to ethambutol is considered reliable, the European Centre for Disease Prevention and Control recommended to consider this and exclusion criterion for the shorter regimen.[26,28–32]

The recently published European Union standards for TB care confirmed this position.[33]

Because resistance to fluoroquinolones and or injectables is a clear contraindication, in settings like former Soviet Union countries where the prevalence of resistance to these drugs ranges between 30% and 45%, the proportion of patients able to benefit from this regimen is very small (10%–30%).[26,30]

Based on these arguments, a recent modeling study estimated that the impact of the shorter regimen on the MDR-TB epidemic will be minor.[34,35]

The 2018 new WHO MDR-TB guidelines are now the 2019 WHO DF-TB consolidated guidelines have recently recommended a shift toward oral MDR-TB regimens, thus adding an element of uncertainty to the future of the shorter regimen. Furthermore, the future possibility of the use of a universal regimen eventually will open additional perspectives.[36]

The 2019 World Health Organization Consolidated Multidrug-resistant Tuberculosis Guideline

The new guideline, based on the evidence from the second global MDR-TB individual data meta-analysis published in 2018,[18] made the historical shift toward a full oral treatment of MDR-TB (see **Table 1** for the latest MDR-TB WHO drug classification).

In the new classification, group A drugs include fluoroquinolones, bedaquiline, and linezolid, whereas group B drugs add on clofazimine and cycloserine or terizidone. Group C drugs include the remaining drugs (ethambutol, delamanid, pyrazinamide, carbapenems, amikacin, ethionamide/prothionamide, and PAS). Whereas bedaquiline, linezolid, and clofazimine have been further promoted, the injectables have been downgraded because of their toxicity, possible lack of efficacy, and worse outcomes; only amikacin is still recommended because it was found to have moderate activity.[20]

The new approach is to use, if possible, all group A drugs and then from group B (and, if necessary, from group C) so as to include a sufficient number of active drugs, greater than 4 active drugs.

The recommended regimen would include at least 4 agents likely to be effective in the first 6 months and 3 drugs in the continuation phase of treatment for a total duration of about 18 months to 20 months, depending on the patient's response.

The recommendations for the shorter regimen's eligibility has been slightly modified: "in MDR/RR-TB patients who have not been previously treated for more than one month with second-line medicines used in the shorter MDR regimen or in whom resistance to fluoroquinolones and second-line injectable agents has been excluded, a shorter MDR-TB regimen of 9–12 months may be used instead of the longer regimens."

The main differences in comparison with the previous guidelines are the clear need for testing and excluding resistance to fluoroquinolones and injectables (the previous wording was "resistance...considered highly unlikely") and the less evident priority assigned to the shorter regimen in view of the STREAM Trial results.[17,24]

OTHER MANAGEMENT CONSIDERATIONS
Diabetes

The current era is one of a diabetic epidemic, and there has some overlap between diabetes and TB, with diabetic patients having a 2-times to 3-times higher risk of developing TB.[37] Diabetic TB patients have been found to generally have greater symptom severity and delayed sputum culture conversion,[38] and a recent meta-analysis demonstrated an association also with MDR-TB.[39,40] Diabetic patients, therefore, should be screened for TB and should be offered preventive therapy; they also should be risk assessed for MDR-TB. Given delays in gastric emptying absorption of TB drugs may be affected, therapeutic drug monitoring may help ensure adequate levels.[41]

Elderly

Elderly patients with MDR-TB tend to have more extensive disease and higher rates of adverse events to therapy, accompanied with worse outcomes and a higher mortality rate; this is perhaps due to a senescent immune system, presence of comorbidities, and drug-drug interactions; a higher suspicion in this cohort is required to avoid transmission of TB in health facilities and elderly care homes and to anticipate the time of diagnosis in order to reduce transmission and improve outcomes.[42–44]

Latent Mycobacterium tuberculosis infection Prophylaxis and Multidrug-resistant Tuberculosis

To date, only observational evidence around the effectiveness of treatment in programmatic settings is available; a recent meta-analysis of 5 studies suggests that treatment of MDR LTBI is effective. Results are impatiently awaited, however, of the first 3 randomized control trials for preventive therapy in contacts of MDR-TB patients for definitive answers regarding composition of regimen and duration.[45]

Surgery and Multidrug-resistant Tuberculosis

Treatment of MDR and XDR-TB patients, despite the new drugs, remains challenging; thoracic surgery, although controversial, similar to the preantibiotic era, continues to remain an option where few options exist. Surgery can act as a therapeutic tool in improving outcomes and obtaining cure, especially when indicated (localized disease) and when there are few available drugs, especially in the continuation phase.[46,47]

Pulmonary Rehabilitation

Patients undergoing surgery most certainly need pulmonary rehabilitation.[47]

Recent evidence suggests that MDR-TB patients, due to extensive disease and long treatment, frequently are left with pulmonary sequelae, such as obstruction and/or restriction, resulting in reduced oxygen saturation, reduced exercise performance, and impairment of quality of life.[48,49]

Pulmonary rehabilitation seems to be effective in these cases.[48,50]

Drug Toxicities: Delamanid and Bedaquiline in Combination

A combination of delamanid and bedaquiline did not seem to potentiate cardiotoxicity in a pooled analysis of 87 patients[48,51]; however, clinical trials need to demonstrate the long-term safety of this pairing, and their unlicensed combined use at present time can be considered (with adequate monitoring) only in patients with no other option.[52]

Central Nervous System Multidrug-resistant Tuberculosis

Central nervous system MDR-TB is extremely challenging to treat and is faced with a higher risk of chronic sequelae and poor clinical outcomes.[53] Unfortunately, the blood barrier penetration of the TB drugs overall is not very good; the drugs that have demonstrated the best brain penetration are pyrazinamide, moxifloxacin, levofloxacin, linezolid, prothionamide, and cycloserine.[53] The new drugs, delamanid and bedaquiline, being highly protein bound, are unlikely to be efficacious against central nervous system disease; a recent case report has demonstrated that no bedaquiline was found in a patient's cerebrospinal fluid.[54]

PROGRAMMATIC MANAGEMENT OF MULTIDRUG-RESISTANT TUBERCULOSIS

The WHO End TB Strategy includes management of MDR-TB as one of the core clinical and public health priorities.[6,55,56] Furthermore, MDR-TB prevention and control is one of the core activities recommended by the WHO to pursue TB Elimination.[57]

In a 2016 review,[55] priority actions have been recommended as having an impact on the MDR/XDR-TB epidemic, including as follows:

1. Prevent development of MDR-TB through high-quality treatment of drug-susceptible TB.
2. Expand rapid testing and detection of drug-resistant TB.
3. Provide immediate access to effective treatment and proper care.
4. Prevent transmission through infection control.
5. Increase political commitment and financing, ensuring adequate diagnosis, treatment, and management for drug-susceptible TB.

Prevent Development of Multidrug-resistant Tuberculosis Through High-quality Treatment of Drug-susceptible Tuberculosis

The strategic approach

An important modeling study[55,58] suggested that cure rates of drug-susceptible cases exceeding 80% can control the MDR-TB epidemic given that rapid diagnosis of new cases is ensured, thus supporting the priority of adequately treating new cases over focusing on failures' management.

The easy principle, in theory, is to limit the creation of new MDR-TB strains of *M tuberculosis* by ensuring high cure rate of new cases, when they are drug susceptible (**Box 1**). The standard regimen for new cases (including 2 months with isoniazid, rifampicin, ethambutol, and pyrazinamide followed by 4 months with isoniazid and rifampicin), if administered with adequate treatment supervision, can achieve a success rate exceeding 95% at the programmatic level.[27] The positive effect of this approach is also to break the chain of transmission, thus contributing to a decline of the overall TB incidence. This approach needs to be complemented with the sterilization of the existing pool of MDR/XDR-TB cases, to alleviate individual suffering as well as prevent further transmission of resistant strains.[27,58] This is possible by improving case detection and cure rates, according to the principles of the Ed TB Strategy.[59]

Outcome of multidrug-resistant tuberculosis and extensively drug-resistant tuberculosis cases Managing MDR and XDR-TB is difficult, however, particularly when the *M tuberculosis* strain has a pattern of resistance beyond rifampicin and isoniazid, the drugs defining MDR-TB.[20,57,60,61]

Box 1
Interventions to prevent drug-resistant TB[102]

There are 5 principal ways to prevent drug-resistant TB:
1. Early detection and high-quality treatment of drug-susceptible TB
2. Early detection and high-quality treatment of drug-resistant TB
3. Effective implementation of infection control measures
4. Strengthening and regulation of health systems
5. Addressing underlying risk factors and social determinants

Globally, according to the WHO report, the treatment success of RR/MDR-TB cases increased from 50% in the 2012 cohort to 55% in the 2015 cohort.[6] A subanalysis of the first large individual-data meta-analysis coordinated by McGill University found that although treatment success was higher in MDR-TB cases (65%), in XDR-TB cases it was as low as 40%, and, in patients harboring strains of *M tuberculosis* with resistances beyond XDR, it was below 20% (a result worse than that observed in the preantibiotic era).[62–64]

The treatment success rates described in the second individual-data meta-analysis for MDR-TB cases was higher,[20] reflecting the more consistent use of linezolid and of new or repurposed drugs in recent cohorts.

This second large study included 12,030 patients from 50 cohorts enrolled in 25 countries. It reported that 7346 achieved treatment success (61%), 1017 failed or relapsed (8%), and 1729 (14%) died. Treatment success was associated with prescription of linezolid, new generation fluoroquinolones (moxifloxacin and levofloxacin), carbapenems, clofazimine, and bedaquiline. In the same study, reduced mortality was associated with the use of linezolid, new fluoroquinolones, and bedaquiline.[20]

Evidence from South Africa confirmed improved outcomes and reduced mortality when bedaquiline was used,[65,66] thus accelerating the movement toward the use full-oral regimens.[17]

How to improve the clinical management of multidrug-resistant tuberculosis and extensively drug-resistant tuberculosis cases? The clinical management of these cases is complex, often requiring a multidisciplinary approach.[48,67] According to the WHO, an important proportion of cases report severe adverse events: 17.2% attributed to linezolid, 14.3% to PAS, 10.3% to amikacin, 9.5% to ethionamide/prothionamide, and 7.8% to cycloserine/terizidone, to mention only some of the drugs recommended by WHO.[17]

Therefore, a multidisciplinary team approach has been recommended to manage these cases, in several countries known as TB Consilium.[48] The idea is that a team including differing and complementary expertise (adult physicians, pediatricians, public health specialists, microbiologists, pharmacologists, surgeons, and so forth) has better chances of identifying the best possible regimen and ensure adequate clinical monitoring and management of adverse events than a single clinician alone.[48] A recent publication described, for some of the known examples of TB Consilia, arguments for and against different approaches and experiences. Although some of them are Internet based and provide real-time answers, others rely on physical meetings or periodic teleconferences or videoconferences.[48] From a programmatic perspective, each national program ideally needs to develop a system, tailored to country-specific needs, able to ensure that at least the more complicated cases (eg, XDR-TB, cases of severe comorbidities, adverse events, and/or needing bedaquiline and delamanid) are discussed in a TB Consilium–like body.

For cases of particular problems, for which specific expertise is not available in the country/center, or in cases where a second opinion can be beneficial, a supranational TB Consilium may be useful. In 2018, a clinical advisory service, promoted by the Global TB Network, called the Global TB Consilium, has been implemented hosted by the World Association for Infectious Diseases and Immunological Disorders (see Web site page: http://www.waidid.org/site/clinicalIntro).

In short, the new service provides free clinical advice within 48 hours, through a team of global renown experts recently selected based on very strict criteria.[48] The service currently operates in English, Russian, Spanish, and Portuguese.[48]

Expand Rapid Testing and Detection of Drug-resistant Tuberculosis

Under the first pillar of the End TB Strategy, the principle that early diagnosis and universal DSTs are necessary is clearly underlined. Resistance to isoniazid and rifampicin can be detected using phenotypic methods on solid culture or liquid-based culture techniques. The main limitation of this approach is that they require long time (2–3 weeks minimum) as well as technical capacity and adequate infection control measures.[55,62,68–71]

Fortunately, new rapid molecular methods based on automated nucleic acid amplification are available to detect M tuberculosis and the mutations usually determine rifampicin resistance. These techniques have several advantages, including rapid turnaround time and lower needs for biosafety/infection control and technical skills of laboratory staff, thus representing a step ahead toward the use of a point-of care test.

GeneXpert MTB/RIFand its new evolution, the GeneXpert MTB/RIF Ultra assay, both recommended by the WHO, allow rapid diagnosis of RR (<2 hours), considered a reliable proxy of MDR.

The test, operating in a closed system (the cartridge), is safe, is automated, prevents further contamination of the sample, and is easy to manage.

Another group of rapid tests (also recommended by WHO) has been developed to detect genetic mutations associated with resistance to fluoroquinolones and injectables, the drugs presently defining XDR-TB.

Although enormous progress has been achieved in scaling-up the use of new rapid diagnostic methods,[72] still an important proportion of MDR-TB cases have no access to these services[6]; ideally, tests should be tiered at point of care; this can then be confirmed at a dedicated center, if confirmed samples are sent to a reference laboratory for DST.

Provide Immediate Access to Effective Treatment and Proper Care

Furthermore, an important proportion of diagnosed cases has no access to adequate treatment or access is delayed due to the difficulty in procuring, distributing, and manage new drugs.[6]

Finally, after more than 40 years of silence, 2 new drugs, bedaquiline and delamanid, have been approved by the United States and the European regulatory authorities for the treatment of MDR-TB in 2012 and 2013, respectively.[55,73,74]

Fortunately, evidence is accumulating on the efficacy and safety of these drugs.[75] Although caution (justifying electrocardiogram monitoring) is necessary, new evidence is accumulating showing the 2 drugs are, in general, well tolerated[76–78] and even their coadministration seems safer than previously thought.[52,76,79–81] New evidence is also accumulating on some of the repurposed drugs like linezolid (now largely used and promoted in group A by the WHO),[17,82,83] clofazimine,[84] and carbapenems.[85–87]

Adequate surveillance of adverse events needs to be in place, particularly for new and repurposed drugs. The WHO advocates for the active TB drug safety monitoring and management approach.[88]

The new challenges are represented by the possibility of offering universal access and social protection to the patients in needs, while ensuring free-of-charge availability of quality drugs to the highest proportion of cases possible as well as optimizing the clinical capacity to offer rapid diagnosis and quality treatment.

Prevention of Transmission Through Infection Control

The importance of infection control within the vision of breaking the chain of transmission is clearly stressed by the WHO End TB Strategy (and by the WHO policy on infection control).[57,89]

In Europe, a survey conducted in 5 references centers and aimed at evaluating how MDR-TB cases were managed, found some drawbacks in the area of infection control (lack of negative pressure ventilation rooms and drawbacks in availability of infection control plans).[90–92] A new audit performed in 2017 found improvement on this aspect.[93]

Recently the WHO Regional Office for Europe published a policy document useful to improve infection control in Europe.[94,95]

Although focused on traditional managerial activities, administrative controls, and environmental controls, the new policy document supports the FAST approach (find cases actively by cough surveillance and rapid molecular sputum testing, separate safely, and treat effectively based on rapid DST), which gave excellent results in several countries, including the Russian Federation. The document also (1) reviews the available evidence on how TB infectiousness evolves in response to effective treatment (and which factors can lower or boost infectiousness); (2) presents policy options on the infectiousness of TB patients relevant to the WHO European Region; (3) defines the limitations in the available evidence; and (4) provides recommendations for further research.

Increase Political Commitment and Financing, Ensuring Adequate Diagnosis, Treatment, and Management for Drug-Susceptible Tuberculosis

The relationship between socioeconomic conditions and TB is well known.[55]

Recently, in evaluating the potential impact of the End TB Strategy, a modeling study has shown that reducing extreme poverty and expanding social protection can reduce the TB incidence by 84.3%.[96–98]

An important aspect of political commitment deserving further discussion is the legal framework, in particular its effect on TB control. Although the WHO recommends reduction of unnecessary hospital admission and a shift toward home-care management in view of the economic, patient-related, and infection control implications, this cannot be done if the health system refunds is based on hospital bed occupancy (as is common in former Soviet Union countries).

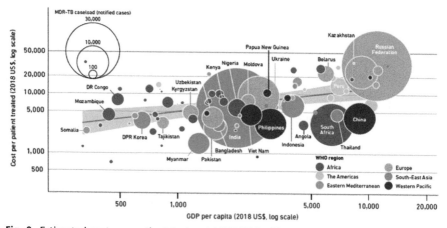

Fig. 9. Estimated cost per patient to treat MDR-TB in 85 countries. [a] Limited to countries with at least 20 patients on second-line treatment in 2017. (*From* Global tuberculosis report 2018. Geneva: World Health Organization; 2018. Licence: CC BY-NC-SA 3.0 IGO. Available on https://apps.who.int/iris/bitstream/handle/10665/274453/9789241565646-eng.pdf?ua=1 Accessed January 15th 2019; with permission.)

In several of these countries, for example, the hospital stay is a standard of care for the intensive phase of treatment (in MDR-TB cases, it can be higher than 200 days) with associated costs ranging from $2935 (Uzbekistan) to $64,250 (Latvia) (**Fig. 9**).[55]

Clearly such an approach prevents these recommendations to be applied.[99,100]

Armenia recently piloted a change in the refund approach, opening the door to an outpatient-driven approach.[101]

Evidently political commitment is necessary to support all the these actions, from adoption of updated guidelines to implementation of adequate infection control measures as well as quality diagnosis and treatment.

The need for updated definitions

Given the recent change in MDR/RR-TB treatment classification, with RR TB treated as MDR-TB and the significant removal of second-line injectables promoting a preferred all-oral regimen, the current definitions for MDR-TB and XDR-TB may require updating.[36]

SUMMARY

Notwithstanding the gradual declines in TB incidence worldwide, MDR/XDR-TB is a growing threat to global health security.

Recent advances in basic and operational research have led to the development and implementation of rapid diagnostic methods for MDR-TB, allowing for increased detection and treatment. New WHO recommendations for use of an all-oral, less toxic treatment regimen provides hope for more patients being enrolled on treatment. Several new drug trials experimenting with multiple combinations of regimens to determine more effective and shorter regimens are ongoing.

Several new technologies are being rolled out and an upscaling of efforts are being made to meet the programmatic challenges of MDR-TB. Achieving control of MDR-TB will require increased political commitment and resources, reducing poverty, improving the quality of housing and sanitation, and resolution of conflicts as well as providing minimum levels of free health care to all.

ACKNOWLEDGMENTS

Sir Zumla acknowledges support from the PANDORA-ID-NET grant from the EDCTP Reg/Grant RIA2016E-1609) is funded by the European and Developing Countries Clinical Trials Partnership (EDCTP2) Programme, which is supported under Horizon 2020, the European Union's Framework Programme for Research and Innovation. A. Zumla is in receipt of a National Institutes of Health Research senior investigator award.

REFERENCES

1. Falzon D, Schünemann HJ, Harausz E, et al. World Health Organization treatment guidelines for drug-resistant tuberculosis, 2016 update. Eur Respir J 2017;49(3):1602308.

2. Fregonese F, Ahuja SD, Akkerman OW, et al. Comparison of different treatments for isoniazid-resistant tuberculosis: an individual patient data meta-analysis. Lancet Respir Med 2018;6:265–75.

3. WHO treatment guidelines for isoniazid-resistant tuberculosis: supplement to the WHO treatment guidelines for drug-resistant tuberculosis. Geneva (Switzerland): World Health Organization; 2018. Licence: CC BY-NC-SA 3.0

IGO. Available at: https://www.who.int/tb/publications/2018/WHO_guidelines_isoniazid_resistant_TB/en/. Accessed January 15, 2019.

4. Medical Research Council. Streptomcin treatment of pulmonary tuberculosis: a Medical Research Council investigation. BMJ 1948;2:769–82.

5. Tiberi S, D'Ambrosio L, De Lorenzo S, et al. Tuberculosis elimination, patients' lives and rational use of new drugs: revisited. Eur Respir J 2016;47(2):664–7.

6. Global tuberculosis report 2018. Geneva (Switzerland): World Health Organization; 2018. Licence: CC BY-NC-SA 3.0 IGO. Available at: https://apps.who.int/iris/bitstream/handle/10665/274453/9789241565646-eng.pdf?ua=1. Accessed January 15, 2019.

7. Price of a Pandemic. Available at: https://docs.wixstatic.com/ugd/309c93_2709b6ff47c946fe97b94a72fdfd94e3.pdf?index=trueand www.globaltbcaucus.org. Accessed January 15, 2019.

8. Sharma A, Hill A, Kurbatova E, et al. Estimating the future burden of multidrug-resistant and extensively drug-resistant tuberculosis in India, the Philippines, Russia, and South Africa: a mathematical modelling study. Lancet Infect Dis 2017. https://doi.org/10.1016/S1473-3099(17)30247-5.

9. Handbook on TB laboratory diagnostic methods for the European Union. Stockholm (Sweden): ECDC: European Centre for Disease Prevention and Control; 2016. Available at: http://ecdc.europa.eu/en/publications/publications/tuberculosis-laboratory-diagnostic-methods-eu.pdf. Accessed April 4, 2019.

10. Use of liquid TB culture and drug susceptibility testing in low- and medium- income settings. Summary report of the Expert Group Meeting on the use of liquid culture media. Geneva (Switzerland): World Health Organization; 2007. Available at: http://www.who.int/tb/laboratory/use_of_liquid_tb_culture_summary_report.pdf. Accessed April 4, 2019.

11. Policy guidance on drug-susceptibility testing (DST) of second-line antituberculosis drugs. Geneva (Switzerland): World Health Organization: The STOPTB department; 2008. WHO/HTM/TB/2008.392; Available at: http://www.who.int/tb/publications/2008/who_htm_tb_2008_392.pdf. Accessed April 4, 2019.

12. Algorithm for laboratory diagnosis and treatment-monitoring of pulmonary tuberculosis and drug-resistant tuberculosis using state-of-the-art rapid molecular diagnostic technologies. Available at: http://www.euro.who.int/__data/assets/pdf_file/0006/333960/ELI-Algorithm.pdf.

13. Expert opinion of the European tuberculosis laboratory initiative core group members for the WHO European region. World Health Organization; 2017. Available at: http://www.euro.who.int/__data/assets/pdf_file/0006/333960/ELI-Algorithm.pdf. Accessed April 4, 2019.

14. Automated real-time nucleic acid amplification technology for rapid and simultaneous detection of tuberculosis and rifampicin resistance: Xpert MTB/RIF assay for the diagnosis of pulmonary and extra- pulmonary TB in adults and children. Policy update. Geneva (Switzerland): World Health Organization; 2011. ISBN: 978 92 4 150633 5. Available at: https://apps.who.int/iris/bitstream/handle/10665/112472/9789241506335_eng.pdf?sequence=1. Accessed April 5, 2019.

15. The use of molecular line probe assays for the detection of resistance to second-line anti-tuberculosis drugs: policy guidance. Geneva (Switzerland): World Health Organization; 2016. WHO/HTM/TB/2016.07; Available at: http://apps.who.int/iris/bitstream/10665/246131/1/9789241510561-eng.pdf. Accessed April 5, 2019.

16. Cabibbe AM, Walker TM, Niemann S, et al. Whole genome sequencing of Mycobacterium tuberculosis. Eur Respir J 2018;52:1801163.

17. Annex III, Flow charts of algorithms for screening and diagnosing tuberculosis (TB) in adults, with modelled yields and predictive values Systematic Screening for Active Tuberculosis: principles and Recommendations. Geneva (Switzerland): World Health Organization; 2013. Accessed April 5, 2019.

18. WHO consolidated guidelines on drug-resistant tuberculosis treatment. Geneva (Switzerland): World Health Organization; 2019. Available at: https://apps.who.int/iris/bitstream/handle/10665/311389/9789241550529-eng.pdf.

19. Tiberi S, Du Plessis N, Walzl G, et al. Tuberculosis: progress and advances in development of new drugs, treatment regimens, and host-directed therapies. Lancet Infect Dis 2018;18:e183–98.

20. Tiberi S, Scardigli A, Centis R, et al. Classifying new anti-tuberculosis drugs: rationale and future perspectives. Int J Infect Dis 2017;56:181–4.

21. Collaborative Group for the Meta-Analysis of Individual Patient Data in MDR-TB treatment–2017, Ahmad N, Ahuja SD, Akkerman OW, et al. Treatment correlates of successful outcomes in pulmonary multidrug-resistant tuberculosis: an individual patient data meta-analysis. Lancet 2018;392:821–34.

22. Van Deun A, Maug AK, Salim MA, et al. Short, highly effective, and inexpensive standardized treatment of multidrug-resistant tuberculosis. Am J Respir Crit Care Med 2010;182(5):684–92.

23. WHO. Global tuberculosis report 2016 2016. Switzerland. Available at: http://apps.who.int/medicinedocs/documents/s23098en/s23098en.pdf.

24. Nunn AJ, Rusen I, Van Deun A, et al. Evaluation of a standardized treatment regimen of anti-tuberculosis drugs for patients with multi-drug-resistant tuberculosis (STREAM): study protocol for a randomized controlled trial. Trials 2014; 15(1):353.

25. Nunn AJ, Philipps P, Meredith S, et al. A trial of a shorter regimen for rifampin-resistant tuberculosis. N Engl J Med 2019. https://doi.org/10.1056/NEJMoa1811867.

26. Cambau E, Viveiros M, Machado D, et al. Revisiting susceptibility testing in MDR-TB by a standardized quantitative phenotypic assessment in a European multicentre study. J Antimicrob Chemother 2015;70:686–96.

27. Sotgiu G, Tiberi S, D'Ambrosio L, et al. Faster for less: the new "shorter" regimen for multidrug-resistant tuberculosis. Eur Respir J 2016;48(5):1503–7.

28. Caminero JA, Scardigli A, van der Werf T, et al. Treatment of drug-susceptible and drug-resistant tuberculosis. In: Migliori GB, Bothamley G, Duarte R, et al, editors. Tuberculosis. 2018. Available at: https://books.ersjournals.com/content/tuberculosis-9781849841009.tab-info.

29. Van Deun A, Chiang CY. Shortened multidrug-resistant tuberculosis regimens overcome low-level fluoroquinolone resistance. Eur Respir J 2017;49(6): 1700223.

30. Heldal E, Van Deun A, Chiang CY, et al. Shorter regimens for multidrug-resistant tuberculosis should also be applicable in Europe. Eur Respir J 2017;49(6): 1700228.

31. van der Werf MJ, Ködmön C, Catchpole M. Shorter regimens for multidrug-resistant tuberculosis should also be applicable in Europe. Eur Respir J 2017; 49(6):1700463.

32. van der Werf MJ, Hollo V, Ködmön C, et al. Eligibility for shorter treatment of multidrug-resistant tuberculosis in the European Union. Eur Respir J 2017; 49(3) [pii:1601992].

33. Munoz-Torrico M, Salazar MA, de Jesús Mohedano Millán M, et al. Eligibility for the shorter regimen for multidrug-resistant tuberculosis in Mexico. Eur Respir J 2018;51(3):1702267.

34. Migliori GB, Sotgiu G, Rosales Klintz S, et al. ERS/ECDC statement: European Union standards for tuberculosis care, 2017 update. Eur Respir J 2018;51(5): 1702678.

35. Kendall EA, Fojo AT, Dowdy DW. Expected effects of adopting a 9 month regimen for multidrug-resistant tuberculosis: a population modelling analysis. Lancet Respir Med 2017;5(3):191–9.

36. Sotgiu G, Migliori GB. Effect of the short-course regimen on the global epidemic of multidrug-resistant tuberculosis. Lancet Respir Med 2017;5(3):159–61.

37. Migliori GB, Global Tuberculosis Network (GTN). Evolution of programmatic definitions used in tuberculosis prevention and care. Clin Infect Dis 2018. https://doi.org/10.1093/cid/ciy990.

38. Dooley KE, Chaisson RE. Tuberculosis and diabetes mellitus: convergence of two epidemics. Lancet Infect Dis 2009;9:737–46.

39. Jiménez-Corona ME, Cruz-Hervert LP, García-García L, et al. Association of diabetes and tuberculosis: impact on treatment and post-treatment outcomes. Thorax 2013;68:214–20.

40. Liu Q, Li W, Xue M, et al. Diabetes mellitus and the risk of multidrug resistant tuberculosis: a meta-analysis. Sci Rep 2017;7(1):1090.

41. Tegegne BS, Mengesha MM, Teferra AA, et al. Association between diabetes mellitus and multi-drug-resistant tuberculosis: evidence from a systematic review and meta-analysis. Syst Rev 2018;7(1):161.

42. Alffenaar JWC, Tiberi S, Verbeeck RK, et al. Therapeutic drug monitoring in tuberculosis: practical application for physicians. Clin Infect Dis 2017;64(1): 104–5.

43. Hao X, Yao L, Sun H, et al. A cohort study on the outcome of multidrug-resistant tuberculosis in elderly patients. Zhonghua Jie He He Hu Xi Za Zhi 2014;37(3): 188–91.

44. Seto J, Wada T, Suzuki Y, et al. *Mycobacterium tuberculosis* transmission among elderly persons, Yamagata Prefecture, Japan, 2009-2015. Emerg Infect Dis 2017;23(3):448–55.

45. Coffman J, Chanda-Kapata P, Marais BJ, et al. Tuberculosis among older adults in Zambia: burden and characteristics among a neglected group. BMC Public Health 2017;17(1):804.

46. Marks SM, Mase SR, Morris SB. Systematic review, meta-analysis, and cost-effectiveness of treatment of latent tuberculosis to reduce progression to multidrug-resistant tuberculosis. Clin Infect Dis 2017;64(12):1670–7.

47. Dara M, Sotgiu G, Zaleskis R, et al. Untreatable tuberculosis: is surgery the answer? Eur Respir J 2015;45(3):577–82.

48. Borisov SE, D'Ambrosio L, Centis R, et al. Outcomes of patients with drug-resistant-tuberculosis treated with bedaquiline -containing regimens and undergoing adjunctive surgery. J Infect 2019;78(1):35–9.

49. Pontali E, Sotgiu G, Tiberi S, et al. Combined treatment of drug-resistant tuberculosis with bedaquiline and delamanid: a systematic review. Eur Respir J 2018; 52(1):1800934.

50. Munoz-Torrico M, Cid-Juarez S, Galicia-Amor S, et al. Sequelae assessment and rehabilitation. In: Migliori GB, Bothamley G, Duarte R, et al, editors. Tuberculosis. 2018. Available at: https://books.ersjournals.com/content/tuberculosis-9781849841009.tab-info.

51. Visca D, Zampogna E, Sotgiu G, et al. Pulmonary rehabilitation is effective in patients with tuberculosis pulmonary sequelae. Eur Respir J 2019;53(3) [pii: 1802184].

52. Pontali E, Sotgiu G, Tiberi S, et al. Cardiac safety of bedaquiline: a systematic and critical analysis of the evidence. Eur Respir J 2017;50:1701462.

53. World Health Organization. WHO best-practice statement on the off-label use of bedaquiline and delamanid for the treatment of multidrug-resistant tuberculosis. Geneva (Switerzland): World Health Organization; 2017. Accessed January 16, 2019.

54. Wilkinson RJ, Rohlwink U, Misra UK, et al. Tuberculous meningitis. Nat Rev Neurol 2017;13(10):581–98. Accessed June 28, 2018.

55. Akkerman OW, Odish OF, Bolhuis MS, et al. Pharmacokinetics of bedaquiline in cerebrospinal fluid and serum in multidrug-resistant tuberculous meningitis. Clin Infect Dis 2016;62:523–4.

56. Matteelli A, Centis R, D'Ambrosio L, et al. WHO strategies for the programmatic management of drug-resistant tuberculosis. Expert Rev Respir Med 2016;10(9): 991–1002.

57. Raviglione M. Evolution of the strategies for control and elimination of tuberculosis. In: Migliori GB, Bothamley G, Duarte R, et al, editors. Tuberculosis. 2018. Available at: https://books.ersjournals.com/content/tuberculosis-9781849841009.tab-info.

58. Lönnroth K, Migliori GB, Abubakar I, et al. Towards tuberculosis elimination: an action framework for low-incidence countries. Eur Respir J 2015;45(4):928–52.

59. Dye C, Williams BG. Criteria for the control of drug-resistant tuberculosis. Proc Natl Acad Sci U S A 2000;97(14):8180–5.

60. Gunther G, van Leth F, Altet N, et al. Beyond multidrug-resistant tuberculosis in Europe: a TBNET study. Int J Tuberc Lung Dis 2015;19(12):1524–7.

61. Borisov SE, Dheda K, Enwerem M, et al. Effectiveness and safety of bedaquiline-containing regimens in the treatment of MDR- and XDR-TB: a multicentre study. Eur Respir J 2017;49(5). https://doi.org/10.1183/13993003.00387-2017.

62. Tiberi S, Pontali E, Tadolini M, et al. Challenging MDR-TB clinical problems- the case for a new Global TB Consilium supporting the compassionate use of new anti-TB drugs. Int J Infect Dis 2019. https://doi.org/10.1016/j.ijid.2019.01.040.

63. Falzon D, Gandhi N, Migliori GB, et al. Resistance to fluoroquinolones and second-line injectable drugs: impact on multidrug-resistant TB outcomes. Eur Respir J 2013;42(1):156–68.

64. Migliori GB, Sotgiu G, Gandhi NR, et al. Drug resistance beyond extensively drug-resistant tuberculosis: individual patient data meta-analysis. Eur Respir J 2013;42(1):169–79.

65. Ahuja SD, Ashkin D, Avendano M, et al. Multidrug resistant pulmonary tuberculosis treatment regimens and patient outcomes: an individual patient data meta-analysis of 9,153 patients. PLoS Med 2012;9(8):e1001300.

66. Schnippel K, Ndjeka N, Maartens G, et al. Effect of bedaquiline on mortality in South African patients with drug-resistant tuberculosis: a retrospective cohort study. Lancet Respir Med 2018;6(9):699–706.

67. Olayanju O, Limberis J, Esmail A, et al. Long-term bedaquiline-related treatment outcomes in patients with extensively drug-resistant tuberculosis from South Africa. Eur Respir J 2018;51(5) [pii:1800544].

68. O'Grady J, Maeurer M, Mwabab P, et al. New and improved diagnostics for detection of drug-resistant pulmonary tuberculosis. Curr Opin Pulm Med 2011;17:134–41.

69. O'Grady J, Bates M, Chilukutu L, et al. Evaluation of the Xpert MTB/RIF assay at a Tertiary Care Referral Hospital in a setting where tuberculosis and HIV infection are highly endemic. Clin Infect Dis 2012;55:1171–8.

70. Pai M, Schito M. Tuberculosis diagnostics in 2015: landscape, priorities, needs, and prospects. J Infect Dis 2015;211(suppl2):S21–8.

71. Catanzaro A, Rodwell TC, Catanzaro DG, et al. Performance comparison of three rapid tests for the diagnosis of drug-resistant tuberculosis. PLoS One 2015;10(8):e0136861.

72. Weyer K, Mirzayev F, Migliori GB, et al. Rapid molecular TB diagnosis: evidence, policy making and global implementation of Xpert MTB/RIF. Eur Respir J 2013; 42(1):252–71.

73. Cox H, Dickson-Hall L, Ndjeka N, et al. Delays and loss to follow-up before treatment of drug-resistant tuberculosis following implementation of Xpert MTB/RIF in South Africa: A retrospective cohort study. PLoS Med 2017;14(2):e1002238.

74. Diacon AH, Pym A, Grobusch M, et al. The diarylquinoline TMC207 for multidrug-resistant tuberculosis. N Engl J Med 2009;360:2397–405.

75. Diacon AH, Donald PR, Pym A, et al. Randomized pilot trial of eight weeks of bedaquiline (TMC207) treatment for multidrug-resistant tuberculosis: long-term outcome, tolerability, and effect on emergence of drug resistance. Antimicrob Agents Chemother 2012;56:3271–6.

76. Migliori GB, Pontali E, Sotgiu G, et al. Combined use of delamanid and bedaquiline to treat multidrug-resistant and extensively drug-resistant tuberculosis: a systematic review. Int J Mol Sci 2017;18(2). https://doi.org/10.3390/ijms18020341.

77. Pontali E, Sotgiu G, D'Ambrosio L, et al. Bedaquiline and multidrug-resistant tuberculosis a systematic and critical analysis of the evidence. Eur Respir J 2016;47(2):394–402.

78. Pontali E, D'Ambrosio L, Centis R, et al. Multidrug-resistant tuberculosis and beyond: an updated analysis of the current evidence on bedaquiline. Eur Respir J 2017;49(3). https://doi.org/10.1183/13993003.00146-2017.

79. Tadolini M, Lingtsang RD, Tiberi S, et al. First case of extensively drug-resistant tuberculosis treated with both delamanid and bedaquiline. Eur Respir J 2016; 48(3):935–8.

80. Maryandyshev A, Pontali E, Tiberi S, et al. Bedaquiline and Delamanid Combination Treatment of 5 Patients with Pulmonary Extensively Drug-Resistant Tuberculosis. Emerg Infect Dis 2017;23(10). https://doi.org/10.3201/eid2310.170834.

81. Ferlazzo G, Mohr E, Laxmeshwar C, et al. Early safety and efficacy of the combination of bedaquiline and delamanid for the treatment of patients with drug-resistant tuberculosis in Armenia, India, and South Africa: a retrospective cohort study. Lancet Infect Dis 2018. Available at: https://doi.org/10.1016/S1473-3099(18)30100-2.

82. Tadolini M, Tiberi S, Migliori GB. Combining bedaquiline and delamanid to treat multidrug-resistant tuberculosis. Lancet Infect Dis 2018;18(5):480–1.

83. Sotgiu G, Pontali E, Migliori GB. Linezolid to treat MDR-/XDR-tuberculosis available evidence and future scenarios. Eur Respir J 2015;45(1):25–9.

84. Sotgiu G, Centis R, D'Ambrosio L, et al. Efficacy, safety and tolerability of linezolid containing regimens in treating MDR- TB and XDR-TB: systematic review and meta-analysis. Eur Respir J 2012;40:1430–42.

85. Dalcolmo M, Gayoso R, Sotgiu G, et al. Effectiveness and safety of clofazimine in multidrug-resistant tuberculosis: a nationwide report from Brazil. Eur Respir J 2017;49(3). https://doi.org/10.1183/13993003.02445-2016.

86. Tiberi S, Sotgiu G, D'Ambrosio L, et al. Comparison of effectiveness and safety of imipenem/clavulanate- versus meropenem/clavulanate-containing regimens in the treatment of MDR- and XDR-TB. Eur Respir J 2016;47(6):1758–66.

87. Tiberi S, Payen MC, Sotgiu G, et al. Effectiveness and safety of meropenem/clavulanate-containing regimens in the treatment of MDR- and XDR-TB. Eur Respir J 2016;47(4):1235–43.

88. Tiberi S, D'Ambrosio L, De Lorenzo S, et al. Ertapenem in the treatment of multidrug-resistant tuberculosis first clinical experience. Eur Respir J 2016; 47(1):333–6.

89. Akkerman O, Aleksa A, Alffenaar JW, et al. Surveillance of adverse events with bedaquiline and delamanid: a global feasibility study. Int J Infect Dis 2019;83:72–6.

90. World Health Organization. WHO policy on infection control in healthcare facilities, congregate settings and households. Geneva (Switzerland): World Health Organization; 2009. Accessed January 20, 2019.

91. Sotgiu G, D'Ambrosio L, Centis R, et al. TB and M/XDR-TB infection control in European TB reference centres: the Achilles' heel? Eur Respir J 2011;38:1221–3.

92. Migliori GB, Sotgiu G, D'Ambrosio L, et al. TB and MDR/XDR-TB in European Union and European Economic Area countries: managed or mismanaged? Eur Respir J 2012;39(3):619–25.

93. Sotgiu G, Centis R, D'ambrosio L, et al. Development of a standardised tool to survey MDR-/XDR-TB case management in Europe. Eur Respir J 2010;36(1):208–11.

94. van der Werf M. ERS/ECDC updated European Union standards of tuberculosis care. Paris: European Respiratory Society Congress; 2018 [abstract: 5326].

95. WHO guidelines on tuberculosis infection prevention and control, 2019 update. Geneva (Switzerland): World Health Organization; 2019. Available at: https://apps.who.int/iris/bitstream/handle/10665/311259/9789241550512-eng.pdf?ua=1&ua=1. Accessed April 5, 2019.

96. Nardell E, Volchenkov G. Transmission control: a refocused approach. In: Migliori GB, Bothamley G, Duarte R, et al, editors. Tuberculosis. 2018. Available at: https://books.ersjournals.com/content/tuberculosis-9781849841009.tab-info.

97. Carter DJ, Glaziou P, Lönnroth K, et al. The impact of social protection and poverty elimination on global tuberculosis incidence: a statistical modelling analysis of Sustainable Development Goal 1. Lancet Glob Health 2018. Available at: https://doi.org/10.1016/S2214-109X(18)30195-5.

98. Migliori GB, Garcia-Basteiro AL. Predicting the effect of improved socioeconomic health determinants on the tuberculosis epidemic. Lancet Glob Health 2018;6:e475–6.

99. Matteelli A, Rendon A, Tiberi S, et al. Tuberculosis elimination: where are we now? Eur Respir Rev 2018;27(148):180035.

100. Davtyan K, Hayrapetyan A, Dara M, et al. Key role of tuberculosis services funding mechanisms in tuberculosis control and elimination. Eur Respir J 2015;45(1): 289–91.

101. Gillini L, Davtyan K, Davtyan H, et al. TB financing in East Europe promotes unnecessary hospital admissions: the case of Armenia. J Infect Dev Ctries 2013; 7(3):289–92.

102. World Health Organization. Companion handbook to the WHO guidelines for the programmatic management of drug-resistant tuberculosis. 2014. Available at: https://www.ncbi.nlm.nih.gov/books/NBK247420/pdf/Bookshelf_NBK247420.pdf.

Antibiotic-Resistant Community-Acquired Bacterial Pneumonia

Jeffery Ho, PhD[a], Margaret Ip, MD[a,b],*

KEYWORDS

- Community-acquired pneumonia • Antimicrobial resistance
- *Streptococcus pneumoniae* • *Mycoplasma pneumoniae* • *Haemophilus influenzae*

KEY POINTS

- Antibiotics are commonly prescribed for respiratory tract infections, including community-acquired pneumonia (CAP), and constitute most antibiotic prescriptions in both ambulatory and hospital care patients.
- There is a changing epidemiology of CAP in the United States and worldwide with an increasing aging population with comorbidities.
- Although the common bacterial pathogens are etiologic agents of CAP globally, geographic differences exist, especially in the Asia Pacific region.
- The prevalence of resistance and their mechanisms of pathogens are important to guide the selection of appropriate antibiotics.
- Advanced technologies with rapid diagnostics may enhance etiologic agent-targeted therapy in future.

INTRODUCTION

Antimicrobial resistance is a global concern, and prudent use of antibiotics is essential to preserve the current armamentarium of effective drugs. Acute respiratory tract infection is the most common reason for antibiotic prescription in adults. Although there have been noticeable declines in the children prescription rate in the United States, antibiotic prescription rates have risen for adults, from approximately 192

Disclosure Statement: M. Ip has received funds and/or self-initiated projects and/or consultancy/advisory boards from Pfizer Corp, MSD, GlaxoSmithKline (HK) Ltd; Belpharma SA, Luxembourg; Novartis Asia Pacific Pharmaceuticals Pte Ltd, and AstraZeneca (HK) Ltd. J. Ho has no conflicts of interest to disclose.
a Department of Microbiology, Faculty of Medicine, Chinese University of Hong Kong, Shatin, Hong Kong; b Department of Microbiology, Chinese University of Hong Kong, Prince of Wales Hospital, Shatin, Hong Kong
* Corresponding author. Department of Microbiology, Chinese University of Hong Kong, Prince of Wales Hospital, Shatin, Hong Kong.
E-mail address: margaretip@cuhk.edu.hk
twitter: @mip_labCU (M.I.)

Infect Dis Clin N Am 33 (2019) 1087–1103
https://doi.org/10.1016/j.idc.2019.07.002
0891-5520/19/© 2019 Elsevier Inc. All rights reserved.

id.theclinics.com

million to 198 million in 2014.[1] Among more than 100 million adult ambulatory care visits annually, approximately 41% of the antimicrobial prescriptions had been prescribed for respiratory conditions, and within hospitals, a major indication for antibiotic use was for community-onset lower respiratory tract infection.[2] Updating the knowledge on the prevalence and resistance of common antimicrobial-resistant pathogens in community-acquired respiratory tract infections (RTI), may pave the way to enhancing appropriate antibiotic use in the treatment of RTI in ambulatory and health care setting.

CHANGING EPIDEMIOLOGY OF COMMUNITY-ACQUIRED PNEUMONIA

Community-acquired pneumonia (CAP) is an important cause of morbidity and mortality worldwide. In the United States, pneumonia accounted for more than 2.6 million hospitalizations per year, ranking it second for all hospital admissions.[3] The incidence of CAP requiring hospitalization has been estimated at 248 cases per 100,000 adults, but increases to 630 per 100,000 adults 65 to 79 years of age, and 1643 cases per 100,000 among those 80 years of age and older.[4] However, a more recent study from University of Louisville, Kentucky in 2017 estimated a higher incidence of 2093 cases per 100,000 of patients aged ≥65 years. Likewise, in Europe, the incidence varied by countries and ranged from 296 per 100,000 in Germany[5] and Hungary,[6] respectively. In a recent review, the incidence of all-cause pneumonia in Europe was 68 to 7000 per 100,000 population, and this varied by country, age group, study, and time period.[7] Besides an increasing incidence with age, other comorbid conditions, such as existing chronic airway,[8,9] obesity,[10] use of proton pump inhibitors,[11] among others, have been associated with increased risks for CAP.[12] Moreover, those 75 years and older with CAP had been associated with up to 2-fold higher risk for death during hospitalization compared with those aged 65 to 74 years, after adjustment for confounders.[13,14] The population aged 65 years and over will be expected to exceed 71.5 million in the United States by 2030. This has almost doubled from 37.3 million in 2006.[15] With the changing demographics in the population of increasing age and those living with comorbid conditions, the potential healthcare burden of CAP is tremendous.

In the Etiology of Pneumonia in the Community (EPIC) study in which 2259 adults with confirmed CAP from hospitals in the US, Streptococcus *pneumoniae* remained the most frequently isolated bacteria in CAP.[4] The etiologies were followed by *Mycoplasma pneumoniae*, *Staphylococcus aureus*, *Legionella pneumophila*, and Enterobacteriaceae.[4] These pathogens are common pathogens of CAP globally, whereas other atypical bacteria, *Chlamydophila pneumoniae* and *Coxiella burnetii*, have also been noted in other countries.[16–19] The prevalence of these bacteria as etiologic agents differs geographically and varies with patient population. Compared with European studies, pathogens such as *Haemophilus influenzae*, *Mycobacterium, tuberculosis*, *M pneumoniae*, and Enterobacteriaceae were more common in Asia.[18] A high incidence of *Klebsiella pneumoniae* is present,[18–20] whereas *Burkholderia pseudomallei* and *Acinetobacter baumanii* are also important causes of CAP in Asia Pacific regions.[21–23] The epidemiology, cause of CAP, and antimicrobial resistance from among the Asia-Pacific region have been comprehensively reviewed.[19] The primary bacterial causes for CAP in different regions worldwide are summarized in **Fig. 1**.[4,19,24–26]

However, more importantly are the antimicrobial resistance patterns of these bacterial pathogens, which vary significantly across various settings within countries and across continents. The prevalence of antimicrobial resistance in *S pneumoniae* and *M pneumoniae* has been documented over the years, impacting on the need

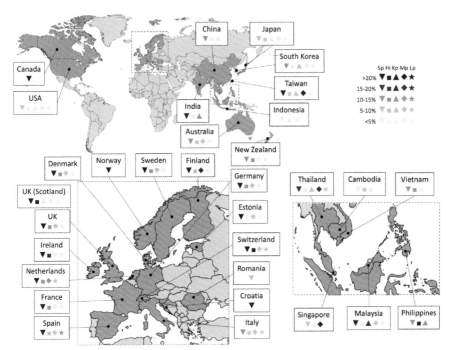

Fig. 1. Geographic distribution of etiologic agents responsible for CAP cases requiring hospitalization.[4,19,24–26] The shape of the marker represents a bacterial species, whereas its blue color shading denotes the percentage of the etiologic agent. Data are not available in countries shaded in gray. Hi, *H influenzae*; Kp, *K pneumoniae*; Lp, *L pneumophila*; Mp, *M pneumoniae*; Sp, *S pneumoniae*.

for more prudent use of antibiotics. In this review, the antimicrobial resistance associated with the common bacteria causing CAP is addressed, and the susceptibilities and mechanisms of resistance are discussed. **Table 1** lists the common bacteria causing CAP and known mechanisms of resistance to antimicrobial resistance phenotypes.

STREPTOCOCCUS PNEUMONIAE

Globally, *S pneumoniae* (SP) remains the most important bacterial pathogen responsible for CAP despite the widespread use of vaccines in the prevention of pneumococcal disease. In the United States, national immunization with protein conjugate vaccine in infants demonstrated the herd effect in protecting adult pneumococcal CAP, such that SP made up only 10% to 15% of all adult CAP hospitalizations in recent studies.[26] In fact, the EPIC study from the Centers for Disease Control and Prevention (CDC) revealed a lower proportion of pneumococcal pneumonia of 5% and all bacterial pneumonia comprising 15% of all CAP cases.[4] Diseases owing to multidrug-resistant (MDR) lineages such as 19A have been significantly reduced in the United States, whereas nonvaccine serotypes became more prevalent.[27,28] A study examining the antimicrobial susceptibilities of 8768 SP from 47 medical centers in the United States revealed that MDR (nonsusceptible to 3 classes of antimicrobial agents) and extensively drug-resistant (nonsusceptible to 5 classes of antimicrobial agents) rates decreased from 25.7% and 12.4% in 2010 to 17.7% and 3.6%, respectively,

Table 1
Common bacteria causing community-acquired pneumonia and known mechanisms of resistance to antimicrobial resistance phenotypes

Organism	Resistance Phenotype	Known Common Mechanism of Resistance	Antimicrobial Agents with Potential In Vitro Activity	Remarks (Reference)
S pneumoniae	Penicillin and β-lactam antibiotics	Mutations of pbp1a, 2b, 2x genes or of non-PBP cell wall synthesis pathways	Penicillins Third-generation cephalosporins, for example, ceftriaxone	Metcalf et al,[34] 2016
	Macrolide resistance	mef/mel genes; mega 2.IVa ermb gene rRNA A2016G mutation	Fluoroquinolones, for example, levofloxacin Linezolid Tigecycline Ceftaroline	Schroeder et al,[31] 2019
	Tetracycline resistance	tetM, tetS genes and others		
	Fluoroquinolone resistance	Mutations at QRDR region of parC, gyrA, (ParE) genes		
H influenzae	Penicillin and β-lactam antibiotics	β-Lactamases, for example, TEM-1, ROB-1	β-Lactam and/or β-lactamase inhibitors, for example, amoxicillin-clavulanate	Barbosa et al,[38] 2011; Mansson et al,[41] 2017
	Ampicillin, first- and second-generation cephalosporins	BLNAR mutation(s) with a.a. substitution of PBP3	Third-generation cephalosporin Fluoroquinolones, for example, levofloxacin	
	Carbapenem (heteroresistance)	Mutation(s) at the ftsI gene (encoding PBP3) Downregulate OMPs AcrAB-TolC efflux pump		Cherkaoui et al,[42] 2017; Cherhaoui et al,[43] 2018
	Macrolide resistance	ermB rRNA L4 Thr121Ser aa substitution		
	Fluoroquinolone resistance	Mutations at QRDR region gyrA and/or parC genes		

M pneumoniae	Macrolide resistance	Domain V of 23S rRNA mutation(s) A-to-G/C at 2063 or 2064 positions	Tetracyclines, fluoroquinolones	
C pneumoniae	NA		Tetracyclines, Fluoroquinolones, macrolides	
L pneumophila	Macrolide resistance	L4, L22 mutations, and domain V of 23S rRNA mutations; Efflux pump encoded by lpeAB genes	Macrolides, for example, clarithromycin; Fluoroquinolones; Rifampicin	Descours et al,[70] 2017; Massip et al,[71] 2017; Vandewalle-Capo et al,[68] 2017; Hennebique et al,[73] 2017
	Fluoroquinolone resistance	Mutations with a.a. substitutions of gyrA gene		
	Rifampicin resistance	Mutations of rpoB gene		Nielsen et al,[67] 2000
S aureus	Methicillin resistance	PBP2a (mecA)	Linezolid; Tigecycline; Ceftaroline	
	Reduced susceptibility or resistance to vancomycin	Alterations in cell wall peptidoglycan (vanA), and/or of regulatory genes agr		
	Macrolide resistance	Erm genes encoding 23S rRNA methylases; Ribosome protection via ABC-F proteins; msrA and mefA genes encoding efflux pump (MFS) transporter; mphC phosphotransferase gene or ereA, ereB esterase genes		
	Fluoroquinolone resistance	Multiple mutations at QRDR with a.a. substitutions of parC and gyrA genes		

(continued on next page)

Table 1
(continued)

Organism	Resistance Phenotype	Known Common Mechanism of Resistance	Antimicrobial Agents with Potential In Vitro Activity	Remarks (Reference)
Enterobacteriaceae (for example, *E coli*, *K pneumoniae*)	Resistance to penicillins, oxyimino-cephalosporins, and monobactams	ESBLs	Carbapenems β-Lactam and/or β-lactamase inhibitors, for example, ceftolozane–tazobactam Aminoglycosides Polymyxins Tigecycline Meropenem-vaborbactam (active against KPC) Ceftazidime-avibactam (active against class A and class Dβ-lactamases, not active against metallo-β-lactamases, eg, NDM) Two-to-three drug combination regimens	Durante-Mangoni et al,[77] 2019
	Carbapenem resistance and resistance to other β-lactam antibiotics	Carbapenemases Ambler class A: serine β-lactamases, for example, KPC and penicillinases; B: metallo-β-lactamases, for example, KPC NDM; D: oxacillinases, for example, OXA-48		
	Resistance to most β-lactam antibiotics, including carbapenems	AmpCβ-lactamases, cell wall porin mutations, efflux pumps		
	Fluoroquinolone resistance	Mutations at QRDR sites of *gyrA* and *parC* genes Plasmid mediated (*qnr* genes)		

Abbreviations: ABC-F, ATP-binding cassette-F; KPC, *Klebsiella pneumoniae* carbapenemase; MFS, major facilitator superfamily; NA, not applicable; NDM, New Delhi metallo-β-lactamase; OMPs, outer membrane porins; QRDR, quinolone-resistant determining region; rRNA, ribosomal RNA.

in 2016.[28] The percentage nonsusceptible to penicillin ($\geq$4 mg/L) and ceftriaxone ($\geq$2 mg/L) was reduced from 13.9% and 9.6% in 2010 to 3.2% and 2.3%, respectively, in 2016. On the other hand, erythromycin nonsusceptibility ($\geq$0.5 mg/L) increased from 41.6% to 46.6% in the same period. The change in percentage susceptibilities is likely the result of vaccine replacement serotypes that were macrolide resistant or MDR phenotypes (eg, 35B, 23A, 23B, and 15B).[28] With the expansion of nonvaccine serotypes, resistance develops especially as selected by the commonly used agents. Resistance development might have been compounded by the use of macrolides regardless of macrolide susceptibility, because it was previously shown in a meta-analysis that the use of macrolide for CAP patients was associated with a reduction in mortality.[29] Domon and colleagues[30] also demonstrated that exposure of macrolide-resistant SP to sublethal concentration of azithromycin or erythromycin reduced the production of pneumolysin through downregulation of pneumolysin gene (*ply*) transcription, thus providing additional explanation for the benefits of macrolides on the clinical outcome in pneumococcal disease. Recently, a novel determinant with specific genomic insertions of the Mega element, Mega-2.Iva and Mega-2.IVc, was associated with high-level macrolide resistance with microbiologically influenced minimum inhibitory concentration (MIC) greater than 16 mg/L. These resistant strains demonstrated a growth fitness advantage over those of the lower-level, mef(E)/mel-mediated phenotypes.[31] Thus, the epidemiology of SP and their resistance profiles are constantly changing and require the need for surveillance.

The US data also contrasted that of the European study in which a high-burden adult pneumococcal CAP was noted despite the use of the 23-valent polysaccharide vaccine.[7] Higher burdens were particularly present in elderly patients with comorbidities. Antimicrobial resistance especially to macrolides is an increasing problem, but there is also much variation between countries within Europe.[32] However, in a recent study, less than 1% of the pneumococci were penicillin resistant.[16] The variations may also relate to the differences in the implementation of pneumococcal vaccines between different countries.

The susceptibilities to levofloxacin, tigecycline, and linezolid remained stable at 98.8%, 99.9%, and 100%, respectively.[28] Ceftaroline was very active against SP in the SENTRY Antimicrobial Surveillance Program in 2015 to 2017 in Europe, Asia Pacific, and Latin America when 1734 of 1736 (99.9%) SP isolates were tested susceptible at the Clinical and Laboratory Standards Institute (CLSI) and Food and Drug Administration (FDA)–susceptible breakpoint of less than 0.5 mg/L, with $MIC_{50/90}$ less than 0.008/0.12 mg/L. Two isolates were nonsusceptible: one each from South Korea and Brazil, both with a ceftaroline MIC 1 mg/L.[33] Currently, the CDC performs whole-genome sequencing of the SP isolates from invasive disease, and it is anticipated that new resistance determinants will be identified and elucidated in the future.[34]

HAEMOPHILUS INFLUENZAE

H influenzae (HI) is an important pathogen causing respiratory tract infections and invasive diseases, including otitis media, meningitis, and sepsis. The introduction of *H influenzae* type b (Hib) vaccination has largely eliminated Hib infections. Remaining are 5 serovars of the encapsulated form, type a to f other than b. Clinical infections caused by the nonencapsulated strains, or non-typeable *H influenzae* (NTHi), also surged in the post-Hib vaccination era.[35] These NTHi strains were highly heterogeneous with multiple subpopulations with distinct core and accessory genes.[36] The elderly and those with chronic obstructive airway diseases were among the most vulnerable groups.

β-LACTAMS-RESISTANT *HAEMOPHILUS INFLUENZAE*

Ampicillin remains the first-line drug of choice for HI infections. Resistance to β-lactams is commonly mediated by production of β-lactamases or altered penicillin-binding protein (PBP) 3, the drug target. The other PBPs have a limited role on relaying drug action in HI. Of 1172 HI isolates obtained from patients with CAP from the SENTRY Antimicrobial Surveillance Program in 2015 to 2017 in Europe, Asia Pacific, and Latin America, all of the HI isolates were susceptible to ceftriaxone (MIC50/90, $\leq$0.015/$\leq$0.015 mg/L), 99.9% were susceptible to meropenem (MIC50/90, 0.06/0.25 mg/L), and 96.9% were susceptible to amoxicillin-clavulanate (MIC50/90, 0.5/2 mg/L).[33]

In a European study, more than 10% of the HI strains were β-lactamase producers.[16] A study from the United States revealed β-lactamase production in 18.7% of HI isolates, and β-lactamase–producing strains exhibited slightly higher ceftaroline MIC values (MIC50/90, 0.015/0.12 mg/L) compared with β-lactamase–negative isolates (MIC50/90, 0.008/0.03 mg/L).[33] Production of TEM-1, TEM-15, and ROB-1 β-lactamases was among the common plasmid-borne resistance mechanisms in HI. These hydrolytic enzymes confer resistance to ampicillin and third-generation cephalosporins.[37] Addition of β-lactamase inhibitors, such as clavulanic acid, to the regimen might not be useful in the case of β-lactamase producers, which had simultaneous amino acid (a.a.) substitution in the transpeptidase domain of PBP3, reducing its binding affinity to ampicillin and other β-lactams. These strains have an ampicillin MIC between 1 and 4 μg/mL, which can easily be missed in routine diagnostic laboratories.[38] Thus, sequencing of *ftsI* gene, which encodes PBP3, has been proposed to be part of the routine antibiotic susceptibility testing in clinical laboratory.[39] Indeed, mutation of the *ftsI* gene is an increasingly recognized mechanism for ampicillin resistance in β-lactamase–negative ampicillin-resistant (BLNAR) strains.[40] Testing 141 HI strains with nucleotide sequence changes in the *ftsI* gene revealed that more than 85% of the isolates had the a.a. substitutions of Asn526Lys, Val547Ile, and Asn569Ser in PBP3.[38,41] Although the virulence of BLNAR strains may vary, infection caused by a certain clone, such as sequence type (ST) 14 NTHi with altered PBP3 type IIb, was associated with a higher hospitalization rate, as compared with other NTHi clonotypes.[41] More alarming is the recent reports of heterogeneous resistance to carbapenems. These strains have gathered several mechanisms together, including modified PBP3, downregulated outer membrane porins, and upregulated AcrAB-TolC multidrug efflux pumps.[42,43] Of 46 imipenem heteroresistant isolates, more than 25 different mutation patterns were observed, highlighting the heterogeneity of NTHi isolates.[42]

NON-β-LACTAM RESISTANCE IN *HAEMOPHILUS INFLUENZAE*

Increasing isolation of BLNAR NTHi led to consideration of alternative drugs other than β-lactams.[44] Mutations of drug targets in combination with reduced drug permeability and enhanced efflux reduced the bacterial susceptibility to other non-β-lactams, such as macrolides and fluoroquinolones. HI with reduced susceptibility to quinolones frequently harbors a.a. substitutions of Ser84Leu and Asp88Tyr in the quinolone-resistance determining regions of GyrA resulting in elevated MIC up to 0.25 μg/mL for tosufloxacin and levofloxacin.[45] Strains with additional a.a. substitutions of Glu88Lys and Ser84Ile in ParC had even higher MIC to levofloxacin of up to 1 μg/mL.[46,47] The mechanisms mediating macrolide resistance include acquisition of resistance determinant *ermB* and target modification in ribosomal RNA proteins L4 of Thr121Ser at position 121 as compared with Rd Kw20, a reference HI standard strain.[43] All in all, resistance or reduced susceptibility to β-lactams, cephems, carbapenems, and other non-β-lactam agents is increasingly reported for HI. Surveillance for these heteroresistant strains should be performed in regions where HI infections are endemic.

MYCOPLASMA PNEUMONIAE

M pneumoniae (MP) is an intracellular organism responsible for CAP, with a higher prevalence seen in young adults and children.[4] Without a peptidoglycan cell wall, MP is intrinsically resistant to β -lactams and glycopeptides. Macrolides remain the first-line drug of choice, whereas tetracyclines and fluoroquinolones are alternative options for pneumonia caused by macrolide-resistant strains.[48,49] The prevalence of macrolide resistance varies across geographic locations. The highest prevalence was seen in China, where 69.2%[50,51] to 85.5%[52,53] of MP isolates had been reported resistant to macrolides. In North America, macrolide resistance ranged from 10% in the United States[54] to 12.1% in Canada[55] and was comparable to the level in South Korea (10.3%).[56] In Italy[57] and Australia,[52] only 1.3% and 3.3% of the MP isolates, respectively, were not susceptible to macrolides.

MACROLIDE-RESISTANT MYCOPLASMA PNEUMONIAE

Strains of MP are classified by genotyping of the P1 adhesin gene and multilocus variable number tandem repeat analysis (MLVA).[49] Common circulating clinical isolates are P1 type 1[52] and MLVA types 4572, 3562, and 3662, for which together accounted for 97% of the MP pneumonia.[49,54] In Hong Kong, the MLVA type 4572 was the major macrolide-resistant MP clone.[58] Resistance to macrolides in MP is commonly caused by point mutations in domain V of the single-copy 23S rRNA gene. Globally, the most common mutation was A-to-G/C transition at 2063 or 2064 position.[59–62] Consistent with the high prevalence of macrolide resistance seen in China, more than 69% of their MP isolates had A2063G mutation.[51,63] In Canada, 12.1% of the 91 MP isolates had A2063G mutation only with 1 isolate harboring A-to-G mutations at both 2063 and 2064 positions.[55] The mutated strains had a high level of resistance to erythromycin among other macrolides with MIC greater than 64 mg/L.[55,60]

Despite increasing reports of macrolide resistance, testing of 91 MP isolates in Canada found that all of them remained sensitive to fluoroquinolones and tetracyclines.[55] In a prospective multicenter observational study conducted in Japan, the macrolide-resistant MP remained highly sensitive to minocycline (MIC90 = 1.0 mg/L) and tosufloxacin (MIC90 = 0.25 mg/L).[64] A fully synthetic fluorocycline TP-271 was in the pipeline and tested effective against macrolide-resistant MP with MIC90 as low as 0.004 mg/L.[65] The use of rapid molecular methods for early detection of macrolide resistance in MP will allow a switch to second-line antibiotics, such as fluoroquinolones, tetracyclines, and fluorocyclines.

CHLAMYDOPHILA PNEUMOPHILA

C pneumophila (CP) is an obligate intracellular bacterial pathogen the entry of which into mucosal epithelial cells is required for intracellular survival. CP is susceptible to antibiotics that interfere with DNA and protein synthesis, including tetracyclines, macrolides, and quinolones, which are the compounds that have been most extensively studied and used for treatment of human infection.[66] The options for treating chlamydial infections have largely remained the same. There are a small number of new drugs currently in preclinical development and early clinical trials that may have a role in the treatment of chlamydial infections.

LEGIONELLA PNEUMOPHILA

L pneumophila (LP) serogroup 1 (sg1) is the major cause of legionnaires' disease, and other serogroups or other *Legionella* species also cause legionellosis. LP infects intra-cellularly, and the mainstay of treatment includes macrolides, fluoroquinolones, and rifampicin, which are able to concentrate intracellularly.[67–69] To date, clarithromycin and cotrimoxazole remain effective against LP strains.[69] Genotyping of LP is conduct-ed by MLVA, revealing that most of the clinical strains (104 out of 105) belong to ST1.[69]

MACROLIDE-RESISTANT *LEGIONELLA PNEUMOPHILA*

The MIC of LP to macrolides is generally lower than that to quinolones,[69] except for occasional reports of higher MIC to moxifloxacin (0.064 mg/L). Resistance to macro-lides is mediated by ribosomal mutations[70] and the presence of a tripartite efflux pump.[68,71] This efflux pump is encoded by lpeAB genes, which are prevalent in L.P. ST1, ST701, ST1335, and related STs, contributing to reduced susceptibility to azi-thromycin, spiramycin, and erythromycin.[68] Mutation of lpeAB genes reduced the MIC of LP to azithromycin from 0.5 mg/L to 0.032 mg/L.[68] Experimental propagation of 12 initially susceptible *L pneumophila* lineages under sublethal concentration of erythromycin or azithromycin revealed the mutational dynamics over the course of resistance development, which was initially driven by mutations in the L4 and L22 ribosomal proteins following changes in the domain V of the 23S rRNA.[70] Solithromy-cin among other ketolides has a considerably lower MIC90 of 0.031 mg/L compared with that of azithromycin (0.25 mg/L) against LP sg1.[72]

FLUOROQUINOLONE AND RIFAMPICIN RESISTANCE IN *LEGIONELLA PNEUMOPHILA*

Resistance to fluoroquinolones in LP is mediated by a.a. substitutions in the DNA gyr-ase, encoded by the gyrA gene.[73] The substitution hotspots include Thr83Ile, Asp87Asn, and Asp87His. These mutations occur in 10% to 13% of respiratory clinical isolates.[73] Interestingly, in infection sites where the local pH is low, finafloxacin ap-pears to be more effective than ciprofloxacin against phagocytosed LP.[74] Similar to other pathogens, rifampicin resistance in LP is probably mediated by rpoB gene sequence mutations. Although literature documenting resistance to this antibiotic class is sparse, a single study comparing the DNA sequence of rpoB gene of pheno-typically resistant LP with rifampicin-resistant *M tuberculosis* revealed 6 single-base mutations in 5 of 6 strains. Nonetheless, the remaining single strain did not contain any mutations as compared with rifampicin-susceptible strains. Thus, other mecha-nisms, besides the *rpoB* gene, may be involved in rifampicin resistance in LP.[67]

STAPHYLOCOCCUS AUREUS

The resistance of *S aureus* (SA) to penicillin was initially due to the production of pen-icillinases, which degrade penicillin in the extracellular space by hydrolyzing the β-lac-tam ring. Methicillin-resistant *S aureus* (MRSA) strains emerged with the production of an altered PBP2a, encoded by *mecA*, which renders the bacteria to be resistant to all other β-lactam antibiotics, with the exception of ceftaroline, which has a higher binding affinity for PBP2a.[75] Community-associated MRSA emerged in the United States and worldwide as a cause of necrotizing pneumonia. MRSA is susceptible to vancomycin, although both heteroresistant (hVISA) and vancomycin-intermediate

Staphylococcus aureus (VISA) have been implicated in cases of vancomycin treatment failure and persistent infection. The reduced susceptibility to vancomycin in both VISA and hVISA strains results from thickening of the cell wall and mutations in or downregulation of several genes, including the accessory gene regulator operon, thought to be driven by prolonged exposure to vancomycin.

Among SA isolates from the Sentry Surveillance Study of community-acquired bacterial pathogens from Europe, Asia, and Latin America in 2015 to 2017, 97.4% (n = 777) were susceptible to ceftaroline (MIC50/90, 0.25/1 mg/L), and susceptibility rates were higher among those from Western (98.0%) and Eastern Europe (100.0%) compared with Asia Pacific (94.0%) and Latin America (95.9%).[33] Oxacillin resistance varied from 31.9% in the Asia Pacific region to 23.7% in Latin America, and 21.7% and 15.0% in Western and Eastern Europe, respectively. All SA isolates were susceptible to linezolid, tigecycline, and vancomycin. Among MRSA isolates (n = 175), ceftaroline susceptibility ranged from 100.0% in European to that of 81.1% in the Asia Pacific region.[33]

ENTEROBACTERIACEAE INCLUDING *KLEBSIELLA PNEUMONIAE*

The emergence and spread of extended spectrum β-lactamases and especially of carbapenemase-producing Enterobacteriaceae worldwide are of particular concern and has limited the choice of therapy. These organisms, particularly with carbapenem-resistant *K pneumoniae* (KP), have mainly been associated with ventilated-, hospital-associated pneumonia, with high mortality,[76] the management of which is detailed in an updated review.[77] The isolation frequency of extended-spectrum β-lactamases (ESBL)-producing *Escherichia coli*, KP, and *Proteus mirabilis* has been detected at rates of 0.5%, 0.2% to 8.7%, and 0%, respectively, in CAP.[78,79] However, with the rapidly increasing carriage rates of ESBL- and carbapenem-resistant *E coli* and KPs from healthy subjects in the community and the isolation of these strains from various environmental sources, there is a potential concern for these MDR organisms to cause CAP in the future.

Other bacteria that are causative agents of CAP in Asian countries, such as *M tuberculosis*, *B pseudomallei*, and *A baumanii*, will not be further discussed, but are referred to in other reviews.[19,22] These causes may need to be considered for travelers who return from these countries and present with CAP.

LIMITATIONS AND MISSING GAPS THAT DESERVE FURTHER STUDIES

The data of CAP surveillance from European countries presented with wide variations across Europe. The lack of surveillance and discrepancies in the surveillance methods in many countries in Asia, including China, make the estimation of the burden of CAP very difficult. The disease burden estimation is also often compounded by the low utilization of microbiologic diagnostics to understand comprehensively the etiologic agents of CAP. Increasingly, rapid diagnostic techniques that identify a broad range of causative organisms enable one to determine the precise etiologic agent and appropriate therapy in the management of CAP. The overuse of antibiotics in the community before investigations in hospitals also yields bias because of the selection for resistant bacteria as well as unreliable resistance profiles for the pathogen concerned.

SUMMARY

CAP poses a significant health challenge and economic burden globally, especially in the current landscape of a dense and aging population. The advancing age with increasing comorbidities add to the predisposing risks to the development of CAP. Moving forward, with the increasing antimicrobial resistance to specific bacterial pathogens, a much larger amount of resources could be invested to improve educational activities to the target population, reduce any modifiable risk factors, and implement preventative measures, including effective vaccinations that may reduce the disease burden, especially in the elderly population. Rapid diagnostics for determination of precise etiologic agents, with appropriate pathogen-specific recommendations to the antibiotic choice in the management of these infections at different settings, should be made available for optimized care.

REFERENCES

1. Antibiotic use in the United States, 2017: antibiotic use by healthcare setting. Available at: https://www.cdc.gov/antibiotic-use/stewardship-report/outpatient.html. Accessed July 1, 2019.
2. Fridkin S, Baggs J, Fagan R, et al. Vital signs: improving antibiotic use among hospitalized patients. MMWR Morb Mortal Wkly Rep 2014;63:194–200.
3. National and regional estimates on hospital use for all patients. Rockville (MD): Agency for Healthcare Research and Quality; 2017. Available at: http://hcupnet.ahrg.gov.
4. Jain S, Self WH, Wunderink RG, et al. Community-acquired pneumonia requiring hospitalization among U.S. adults. N Engl J Med 2015;373:415–27.
5. Ewig S, Birkner N, Strauss R, et al. New perspectives on community-acquired pneumonia in 388 406 patients. Results from a nationwide mandatory performance measurement programme in healthcare quality. Thorax 2009;64:1062–9.
6. Tichopad A, Roberts C, Gembula I, et al. Clinical and economic burden of community-acquired pneumonia among adults in the Czech Republic, Hungary, Poland and Slovakia. PLoS One 2013;8:e71375.
7. Torres A, Cillóniz C, Blasi F, et al. Burden of pneumococcal community-acquired pneumonia in adults across Europe: a literature review. Respir Med 2018;137:6–13.
8. Williams NP, Coombs NA, Johnson MJ, et al. Seasonality, risk factors, and burden of community-acquired pneumonia in COPD patients: a population database study using linked healthcare records. Int J Chron Obstruct Pulmon Dis 2017;12:313–22.
9. Pasquale CB, Vietri J, Choate R, et al. Patient-reported consequences of community-acquired pneumonia in patients with chronic obstructive pulmonary disease. Chronic Obstr Pulm Dis 2019;6:132–44.
10. Frasca D, McElhaney J. Influence of obesity on pneumococcus infection risk in the elderly. Front Endocrinol 2019;10:71.
11. Cohen SM, Lee HJ, Leiman DA, et al. Associations between community-acquired pneumonia and proton-pump inhibitors in the laryngeal/voice-disordered population. Otolaryngol Head Neck Surg 2019;160:519–25.
12. Torres A, Blasi F, Dartois N, et al. Which individuals are at increased risk of pneumococcal disease and why? Impact of COPD, asthma, smoking, diabetes, and/or chronic heart disease on community-acquired pneumonia and invasive pneumococcal disease. Thorax 2015;70:984–9.
13. Corrado RE, Lee D, Lucero DE, et al. Burden of adult community-acquired, healthcare-associated, hospital-acquired, and ventilator-associated pneumonia, New York City, 2010 to 2014. Chest 2017;152:930–42.
14. Olasupo O, Xiao H, Brown JD. Relative clinical and cost burden of community-acquired pneumonia hospitalizations in older adults in the United States–a cross-sectional analysis. Vaccines 2018;6:E59.

15. Peyrani P, Mandell L, Torres A, et al. The burden of community-acquired bacterial pneumonia in the era of antibiotic resistance. Expert Rev Respir Med 2019;13: 139–52.
16. Leven M, Coenen S, Loens K, et al. Aetiology of lower respiratory tract infection in adults in primary care: a prospective study in 11 European countries. Clin Microbiol Infect 2018;24:1158–63.
17. Cilloniz C, Cardozo C, Garcia-Vidal C. Epidemiology, pathophysiology and microbiology of community-acquired pneumonia. Ann Res Hosp 2018;2:1–11.
18. Peto L, Nadjm B, Horby P, et al. The bacterial aetiology of adult community-acquired pneumonia in Asia: a systematic review. Trans R Soc Trop Med Hyg 2014;108:326–37.
19. Song JH, Huh K, Chung RY. Community-acquired pneumonia in the Asia-Pacific region. Semin Respir Crit Care Med 2016;37:839–54.
20. Lui G, Ip M, Lee N, et al. The role of atypical pathogens among adult hospitalized patients with community-acquired pneumonia. Respirology 2009;14:1098–105.
21. Hui DS, Ip M, Ling T, et al. A multicentre surveillance study on the characteristics, bacterial aetiologies and in vitro antibiotic susceptibilities in patients with acute exacerbations of chronic bronchitis. Respirology 2011;16(3):532–9.
22. Patamatamkul S, Klungboonkrong V, Praisarnti P, et al. A case-control study of community-acquired *Acineobacter baumannii* pneumonia and melioidosis pneumonia in northeast Thailand: an emerging fatal disease with unique clinical features. Diagn Microbiol Infect Dis 2017;87:79–86.
23. Musher DM, Thorner AR. Community-acquired pneumonia. N Engl J Med 2014; 371:1619–28.
24. Gadsby NJ, Russell CD, McHugh MP, et al. Comprehensive molecular testing for respiratory pathogens in community-acquired pneumonia. Clin Infect Dis 2016; 62:817–23.
25. Welte T, Torres A, Nathwani D. Clinical and economic burden of community-acquired pneumonia among adults in Europe. Thorax 2012;67:71–9.
26. Musher DM, Abers MS, Barlett JG. Evolving understanding of the causes of pneumonia in adults, with special attention to the role of pneumococcus. Clin Infect Dis 2017;65:1736–44.
27. Lo SW, Gladstone RA, van Tonder AJ, et al. Global Pneumococcal Sequencing Consortium. Pneumococcal lineages associated with serotype replacement and antibiotic resistance in childhood invasive pneumococcal disease in the post-PCV13 era: an international whole-genome sequencing study. Lancet Infect Dis 2019;19:759–69.
28. Pfaller MA, Mendes RE, Duncan LR, et al. In vitro activities of ceftaroline and comparators against *Streptococcus pneumoniae* isolates from U.S. hospitals: results from seven years of the AWARE surveillance program (2010 to 2016). Antimicrob Agents Chemother 2018;62 [pii:e01555-17].
29. Sligl WI, Asadi L, Eurich DT, et al. Macrolides and mortality in critically ill patients with community-acquired pneumonia: a systematic review and meta-analysis. Crit Care Med 2014;42:420–32.
30. Domon H, Maekawa T, Yonezawa D, et al. Mechanism of macrolide-induced inhibition of pneumolysin release involves impairment of autolysin release in macrolide-resistant Streptococcus pneumoniae. Antimicrob Agents Chemother 2018;62 [pii:e00161-18].
31. Schroeder MR, Lohsen S, Chancey ST, et al. High-level macrolide resistance due to the mega element [mef(E)/mel] in *Streptococcus pneumoniae*. Front Microbiol 2019;10:688.

32. European Antimicrobial Resistance Surveillance System (EARSS). Available at: https://ecdc.europa.eu/sites/portal/files/documents/AMR-surveillance-Europe-2016.pdf. Accessed July 1, 2019.

33. Sader HS, Flamm RK, Streit JM, et al. Antimicrobial activity of ceftaroline and comparator agents tested against organisms isolated from patients with community-acquired bacterial pneumonia in Europe, Asia, and Latin America. Int J Infect Dis 2018;77:82–6.

34. Metcalf BJ, Chochua S, Gertz RE Jr, et al. Active Bacterial Core Surveillance Team. Using whole genome sequencing to identify resistance determinants and predict antimicrobial resistance phenotypes for year 2015 invasive pneumococcal disease isolates recovered in the United States. Clin Microbiol Infect 2016; 22:1002.e1-8.

35. Suga S, Ishiwada N, Sasaki Y, et al. A nationwide population-based surveillance of invasive Haemphilus influenzae diseases in children after the introduction of the Haemophilus influenzae type b vaccine in Japan. Vaccine 2018;36:5678–84.

36. Pinto M, Gonzalez-Diaz A, Machado MP, et al. Insights into the population structure and pan-genome of Haemophilus influenzae. Infect Genet Evol 2019;67: 126–35.

37. Sondergaard A, Norskov-Lauritsen N. Contribution of PBP3 substitutions and TEM-1, TEM-15, and ROB-1 beta-lactamases to cefotaxime resistance in Haemophilus influenzae and Haemophilus parainfluenzae. Microb Drug Resist 2016;22: 247–52.

38. Barbosa AR, Giufre M, Cerquetti M, et al. Polymorphism in ftsI gene and β-lactam susceptibility in Portuguese Haemophilus influenzae strains: clonal dissemination of β-lactamase-positive isolates with decreased susceptibility to amoxicillin-clavulanic acid. J Antimicrob Chemother 2011;66:788–96.

39. Schotte L, Wautier M, Martiny D, et al. Detection of beta-lactamase-negative ampicillin resistance in Haemophilus influenzae in Belgium. Diagn Microbiol Infect Dis 2019;93:243–9.

40. Garcia-Cobos S, Arroyo M, Perez-Vazquez M, et al. Isolates of β-lactamase-negative ampicillin-resistant Haemophilus influenzae causing invasive infections in Spain remain susceptible to cefotaxime and imipenem. J Antimicrob Chemother 2014;69:111–6.

41. Mansson V, Skaare D, Riesbeck K, et al. The spread and clinical impact of ST144CC-PBP3 type IIb/A, a clonal group of non-typeable Haemophilus influenzae with chromosomally mediated β-lactam resistance–a prospective observational study. Clin Microbiol Infect 2017;23:209.e1-7.

42. Cherkaoui A, Diene SM, Renzoni A, et al. Imipenem heteroresistance in nontypeable Haemophilus influenzae is linked to a combination of altered PBP3, slow drug influx, and direct efflux regulation. Clin Microbiol Infect 2017;23:118.

43. Cherkaoui A, Gaia N, Baud D, et al. Molecular characterization of fluoroquinolones, macrolides, and imipenem resistance in Haemophilus influenzae: analysis of the mutations in QRDRs and assessment of the extent of the AcrAB-TolC-mediated resistance. Eur J Clin Microbiol Infect Dis 2018;37: 2201–10.

44. Han MS, Jung HJ, Lee HJ, et al. Increasing prevalence of group III penicillin-binding protein 3 mutations conferring high-level resistance to beta-lactams among nontypeable Haemophilus influenzae isolates from children in Korea. Microb Drug Resist 2019;25:567–76.

45. Ubukata K, Morozumi M, Sakuma M, et al. Genetic characteristics and antibiotic resistance of *Haemophilus influenzae* isolates from pediatric patients with acute otitis media after introduction of 13-valent pneumococcal conjugate vaccine in Japan. J Infect Chemother 2019;25(9):720–6.

46. Chen D, Wen S, Feng D, et al. Microbial virulence, molecular epidemiology and pathogenic factors of fluoroquinolones-resistant *Haemophilus influenzae* infections in Guangzhou, China. Ann Clin Microbiol Antimicrob 2018;23:41.

47. Tanaka E, Hara N, Wajima T, et al. Emergence of *Haemophilus influenzae* with low susceptibility to quinolones and persistence in tosufloxacin treatment. J Glob Antimicrob Resist 2019;18:104–8.

48. Hanada S, Morozumi M, Takahashi Y, et al. Community-acquired pneumonia caused by macrolide-resistant *Mycoplasma pneumoniae* in adults. Intern Med 2014;53:1675–8.

49. Rodriguez N, Mondeja B, Sardinas R, et al. First detection and characterization of macrolide-resistant *Mycoplasma pneumoniae* strains in Cuba. Int J Infect Dis 2019;80:115–7.

50. Yu HX, Zhao MM, Pu ZH, et al. A study of community-acquired *Mycoplasma pneumoniae* in Yantai, China. Colomb Med (Cali) 2018;49:160–3.

51. Guo DX, Hu WJ, Wie R, et al. Epidemiology and mechanism of drug resistance of *Mycoplasma pneumoniae* in Beijing, China: a multi-center study. Bosn J Basic Med Sci 2019;19:288–96.

52. Xue G, Wang Q, Yan C, et al. Molecular characterizations of PCR-positive *Mycoplasma pneumoniae* specimens collected from Australia and China. J Clin Microbiol 2014;52:1478–82.

53. Qu J, Yu X, Liu Y, et al. Specific multilocus variable-number tandem-repeat analysis genotypes of Mycoplasma pneumoniae are associated with diseases severity and macrolide susceptibility. PLoS One 2013;8:e82174.

54. Diaz MH, Benitez AJ, Winchell JM. Investigations of *Mycoplasma pneumoniae* infections in the United States: trends in molecular typing and macrolide resistance from 2006 to 2013. J Clin Microbiol 2015;53:124–30.

55. Eshaghi A, Memari N, Tang P, et al. Macrolide-resistant *Mycoplasma pneumoniae* in humans, Ontario, Canada, 2010-2011. Emerg Infect Dis 2013;19:1525–7.

56. Kim YJ, Shin KS, Lee KH, et al. Clinical characteristics of macrolide-resistant Mycoplasma pneumoniae from children in Jeju. J Korean Med Sci 2017;32:1642–6.

57. Loconsole D, De Robertis AL, Mallamaci R, et al. First description of macrolide-resistant *Mycoplasma pneumoniae* in adults with community-acquired pneumonia in Italy. Biomed Res Int 2019;2019:7168949.

58. Ho PL, Law PY, Chan BW, et al. Emergence of macrolide-resistant *Mycoplasma pneumoniae* in Hong Kong is linked to increasing macrolide resistance in multilocus variable-number tandem-repeat analysis type 4-5-7-2. J Clin Microbiol 2015;53:3560–4.

59. Caballero Jde D, del Campo R, Mafe Mdel C, et al. First report of macrolide resistance in a *Mycoplasma pneumoniae* isolate causing community-acquired pneumonia in Spain. Antimicrob Agents Chemother 2014;58:1265–6.

60. Dumke R, Stolz S, Jacobs E, et al. Molecular characterization of macrolide resistance of a *Mycoplasma pneumoniae* strain that developed during therapy of a patient with pneumonia. Int J Infect Dis 2014;29:197–9.

61. Copete AR, Aguilar YA, Rueda ZV, et al. Genotyping and macrolide resistance of *Mycoplasma pneumoniae* identified in children with community-acquired pneumonia in Medellin, Colombia. Int J Infect Dis 2018;66:113–20.

62. Matsumoto M, Nagaoka K, Suzuki M, et al. An adult case of severe life-threatening *Mycoplasma pneumoniae* pneumonia due to a macrolide-resistant strain, Japan: a case report. BMC Infect Dis 2019;19:204.

63. Wu PS, Chang LY, Lin HC, et al. Epidemiology and clinical manifestations of children with macrolide-resistant Mycoplasma pneumoniae pneumonia in Taiwan. Pediatr Pulmonol 2013;48:904–11.

64. Ishiguro N, Koseki N, Kaiho M, et al. Therapeutic efficacy of azithromycin, clarithromycin, minocycline and tosufloxacin against macrolide-resistant and macrolide-sensitive *Mycoplasma pneumoniae* in pediatric patients. PLoS One 2017;12:e0173635.

65. Grossman TH, Fyfe C, O'Briend W, et al. Fluorocycline TP-271 is potent against complicated community-acquired bacterial pneumonia pathogens. mSphere 2017;2:e4–17.

66. Kohlhoff SA, Hammerschlag MR. Treatment of chlamydial infections: 2014 update. Expert Opin Pharmacother 2015;16:205–12.

67. Nielsen K, Hindersson P, Hoiby N, et al. Sequencing of the rpoB gene in *Legionella pneumophila* and characterization of mutations associated with rifampin resistance in *Legionellaceae*. Antimicrob Agents Chemother 2000; 44:2679–83.

68. Vandewalle-Capo M, Massip C, Descours G, et al. Minimal inhibitory concentration distribution among wild-type strains of *Legionella pneumophila* identifies a subpopulation with reduced susceptibility to macrolides owing to efflux pump genes. Int J Antimicrob Agents 2017;50:684–9.

69. Sharaby Y, Nitzan O, Brettar I, et al. Antimicrobial agent susceptibilities of *Legionella pneumophila* MLVA-8 genotypes. Sci Rep 2019;9:6138.

70. Descours G, Ginevra C, Jacotin N, et al. Ribosomal mutations conferring macrolide resistance in *Legionella pneumophila*. Antimicrob Agents Chemother 2017; 61 [pii:e02188-16].

71. Massip C, Descours G, Ginevra C, et al. Macrolide resistance in *Legionella pneumophila*: the role of LpeAB efflux pump. J Antimicrob Chemother 2017;72: 1327–33.

72. Mallegol J, Fernandes P, Melano RG, et al. Antimicrobial activity of solithromycin against clinical isolates of *Legionella pneumophila* serogroup 1. Antimicrob Agents Chemother 2014;58:909–15.

73. Hennebique A, Bidart M, Jarraud S, et al. Digital PCR for detection and quantification of fluoroquinolone resistance in *Legionella pneumophila*. Antimicrob Agents Chemother 2017;61 [pii:e00628-17].

74. Lemaire S, van Bambeke F, Tulkens PM. Activity of finafloxacin, a novel fluoroquinolone with increased activity at acid pH, towards extracellular and intracellular *Staphylococcus aureus, Listeria monocytogenes*, and *Legionella pneumophila*. Int J Antimicrob Agents 2011;38:52–9.

75. Villegas-Estrada A, Lee M, Hesek D, et al. Co-opting the cell wall in fighting methicillin-resistant *Staphylococcus aureus*: potent inhibition of PBP 2a by two anti-MRSA beta-lactam antibiotics. J Am Chem Soc 2008;130:9212–3.

76. Gu D, Dong N, Zheng Z, et al. A fatal outbreak of ST11 carbapenem-resistant hypervirulent *Klebsiella pneumoniae* in a Chinese hospital: a molecular epidemiological study. Lancet Infect Dis 2018;18(1):37–46.

77. Durante-Mangoni E, Andini R, Zampino R. Management of carbapenem-resistant Enterobacteriaceae infections. Clin Microbiol Infect 2019;25(8):943–50.
78. Horie H, Ito I, Konishi S, et al. Isolation of ESBL-producing bacteria from sputum in community-acquired pneumonia or healthcare-associated pneumonia does not indicate the need for antibiotics with activity against this class. Intern Med 2018;57:487–95.
79. Ma HM, Hui DS, Lui GC, et al. Risk factors for drug-resistant bacterial pneumonia in older patients hospitalized with pneumonia in a Chinese population. QJM 2013; 106:823–9.

Antibiotic-Resistant Enteric Infections

Sadia Shakoor, MBBS[a,b], James A. Platts-Mills, MD[c], Rumina Hasan, MBBS, PhD[d,e],*

KEYWORDS

- Antibiotic resistance • Azithromycin • *Salmonella* • *Shigella* • *Campylobacter*
- Diarrhea • Enteric fever • OneHealth

KEY POINTS

- Antibiotic resistance among diarrheal and enteric pathogens is increasing and spreading globally owing to convergence of multiple risk factors among populations.
- Widespread ciprofloxacin resistance among diarrheal pathogens has rendered this antibiotic virtually ineffective in infectious diarrhea and enteric fever syndromes in high-burden regions.
- Azithromycin has emerged as an affective empiric treatment of enteric infections, except in populations with specific risk factors, such as men who have sex with men in *Shigella* endemic regions.
- Emergence of plasmidborne extended-spectrum beta lactamases in enteric fever is an alarming development and needs urgent control measures.
- Development and evaluation of pathogen-specific vaccines is needed, followed by strategic implementation in high-burden countries and regions. However, this should not distract from population-level measures of water, sanitation, and hygiene improvement, which have wider benefits.

INTRODUCTION

Enteric infections claimed an estimated 1.7 million lives in 2017 globally, with the highest burden in low-income and middle-income countries (LMICs) and at extremes of age.[1] This estimate includes systemic infections, that is, typhoid and paratyphoid,

Disclosures: Authors have no commercial or financial conflicts of interest.
[a] Pathology and Laboratory Medicine, Aga Khan University, Stadium Road, PO Box 3500, Karachi 74800, Pakistan; [b] Pediatrics and Child Health, Aga Khan University, Stadium Road, PO Box 3500, Karachi 74800, Pakistan; [c] Division of Infectious Diseases and International Health, University of Virginia, 200 Jeanette Lancaster Way, Charlottesville, VA 22903, USA; [d] Department of Pathology and Laboratory Medicine, Aga Khan University, Stadium Road, PO Box 3500, Karachi 74800, Pakistan; [e] Faculty of Infectious and Tropical Disease, London School of Hygiene and Tropical Medicine, Keppel Street, Bloomsbury, London WC1E 7HT, UK
* Corresponding author. Department of Pathology and Laboratory Medicine, Aga Khan University, Stadium Road, PO Box 3500, Karachi 74800, Pakistan.
E-mail address: Rumina.hasan@aku.edu

Infect Dis Clin N Am 33 (2019) 1105–1123
https://doi.org/10.1016/j.idc.2019.05.007
0891-5520/19/© 2019 Elsevier Inc. All rights reserved.

and typhoid alone claims hundreds of thousands of lives each year, mostly in Asia and sub-Saharan Africa.[2] Although observed incidence and mortality from enteric infections are highest among children and those older than 70 years, the epidemiology is changing,[1] and risk factors other than age are emerging. As efforts continue to reduce mortality among children, and to improve water, sanitation, and hygiene (WASH) measures and universal access to health care, new challenges have emerged. Among these is the rise in rates of antimicrobial resistance (AMR) in localized and/or invasive disease caused by enteric pathogens whereby antibiotics are absolute or relative indications,[3,4] such as *Salmonella enterica* serovars Typhi and Paratyphi, *Shigella* spp, *Campylobacter* spp, *Vibrio cholerae*, and diarrheagenic *Escherichia coli* (DEC), nontyphoidal salmonellae (NTS), *Clostridium difficile*, *Helicobacter pylori*, *Giardia* spp, and *Cryptosporidium* spp.

Emerging enteric infections reported by the Program for Monitoring Emerging Diseases (ProMED-mail) over the past 10 years (2009–2019) have identified emerging resistance in the following pathogens: *S enterica* (both typhoidal and nontyphoidal), DEC, *Shigella* spp, *Campylobacter* spp, and *Vibrio* spp.[5] Reports highlight the importance of infections in special populations and epidemiologic modifiers in high-risk groups. Resistance also has been reported with increasing frequency in *H pylori*.[6] **Table 1** describes the most important enteric pathogens for which antimicrobial therapy can be required and outlines pertinent phenotypic and genotypic AMR features, risk factors, current treatment recommendations for resistant strains, and available vaccines.[7–65]

A large proportion of emerging infections is caused by drug-resistant bacteria owing to the survival benefit in environments contaminated with antibiotics and antibiotic residues. Enteric bacteria are naturally adapted to such survival and spread in microbe-rich intestinal environments, and following continued shedding in fecal matter, survival in sewage and "brown water."[66]

Notably, emergence of extended-spectrum beta-lactamase (ESBL) carrying *Salmonella* Typhi (*S* Typhi) in Pakistan,[25] and that of azithromycin-resistant *Shigella* spp among men who have sex with mean (MSM)[34] has narrowed treatment options. Widespread ciprofloxacin resistance among all diarrheal and enteric pathogens has led to the ineffectiveness of this antibiotic in infectious diarrhea and enteric fever.[8,13,16,17,19–21,31,32,40,44] *H pylori* presents a unique challenge with respect to increasing antibiotic resistance and ineffective treatment regimens leading to intractable gastrointestinal illness, economic loss, and long-term morbidity.[54–57] Drug resistance is rarely observed in vitro in parasitic infections; however, clinical resistance and treatment failure have been reported.[60–65]

Although pathogen-specific risk factors may be modifiable, and treatment and preventive strategies may be used in areas with high burden, there are overarching factors at play that can be improved on to reduce the burden of enteric infections, and prevent the emergence of highly resistant phenotypes.

FACTORS CONTRIBUTING TO THE EMERGENCE OF ANTIBIOTIC-RESISTANT ENTERIC INFECTIONS

AMR in enteric pathogens is largely acquired by horizontal gene transfer (HGT) through exchange of resistance-determining mobile genetic elements (MGEs) carried on plasmids or chromosomes of bacteria belonging to different taxonomic groups.[67] Such exchange occurs in natural reservoirs or microbial ecosystems that serve as reservoirs of antibiotic-resistance genes (ARGs). The ARG pool is maintained in environments with high selective pressure exerted by contaminating antibiotic and antibiotic

Table 1

Details of enteric pathogens with recognized and emerging antibiotic resistance: risk factors for antibiotic resistance, antibiotic-resistance genes responsible (where applicable), regions reporting resistance, treatment recommendations for infections, and vaccines available

Enteric Pathogen	Population-Specific Risk Factors for Drug Resistance or Treatment Failure	Emerging/Reemerging Resistance Antibiotic [Drug-Resistance Gene]	Regions Reporting Resistance in Past 10 y	Current Recommendation for Antibiotic Therapy	Vaccines	References
Salmonella enterica						
NTS (*Salmonella* Typhimurium, *Salmonella* Enteritidis, *Salmonella* Agona, *Salmonella* Choleraseus, *Salmonella* Virchow, *Salmonella* Heidelberg, *Salmonella* Montevideo, *Salmonella* Corvalis, *Salmonella* Newport, etc.)	Residence in or travel to regions with high rates of antimicrobial resistance, poor access to safe water adequate sanitation. Exposure to infected food and animals. Immunocompromised individuals, HIV, extremes of age and malnutrition	Fluoroquinolones [Plasmid mediated *qnr* or quinolone resistance-determining region (QRDR) *gyrA*, *parC*] Third and fourth generation cephalosporins [*bla* CTX-M, on Inc plasmids, *bla*-CMY *bla*-TEM, *bla*-OXA] Carbapenems (*ompC* overexpression, *bla*-VIM, *bla*-NDM, *bla*-IMP) Azithromycin [*mphA*, *mphB*, *mefB*] Colistin [*mcr* gene mutations]	Asia, Africa, Americas, Europe Asia, Africa, Americas, Europe Asia, Europe Asia, Europe Europe, Africa, Asia, Australia	Recommendations vary. Antibiotic treatment recommended for infants and young infants and the immunocompromised, but rarely culture-guided. Diarrhea in older children and adults usually self-limiting. Culture-guided antibiotic treatment for invasive disease.	Vaccines candidates for *S* Typhimurium and *S* Dublin in development.	7–16

(continued on next page)

Table 1
(continued)

Enteric Pathogen	Population-Specific Risk Factors for Drug Resistance or Treatment Failure	Emerging/Reemerging Resistance Antibiotic [Drug-Resistance Gene]	Regions Reporting Resistance in Past 10 y	Current Recommendation for Antibiotic Therapy	Vaccines	References
Salmonella Typhi	Children and young adults; Residence in or travel to regions with high rates of resistance; Exposure to infected food or water	Fluoroquinolones: Ciprofloxacin [QRDR; (gyrA, gyrB, parC)], lasmidborne qnr genes; efflux pumps. Extended-spectrum cephalosporins ESBL [bla-SHV bla-TEM-1; bla-CTX-M] H58 lineage of S Typhi a highly transmissible clade that can harbor a complex multidrug resistance (MDR) element residing either on transmissible IncHI1 plasmids or within multiple chromosomal integration sites. Azithromycin [mefA, ermB]	Africa Asia United States Asia Asia	Culture and susceptibility-guided treatment preferred. Fluoroquinolones in areas with low resistance. In South Asia with high fluoroquinolone resistance, 3rd generation cephalosporins are recommended. For ESBL-producing (XDR) S Typhi, azithromycin is used, but no trials or recommended duration of therapy.	Injectable typhoid conjugate vaccine (TCV); for 6 mo to 45 y of age. Injectable unconjugated polysaccharide vaccine (Vi-PS vaccine) 2 y and older. Oral live attenuated Ty21a vaccine older than 6 y.	17-27
Salmonella Paratyphi A		Fluoroquinolones [QRDR; (gyrA, gyrB)] Third-generation cephalosporins Azithromycin, failure to respond	Asia Asia Travelers from Asia	As for S Typhi, although extensive resistance has not been reported in S Paratyphi A to date.	No vaccine licensed to date.	17,21,28-30

Organism	Risk factors	Resistance (genes)	Region	Treatment	Vaccine	Ref
Shigella spp	Children under 5 in LMIC MSM HIV	Ciprofloxacin [gyrA] Azithromycin [mphA, ermB] Ceftriaxone resistance (ESBL) [blaCTX-M] Coresistance ESBL and azithromycin genes on IncF plasmid	South Asia Americas, Australia, Europe Asia, Africa, Europe, Americas	Azithromycin; where available, culture and susceptibility testing recommended.	Shigella sonnei O antigen and outer membrane vesicle vaccines in trials, other approaches in development.	31–37
Campylobacter spp (Campylobacter jejunil Campylobacter coli)	Residence in or travel to regions with high rates of resistant Campylobacter in poultry	Fluoroquinolones (ciprofloxacin/levofloxacin) [gyrA, QRDR; cmeABC efflux pump gene cmeR–cmeABC in the presence of gyrA mutations] Macrolides (erythromycin/azithromycin) [23srRNA gene, ermB gene] Genes may be carried on a transposable multidrug resistance genomic island (MDRGI)	Americas, Europe, Asia, Africa	Most infections self-limiting, antibiotics indicated in immunocompromised patients, and in those with persistent or extraintestinal infections.	Vaccine candidates for human and animal use; killed whole cell and subunit, vaccines unsuccessful in phase 1; glycoconjugate vaccines to enter phase 1 trial.	38–42
DEC						
EHEC	Residence in high-income country	ESBL in O104:H4 Azithromycin O106:H18 and O26:H11 [mphA, ermB]	Europe	Antibiotics not recommended but azithromycin, rifaximin, and carbapenems (and even fosfomycin) may have some effect without inducing shiga toxin (stx) production.	Two types of commercial vaccines for cattle but no regulatory requirements to vaccinate.	43–45

(continued on next page)

Table 1
(continued)

Enteric Pathogen	Population-Specific Risk Factors for Drug Resistance or Treatment Failure	Emerging/Reemerging Resistance Antibiotic [Drug-Resistance Gene]	Regions Reporting Resistance in Past 10 y	Current Recommendation for Antibiotic Therapy	Vaccines	References
EAEC/ETEC	*Travel destinations in LMICs*	Ciprofloxacin [*gyrA, parC, qnr*] ESBL [*bla*-CTX-M; *bla*-DHA, *bla*-CMY] Azithromycin [*mphA, ermB*]	Asia, Africa	Azithromycin, rifaximin/ rifamycin.	ETEC vaccine in trials.	46–50
Vibrio cholerae		Ciprofloxacin [*qnr* genes on SXT element] Azithromycin [23srRNA gene; mobile elements/IncA plasmids carrying *ereAB, erm* B, *mphA, mefE* genes] Carbapenems [*bla*-oxa gene, *bla*NDM-1]	Asia, Africa, Europe Asia Europe, Asia	Antibiotics not the mainstay of treatment but are adjunctive to supportive and rehydration therapy.	Oral cholera vaccines; Vaccine efficacy low in younger children.	51–53
Helicobacter pylori	*Pediatric age group, cag A negative strains, previous treatment of H pylori infection, high population volume of antibiotic consumption*	Clarithromycin [point mutations in 23srRNA gene: A2143G/A2142G/A2142C] Levofloxacin [*gyrA*] Metronidazole [mutations in *rdxA* gene]	Asia, America, Europe	First line clarithromycin containing regimens in regions with <15% clarithromycin resistance; molecular resistance detection if region has >15% resistance. Second-line regimens with levofloxacin; metronidazole.	None.	54–57

Antibiotic-Resistant Enteric Infections **1111**

Organism	Risk factors	Resistance	Geographic	Treatment	Alternative	Ref
Clostridium difficile	*Previous treatment with metronidazole*	Metronidazole clinical resistance; susceptibility testing is challenging, and often not performed but reduced susceptibility has been reported		Metronidazole for mild to moderate infections; fidaxomicin and vancomycin for severe infections.	None.	58,59
Giardia lamblia (syn. *intestinalis, duodenalis*)	*Repeated Giardia infections, immunocompromised status*	Metronidazole clinical resistance (nitroimidazole refractory giardiasis) has been reported; in vitro resistance not reported; resistant cell lines have downregulated *G lamblia* nitroreductase 1 (GlNR1) due to mutation of *NR1* gene	Asia, Europe	Metronidazole; no guidelines for treatment refractory giardiasis.	None.	60-62
Cryptosporidium spp	*Immunocompromised state Children with HIV infection*	Nitazoxanide; no resistance but rather a lack of therapeutic efficacy in immunocompromised state	Africa, Europe	Rehydration, immune restoration; antiretroviral therapy in HIV infection.	None.	63-65

Abbreviations: DEC, diarrheagenic *Escherichia coli;* EAEC, enteroaggregative *E coli;* EHEC, enterohemorrhagic *E coli;* ESBL, extended spectrum beta-lactamase; ETEC, enterotoxigenic *E coli;* HIV, human immunodeficiency virus; LMIC, low and middle-income countries; MSM, men who have sex with men; NTS, nontyphoidal salmonellae; XDR, extensively drug resistant.

residue,[68] leftovers of human and veterinary use. Facilitating conditions, such as nutrient limitation, biofilms, and physicochemical stress, are thought to be responsible for exchange of MGEs in these natural ecosystems.[69] Unrestricted use of antibiotics in humans, animals, agriculture, food production and packaging, and presence of residues in sewage are thus responsible for HGT among bacteria. Studies have shown that resistance determinants present in human pathogens are acquired from environmental bacteria.[70] Enteric bacteria are adapted for survival in aquatic environments and have been found in wastewater and sewage. Inadequate sanitation leads to contamination of irrigation water, soil, and even drinking water, thus providing an opportunity for environmental and pathogenic bacteria to exchange genetic material and acquire new virulence and resistance determinants.[71]

Plasmids and MGEs can carry multiple resistance determinants[72]; bacterial exchange can therefore result in acquisition of multiple resistance genes by pathogenic bacteria. Multidrug-resistant bacterial strains thus "created" have a survival advantage in pharmaceutically polluted environments, and are fit to multiply and propagate under such conditions. An example of emerging resistance is the acquisition of plasmidborne resistance determinants for cephalosporin and quinolone resistance by the pathogenic S Typhi.[25] Analysis of sequencing data has suggested the exchange occurred between environmental E coli and S Typhi perhaps in an aquatic environment resulting from sewage contamination of drinking water. Inadequate WASH infrastructure further helps propagate these infections through a continuous cycle of fecal shedding and contamination of useable water.[73]

Several of the enteric human pathogens, including Campylobacter spp, selected DEC, and NTS are also zoonoses. As human population expands and food demands increase, interaction between humans and food animals also increases, thereby facilitating emergence and reemergence of zoonotic species as pathogens. Evidence from analyses of transmission and emergence risk of human pathogens have revealed that zoonotic infections have greater emergence potential[74,75]; AMR in food animals and companion animals is therefore by extension a risk factor for AMR emergence. AMR risk assessment and control therefore requires an integrated "OneHealth" approach that accounts for AMR in humans, animals, and the environment.[76]

Spread of multidrug-resistant enteric bacteria is facilitated by poor hygiene and other factors responsible for feco-oral transmission of pathogens (including high transmissibility and low infectious doses) within communities. Childhood malnutrition, although a direct consequence of enteric infections, is also a risk factor for infections, as well as for AMR.[77] AMR may contribute to prolonged fecal shedding of enteric pathogens,[78] facilitating human-to-human transmission, especially if hygiene and sanitation measures are poor.

Among the principal drivers of enteric disease transmission is the capacity for direct person-to-person transmission. Enteric infections are not restricted to foodborne and waterborne routes, but also can be transmitted through anorectal sexual contact. Sexually transmitted enteric infections include shigellosis, campylobacteriosis, amebiasis, and giardiasis.[79] Increasing AMR in Shigella spp, global travel, and high transmissibility following sexual contact has triggered a global epidemic of multidrug-resistant Shigella spp among MSM. Global spread of AMR, irrespective of transmission routes, is facilitated by travel and trade. Centralized mass food production with requisite use of antibiotics either as growth promoters or as therapeutic agents, unhygienic standards of production, and lack of regulatory oversight lead to global export of contaminated retail meat, fish, poultry and related products.[80] The resulting spread of enteric infections and AMR though the food chain has become an economically and politically charged debate in need of urgent solutions. **Box 1** highlights the principal risk factors for emergence and propagation of antibiotic-resistant enteric pathogens.

CHALLENGES OF ANTIMICROBIAL RESISTANCE SURVEILLANCE IN ENTERIC INFECTIONS

Population surveillance of enteric pathogens and associated AMR is dependent on the availability of and access to microbiological diagnosis. In high-burden countries, where laboratory diagnostics may not always be available, etiologies of most acute diarrheal episodes as well as enteric illnesses, remain undetermined. Improving accessibility of affordable pathogen-specific rapid diagnostic assays at the primary care is now a possibility with accurate antigen detection assays for *V cholerae* O1 and O139, and *S flexneri* 2a[81]; however, such culture-independent diagnostic tests (CIDTs) do not detect AMR.[82]

Culture-based diagnosis may be performed especially on dysenteric stools, at district or national level laboratories, but sensitivities of such assays is limited.[83] CIDTs commonly used for *H pylori* also do not detect AMR, however, polymerase chain reaction (PCR)-based hybridization assays with the ability to detect clarithromycin resistance can be performed on either stool or invasive biopsy samples.[84] Given the increasing importance of AMR surveillance and its association with emerging strains and outbreaks, there is a need to develop more pathogen-specific CIDTs, which can detect AMR.

AMR surveillance in foodborne and zoonotic enteric pathogens in LMICs is further limited by lack of veterinary diagnostic facilities and food safety measures requiring routine detection of pathogens in retail meat and packaged food.[85] OneHealth AMR surveillance networks have been proposed with integration of human and animal consumption and resistance data, and environmental surveillance; however, current surveillance systems, especially in LMICs are limited in both quality and capacity to create and maintain such networks.[86] **Box 2** summarizes major challenges in performing AMR surveillance of enteric pathogens.

PUBLIC HEALTH AND ECONOMIC COSTS OF ANTIMICROBIAL RESISTANCE IN ENTERIC INFECTIONS

Ciprofloxacin, previously the antibiotic of choice in dysentery and diarrhea of bacterial etiology, as well as in enteric fever, is not only longer universally effective, but due to

---

Box 1
Risk factors identified for emerging antimicrobial resistance (AMR) in enteric infections

Emergence of AMR in enteric pathogens
  Exchange of mobile genetic elements among intestinal and environmental microbiome
  Inadequate water, sanitation, and hygiene (WASH) measures
  Presence of antibiotics and antibiotic residues in aquatic environments
  Zoonotic reservoir

Propagation of resistant enteric pathogens
  Poor hygiene and inadequate WASH measures
  Childhood malnutrition
  Unhygienic food production
  Population antibiotic overuse/misuse
  Emerging transmission routes facilitating direct contact spread (sexual contact)
  Travel and trade
  Lack of effective antibiotics to treat emerging AMR diseases

> **Box 2**
> **Challenges of AMR surveillance in enteric infections**
>
> Limited laboratory capacity in high-burden regions
>
> Lack of point-of-care or point-of-need diagnostic tests
>
> Inability of culture-independent diagnostic tests to identify AMR
>
> Inherent low sensitivity of culture-dependent diagnostic tests
>
> Lack of integrated "OneHealth" surveillance systems

very high resistance rates, is no longer the recommended empiric antibiotic. Emergence of resistance to third-generation cephalosporins and macrolides such as erythromycin and azithromycin has left no empiric choices that are universally effective. Although this is not unusual, as resistance is a naturally occurring phenomenon, the survival fitness of antibiotic-resistant strains of pathogens have triggered global spread through several routes: travel, emerging epidemiologic niches, intensive farming, centralized mass food production, and trade. Consequently, the epidemiology of enteric infectious syndromes has received a renewed focus due to emerging AMR, necessitating investment in new preventive strategies, such as safe food production and vaccines. However, poor sanitation and unsafe water continue to be major risk factors of AMR and enteric infections in LMICs, in which most antibiotic resistance originates.[25,87] In these settings, economic incentives to invest in improving WASH, nutrition, and health access are likely to be of longer-term benefit.

The economic costs of foodborne and waterborne enteric infections are extensive. These include direct costs of treatment, health care personnel, and diagnostic testing.[88,89] Indirect costs include long-term morbidity resulting in loss of productivity and emotional costs resulting from illness and health care–related financial burdens. The attributable costs of AMR in enteric infections are difficult to determine without accurate estimates of the burden of AMR in enteric infections; however, more broadly it has been estimated that more than 700,000 people die of resistant infections annually. and by 2050 this this could escalate to 10 million deaths annually if AMR continues to spread unchecked.[90] Estimation of the direct and indirect economic costs of AMR is essential to steer investments toward high-impact strategies. Direct and indirect costs of enteric infections, particularly foodborne enteric infections, have been estimated in numerous high-income settings.[89,91] However, in LMICs where access to health care is limited and medical services are fragmented, such estimates are difficult, as LMICs have limited budgets to invest in the health of their populations, and as a result, out of patient-pocket expenditures are high.

Three examples of AMR in enteric infections, each with a unique predominant risk factor for emergence are highlighted: extensively drug resistant (XDR) *S* Typhi emergence due to contaminated sewage and poor WASH measures in an LMIC setting, global emergence and spread of multidrug-resistant *Shigella* spp in MSM, and chromosomal resistance in *H pylori* due to antibiotic overuse in populations.

Notable Emerging Antimicrobial Resistance in Enteric Pathogens

Extended-spectrum beta-lactamase producing–Salmonella Typhi
S Typhi causes a severe systemic illness, the true burden of which is difficult to estimate due to inaccuracy of clinical signs and symptoms as well as laboratory diagnostics. However, the pathogen causes a high burden of systemic illness especially in

South and Southeast Asia; as many as 21 million cases occur annually, resulting in an estimated 116,800 deaths.[1,92] The emergence of ciprofloxacin resistance in the late 1990s was cause for great concern, as treatment options diminished against the multidrug-resistant phenotype (ie, S Typhi resistant to ampicillin, co-trimoxazole, and chloramphenicol).[17,19,20] Third-generation cephalosporins were widely used to treat enteric fever in Asia; however, the recent emergence and spread of XDR S Typhi in Pakistan has significantly limited available treatment options.[25] Moreover, currently prescribed antibiotics against this strain, carbapenems and azithromycin, have not been systematically evaluated in enteric fever in controlled trials. Consequently, optimal treatment duration, fever clearance times, and duration of shedding and impact on possible chronic carriage are unknown for such strains when treated with azithromycin and carbapenems. Emergence of antibiotic resistance has also increased the cost of treatment of typhoid fever.[93]

Azithromycin-resistant and extended-spectrum beta-lactamase–carrying Shigella species

The epidemiology of antibiotic-resistant emerging and reemerging shigellosis is complex owing to the several co-circulating species, serotypes, and biotypes of Shigella spp.[94] Recent travel and emerging transmission routes have muddled the picture further. In settings with high rates of ampicillin and co-trimoxazole–resistant Shigella spp, empiric treatment of dysentery with fluoroquinolones, or azithromycin was advocated.[95] Ciprofloxacin-resistant Shigella spp emerged in the late 1990s and spread throughout Asia in the first decade of this century.[32] S flexneri and Shigella sonnei are the predominant species in these regions; however, Shigella dysentriae resistant to fluoroquinolones have also been reported. Multidrug-resistant Shigella spp have emerged with multiple cumulative resistance mechanisms, and with coresistance to macrolides and third-generation cephalosporins.[36] The emergence and rapid spread of azithromycin-resistant, ciprofloxacin-resistant, and ceftriaxone-resistant Shigella spp in MSM is of particular concern owing to its rapid spread resulting from direct sexual contact.[34] This event is of particular concern, as it has occurred in regions previously nonendemic for shigellosis. Higher rates of ESBL-producing and cephalosporin-resistant Shigella spp were reported from Asia than from Europe and Americas as per a systematic review of data from 1998 to 2012.[35] However, due to the rise of shigellosis among MSM, high rates of resistance to third-generation cephalosporins and azithromycin are now also observed in Europe, America, and Australia, in MSM and individuals positive for human immunodeficiency virus.[34,36]

Emergence and rapid spread of ciprofloxacin, azithromycin, and cephalosporin resistance has complicated recommendations for empiric treatment of shigellosis,[31] and it has become increasingly important to establish diagnosis and perform susceptibility testing to detect resistance and modify treatment. Inherent problems with this approach are the lower sensitivity of culture-based diagnosis, inability of PCR-based diagnosis to identify resistance, and inaccessibility and high cost of sequencing-based diagnosis, which can predict susceptibilities.[96,97] Moreover, azithromycin resistance surveillance remains problematic owing to lack of standard guidelines to guide clinical resistance detection and therapy.[98]

Clarithromycin resistance in Helicobacter pylori

High resistance rates in H pylori have been associated with pediatric age group, cagA-negative strains, and high volume of consumption of the related antibiotic group in populations.[55] Over the past few years, escalating reports of clinical failure with the triple antibiotic therapy regimen and increasing antibiotic resistance rates have prompted several consensus reports for the treatment of *H pylori* infections.[56,99,100] A principal driver is clarithromycin resistance, which has increased in the past 10 to 15 years. Majority reports on clarithromycin resistance have shown a clear impact of rising clarithromycin resistance on the efficacy of therapeutic regimens.[101] Resistance to clarithromycin decreases the efficacy of treatment regimens, including the novel concomitant, hybrid, and sequential therapeutic regimens.[55,56] In regions with high *H pylori* seropositivity and high infection rates, resistance rates against clarithromycin now exceed the minimum 15% to qualify for primary susceptibility testing before treatment is initiated with a macrolide-containing regimen.[56]

Although fluoroquinolones are frequently used in alternative regimens, the body of literature pertaining to susceptibility testing and resistance rates is not very vast. However, resistance rates ranging between 20% and 30% have been reported from the United States, China, Portugal, and Italy.[55] Second-line regimens containing levofloxacin as part of quadruple therapy are recommended; however, in case of failure of these regimens, culture and susceptibility testing to determine fluoroquinolone and rifabutin susceptibilities.[55,56] Metronidazole resistance is also known to occur and affect therapeutic efficacy; however, there is poor correlation between in vitro and clinical resistance, and resistance may be partially overcome by increasing dosages.

PREVENTION STRATEGIES

Antibiotics are a shared resource, and the social costs of AMR are greater than individual costs and affect the poor and vulnerable disproportionally.[73] AMR is therefore a societal and ecological issue requiring ecological and societal solutions.[102] As resistance emerges in enteric pathogens as a result of the complex interaction between environmental contaminants and pathogenic bacteria, implementation of optimal WASH measures is integral as a prevention strategy for AMR, and is also a time-honored approach for the prevention of enteric infections. However, improving WASH is often not within the purview of health authorities alone, and requires multisectoral political commitment. To ensure an all-encompassing preventive and control strategy for AMR as well as enteric infections, a OneHealth approach is ideal.[103] This collaborative and multisectoral approach works at global as well as local levels, and centers on collective surveillance, readiness, and improvement of human, animal, and environmental health, as well as industry and civil society.[104,105]

Universal access to health care and reliable diagnostics is essential to AMR prevention.[106] However, given the wide-ranging scope of activities essential to prevention of AMR as well as enteric infections, it is imperative to invest in the health of populations in addition to health care of the sick. Because communities and populations hold agency over their collective health, investing in health education and community-centered outcomes (hygiene, sanitation, adequate nutrition, reduced antibiotic use, and safe sex) is likely to lead to both sustainable and long-term benefits.

The prevention of enteric infections has seen unprecedented advancements in the production, testing, and implementation of vaccines. Vaccines field tested and marketed for human use include those against *S* Typhi, and *V. cholerae* O1/O139, and vaccines against *S flexneri* 2a and enterotoxogenic *E coli* are in phase II trials.[37] Two glycoconjugated typhoid vaccines are commercially available, one of which has received prequalification by the World Health Organization,[27] and these are effective against children older than 6 months. Vaccines are also plausible alternatives for antibiotics in food animals, thus reducing antibiotic consumption and preventing AMR.[107] Although vaccination is not a substitute for WASH preventive strategies, vaccination can be a novel tool to prevent AMR through lowering the need for antibiotics in the populations at large.[108] However, WASH measures have lagged significantly behind vaccine development and implementation, and continued efforts for vaccine development and testing should not divert focus from funding and investments in WASH measures.

EMERGING AND NOVEL TREATMENT STRATEGIES

Probiotics have been reported to reduce the duration of diarrhea in children,[109] and some guidelines also recommend routine use of *Lactobacillus rhamnosus GG* or *Saccharomyces boulardii* as adjuncts to rehydration therapy,[4] although evidence generated differs by setting and disease severity. Evidence also does not support use of probiotics as replacements for antibiotic therapy in moderate to severe diarrhea, and pathogen-specific data are lacking, making the impact of probiotics on AMR prevention uncertain. Development of recombinant probiotics containing target genes from pathogenic bacteria have shown promise in initial studies but have not entered clinical testing.[110] If proven effective and safe, this strategy can potentially eliminate the need for antibiotics in acute diarrhea.

The nonabsorbable antibiotics rifaximin and rifamycin are effective in moderate to severe traveler's diarrhea (TD) but have no effect on invasive infections. It is noteworthy, however, that use of rifamycin in TD has shown lower rates of resistance in gut microbiota after treatment when compared with ciprofloxacin treatment.[111] Pathogen-specific and syndrome-specific guidelines to replace azithromycin with rifamycin or rifaximin could prevent azithromycin overuse and protect other pathogens from developing resistance to this antibiotic through decrease in selective pressure.

SUMMARY

As development and sustainability become the modern paradigms in global health, the emergence of AMR represents a massive challenge. Prevention strategies for enteric infections, such as improvement of population health, sanitation, and vaccination, are also effective against AMR, and synergistic outcomes of independent efforts are likely. However, enhanced focus on and investment in WASH strategies is needed in high enteric infection burden and high AMR burden LMICs to reduce the public health and economic burden resulting from resistant enteric infections.

REFERENCES

1. Roth GA, Abate D, Abate KH, et al. Global, regional, and national age-sex-specific mortality for 282 causes of death in 195 countries and territories, 1980–2017: a systematic analysis for the Global Burden of Disease Study 2017. Lancet 2018;392(10159):1736–88.
2. Stanaway JD, Reiner RC, Blacker BF, et al. The global burden of typhoid and paratyphoid fevers: a systematic analysis for the Global Burden of Disease Study 2017. Lancet Infect Dis 2019. https://doi.org/10.1016/S1473-3099(18)30685-6 [pii:S1473-3099(18)30685-30686].
3. Pernica JM, Steenhoff AP, Welch H, et al. Correlation of clinical outcomes with multiplex molecular testing of stool from children admitted to hospital with gastroenteritis in Botswana. J Pediatric Infect Dis Soc 2016;5(3):312–8.
4. Guarino A, Ashkenazi S, Gendrel D, et al. European Society for Pediatric Gastroenterology, Hepatology, and Nutrition/European Society for Pediatric Infectious Diseases evidence-based guidelines for the management of acute

gastroenteritis in children in Europe: update 2014. J Pediatr Gastroenterol Nutr 2014;59(1):132–52.

5. ISID ProMED-mail. Brookline, MS, USA; International Society for Infectious Diseases. Available at: http://www.promedmail.org. Accessed April 2, 2019.

6. Savoldi A, Carrara E, Graham DY, et al. Prevalence of antibiotic resistance in *Helicobacter pylori*: a systematic review and meta-analysis in World Health Organization regions. Gastroenterology 2018;155(5):1372–82.e17.

7. Haselbeck AH, Panzner U, Im J, et al. Current perspectives on invasive nontyphoidal *Salmonella* disease. Curr Opin Infect Dis 2017;30(5):498–503.

8. Crump JA, Sjölund-Karlsson M, Gordon MA, et al. Epidemiology, clinical presentation, laboratory diagnosis, antimicrobial resistance, and antimicrobial management of invasive *Salmonella* infections. Clin Microbiol Rev 2015;28(4): 901–37.

9. Neuert S, Nair S, Day MR, et al. Prediction of phenotypic antimicrobial resistance profiles from whole genome sequences of non-typhoidal *Salmonella enterica*. Front Microbiol 2018;9:592.

10. Kariuki S, Gordon MA, Feasey N, et al. Antimicrobial resistance and management of invasive *Salmonella* disease. Vaccine 2015;33(Suppl 3):C21–9.

11. Carnevali C, Morganti M, Scaltriti E, et al. Occurrence of mcr-1 in colistin-resistant *Salmonella enterica* isolates recovered from humans and animals in Italy, 2012 to 2015. Antimicrob Agents Chemother 2016;60(12):7532–4.

12. Doumith M, Godbole G, Ashton P, et al. Detection of the plasmid-mediated mcr-1 gene conferring colistin resistance in human and food isolates of *Salmonella enterica* and *Escherichia coli* in England and Wales. J Antimicrob Chemother 2016;71(8):2300–5.

13. Vlieghe ER, Phe T, De Smet B, et al. Azithromycin and ciprofloxacin resistance in *Salmonella* bloodstream infections in Cambodian adults. PLoS Negl Trop Dis 2012;6(12):e1933.

14. Nair S, Ashton P, Doumith M, et al. WGS for surveillance of antimicrobial resistance: a pilot study to detect the prevalence and mechanism of resistance to azithromycin in a UK population of non-typhoidal *Salmonella*. J Antimicrob Chemother 2016;71(12):3400–8.

15. Arnott A, Wang Q, Bachmann N, et al. Multidrug-resistant *Salmonella enterica* 4,[5], 12: i:-Sequence Type 34, New South Wales, Australia, 2016–2017. Emerg Infect Dis 2018;24(4):751–3.

16. Wen SC, Best E, Nourse C. Non-typhoidal *Salmonella* infections in children: review of literature and recommendations for management. J Paediatr Child Health 2017;53(10):936–41.

17. Pokharel BM, Koirala J, Dahal RK, et al. Multidrug-resistant and extended-spectrum beta-lactamase (ESBL)-producing *Salmonella enterica* (serotypes Typhi and Paratyphi A) from blood isolates in Nepal: surveillance of resistance and a search for newer alternatives. Int J Infect Dis 2006;10(6):434–8.

18. Lynch MF, Blanton EM, Bulens S, et al. Typhoid fever in the United States, 1999-2006. JAMA 2009;302(8):859–65.

19. Smith AM, Govender N, Keddy KH. Quinolone-resistant salmonella typhi in South Africa, 2003–2007. Epidemiol Infect 2010;138(1):86–90.

20. Yanagi D, de Vries GC, Rahardjo D, et al. Emergence of fluoroquinolone-resistant strains of *Salmonella enterica* in Surabaya, Indonesia. Diagn Microbiol Infect Dis 2009;64(4):422–6.

21. Song Y, Roumagnac P, Weill FX, et al. A multiplex single nucleotide polymorphism typing assay for detecting mutations that result in decreased

fluoroquinolone susceptibility in *Salmonella enterica* serovars Typhi and Paratyphi A. J Antimicrob Chemother 2010;65(8):1631–41.

22. Crump JA, Mintz ED. Global trends in typhoid and paratyphoid fever. Clin Infect Dis 2010;50(2):241–6.

23. Al Naiemi N, Zwart B, Rijnsburger MC, et al. Extended-spectrum-beta-lactamase production in a *Salmonella enterica* serotype Typhi strain from the Philippines. J Clin Microbiol 2008;46(8):2794–5.

24. Wong VK, Baker S, Pickard DJ, et al. Phylogeographical analysis of the dominant multidrug-resistant H58 clade of *Salmonella* Typhi identifies inter- and intracontinental transmission events. Nat Genet 2015;47(6):632–9.

25. Klemm EJ, Shakoor S, Page AJ, et al. Emergence of an extensively drug-resistant *Salmonella enterica* serovar Typhi clone harboring a promiscuous plasmid encoding resistance to fluoroquinolones and third-generation cephalosporins. MBio 2018;9(1) [pii:e00105-e00118].

26. Ahsan S, Rahman S. Azithromycin resistance in clinical isolates of *Salmonella enterica* serovars Typhi and paratyphi in Bangladesh. Microb Drug Resist 2019;25(1):8–13.

27. World Health Organization. Typhoid vaccines: WHO position paper, March 2018–recommendations. Vaccine 2019;37(2):214–6.

28. Gandra S, Mojica N, Klein EY, et al. Trends in antibiotic resistance among major bacterial pathogens isolated from blood cultures tested at a large private laboratory network in India, 2008–2014. Int J Infect Dis 2016;50:75–82.

29. Fernando S, Molland JG, Gottlieb T. Failure of oral antibiotic therapy, including azithromycin, in the treatment of a recurrent breast abscess caused by *Salmonella enterica* serotype Paratyphi A. Pathog Glob Health 2012;106(6):366–9.

30. Molloy A, Nair S, Cooke FJ, et al. First report of *Salmonella enterica* serotype paratyphi A azithromycin resistance leading to treatment failure. J Clin Microbiol 2010;48(12):4655–7.

31. Kotloff KL, Riddle MS, Platts-Mills JA, et al. Shigellosis. Lancet 2018;391(10122):801–12.

32. The HC, Baker S. Out of Asia: the independent rise and global spread of fluoroquinolone-resistant *Shigella*. Microb Genom 2018;4(4). https://doi.org/10.1099/mgen.0.000171.

33. Puzari M, Sharma M, Chetia P. Emergence of antibiotic resistant *Shigella* species: a matter of concern. J Infect Public Health 2018;11(4):451–4.

34. Baker KS, Dallman TJ, Ashton PM, et al. Intercontinental dissemination of azithromycin-resistant shigellosis through sexual transmission: a cross-sectional study. Lancet Infect Dis 2015;15(8):913–21.

35. Gu B, Zhou M, Ke X, et al. Comparison of resistance to third-generation cephalosporins in *Shigella* between Europe-America and Asia-Africa from 1998 to 2012. Epidemiol Infect 2015;143(13):2687–99.

36. Ingle DJ, Easton M, Valcanis M, et al. Co-circulation of multidrug-resistant *Shigella* among men who have sex with men, Australia. Clin Infect Dis 2019. https://doi.org/10.1093/cid/ciz005.

37. Riddle MS, Chen WH, Kirkwood CD, et al. Update on vaccines for enteric pathogens. Clin Microbiol Infect 2018;24(10):1039–45.

38. Post A, Martiny D, van Waterschoot N, et al. Antibiotic susceptibility profiles among *Campylobacter* isolates obtained from international travelers between 2007 and 2014. Eur J Clin Microbiol Infect Dis 2017;36(11):2101–7.

39. Kaakoush NO, Castaño-Rodríguez N, Mitchell HM, et al. Global epidemiology of *Campylobacter* infection. Clin Microbiol Rev 2015;28(3):687–720.

40. Sproston EL, Wimalarathna HM, Sheppard SK. Trends in fluoroquinolone resistance in *Campylobacter*. Microb Genom 2018;4(8). https://doi.org/10.1099/mgen.0.000198.

41. Schiaffino F, Colston JM, Paredes-Olortegui M, et al. Antibiotic resistance of *Campylobacter* species in a pediatric cohort study. Antimicrob Agents Chemother 2019;63(2) [pii:e01911-e01918].

42. Hansson I, Sandberg M, Habib I, et al. Knowledge gaps in control of *Campylobacter* for prevention of campylobacteriosis. Transbound Emerg Dis 2018; 65(Suppl 1):30–48.

43. Mir RA, Kudva IT. Antibiotic-resistant Shiga toxin-producing *Escherichia coli*: an overview of prevalence and intervention strategies. Zoonoses Public Health 2019;66(1):1–13.

44. Zeighami H, Haghi F, Hajiahmadi F, et al. Multi-drug-resistant enterotoxigenic and enterohemorrhagic *Escherichia coli* isolated from children with diarrhea. J Chemother 2015;27(3):152–5.

45. Jost C, Bidet P, Carrère T, et al. Susceptibility of enterohaemorrhagic *Escherichia coli* to azithromycin in France and analysis of resistance mechanisms. J Antimicrob Chemother 2016;71(5):1183–7.

46. Guiral E, Quiles MG, Muñoz L, et al. Emergence of resistance to quinolones and β-lactam antibiotics in enteroaggregative and enterotoxigenic *Escherichia coli* causing traveler's diarrhea. Antimicrob Agents Chemother 2019;63(2) [pii: e01745-18].

47. Steffen R. Epidemiology of travellers' diarrhea. J Travel Med 2017; 24(suppl_1):S2–5.

48. Tribble DR. Resistant pathogens as causes of traveller's diarrhea globally and impact (s) on treatment failure and recommendations. J Travel Med 2017; 24(suppl_1):S6–12.

49. Taylor DN, Hamer DH, Shlim DR. Medications for the prevention and treatment of travellers' diarrhea. J Travel Med 2017;24(suppl_1):S17–22.

50. Do Nascimento V, Day MR, Doumith M, et al. Comparison of phenotypic and WGS-derived antimicrobial resistance profiles of enteroaggregative Escherichia coli isolated from cases of diarrhoeal disease in England, 2015–16. J Antimicrob Chemother 2017;72(12):3288–97.

51. Bier N, Schwartz K, Guerra B, et al. Survey on antimicrobial resistance patterns in *Vibrio vulnificus* and *Vibrio cholerae* non-O1/non-O139 in Germany reveals carbapenemase-producing *Vibrio cholerae* in coastal waters. Front Microbiol 2015;6:1179.

52. Wang R, Liu H, Zhao X, et al. IncA/C plasmids conferring high azithromycin resistance in *Vibrio cholerae*. Int J Antimicrob Agents 2018;51(1):140–4.

53. Weil AA, Ryan ET. Cholera: recent updates. Curr Opin Infect Dis 2018;31(5): 455–61.

54. Agudo S, Pérez-Pérez G, Alarcón T, et al. High prevalence of clarithromycin-resistant *Helicobacter pylori* strains and risk factors associated with resistance in Madrid, Spain. J Clin Microbiol 2010;48(10):3703–7.

55. Thung I, Aramin H, Vavinskaya V, et al. The global emergence of *Helicobacter pylori* antibiotic resistance. Aliment Pharmacol Ther 2016;43(4):514–33.

56. Malfertheiner P, Megraud F, O'morain CA, et al. Management of *Helicobacter pylori* infection—the Maastricht V/Florence consensus report. Gut 2017; 66(1):6–30.

57. Siddique O, Ovalle A, Siddique AS, et al. *Helicobacter pylori* infection: an update for the internist in the age of increasing global antibiotic resistance. Am J Med 2018;131(5):473–9.

58. Chatedaki C, Voulgaridi I, Kachrimanidou M, et al. Antimicrobial susceptibility and mechanisms of resistance of Greek *Clostridium difficile* clinical isolates. J Glob Antimicrob Resist 2019;16:53–8.

59. Gonzales-Luna A, Shen WJ, Dotson K, et al. Increased clinical failure rates associated with reduced metronidazole susceptibility in *Clostridioides difficile*. Open Forum Infect Dis 2018;5(Suppl 1):S255–6.

60. Carter ER, Nabarro LE, Hedley L, et al. Nitroimidazole-refractory giardiasis: a growing problem requiring rational solutions. Clinical Microbiology and Infection. Clin Microbiol Infect 2018;24(1):37–42.

61. Requena-Méndez A, Goñi P, Lóbez S, et al. A family cluster of giardiasis with variable treatment responses: refractory giardiasis in a family after a trip to India. Clin Microbiol Infect 2014;20(2):O135–8.

62. Nabarro LE, Lever RA, Armstrong M, et al. Increased incidence of nitroimidazole-refractory giardiasis at the Hospital for Tropical Diseases, London: 2008–2013. Clin Microbiol Infect 2015;21(8):791–6.

63. Amadi B, Mwiya M, Sianongo S, et al. High dose prolonged treatment with nitazoxanide is not effective for cryptosporidiosis in HIV positive Zambian children: a randomised controlled trial. BMC Infect Dis 2009;9:195.

64. Costa D, Razakandrainibe R, Sautour M, et al. Human cryptosporidiosis in immunodeficient patients in France (2015–2017). Exp Parasitol 2018;192:108–12.

65. Shoultz DA, de Hostos EL, Choy RK. Addressing cryptosporidium infection among young children in low-income settings: the crucial role of new and existing drugs for reducing morbidity and mortality. PLoS Negl Trop Dis 2016;10(1): e0004242.

66. McFeters GA, Stuart DG. Survival of coliform bacteria in natural waters: field and laboratory studies with membrane-filter chambers. Appl Microbiol 1972;24(5): 805–11.

67. Perry J, Wright G. The antibiotic resistance "mobilome": searching for the link between environment and clinic. Front Microbiol 2013;4:138.

68. Kristiansson E, Fick J, Janzon A, et al. Pyrosequencing of antibiotic-contaminated river sediments reveals high levels of resistance and gene transfer elements. PLoS One 2011;6(2):e17038.

69. Lorenz MG, Wackernagel W. Bacterial gene transfer by natural genetic transformation in the environment. Microbiol Rev 1994;58(3):563–602.

70. von Wintersdorff CJ, Penders J, van Niekerk JM, et al. Dissemination of antimicrobial resistance in microbial ecosystems through horizontal gene transfer. Front Microbiol 2016;7:173.

71. Byarugaba DK. A view on antimicrobial resistance in developing countries and responsible risk factors. Int J Antimicrob Agents 2004;24(2):105–10.

72. Carattoli A. Plasmids and the spread of resistance. Int J Med Microbiol 2013; 303(6–7):298–304.

73. Okeke IN, Aboderin OA, Byarugaba DK, et al. Growing problem of multidrug-resistant enteric pathogens in Africa. Emerg Infect Dis 2007;13(11):1640–6.

74. Cleaveland S, Laurenson MK, Taylor LH. Diseases of humans and their domestic mammals: pathogen characteristics, host range and the risk of emergence. Philos Trans R Soc Lond B Biol Sci 2001;356(1411):991–9.

75. Taylor LH, Latham SM, Woolhouse ME. Risk factors for human disease emergence. Philos Trans R Soc Lond B Biol Sci 2001;356(1411):983–9.

76. Queenan K, Häsler B, Rushton J. A One Health approach to antimicrobial resistance surveillance: is there a business case for it? Int J Antimicrob Agents 2016; 48(4):422–7.

77. Walson JL, Berkley JA. The impact of malnutrition on childhood infections. Curr Opin Infect Dis 2018;31(3):231–6.

78. Gopinath S, Carden S, Monack D. Shedding light on *Salmonella* carriers. Trends Microbiol 2012;20(7):320–7.

79. Mitchell H, Hughes G. Recent epidemiology of sexually transmissible enteric infections in men who have sex with men. Curr Opin Infect Dis 2018;31(1):50–6.

80. George A. Antimicrobial resistance, trade, food safety and security. One Health 2017;5:6–8.

81. Gonzalez MD, McElvania E. New developments in rapid diagnostic testing for children. Infect Dis Clin North Am 2018;32(1):19–34.

82. Fang FC, Patel R. 2017 Infectious Diseases Society of America infectious diarrhea guidelines: a view from the clinical laboratory. Clin Infect Dis 2017;65(12): 1974–6.

83. Van Lint P, De Witte E, Ursi JP, et al. A screening algorithm for diagnosing bacterial gastroenteritis by real-time PCR in combination with guided culture. Diagn Microbiol Infect Dis 2016;85(2):255–9.

84. Xuan SH, Wu LP, Zhou YG, et al. Detection of clarithromycin-resistant *Helicobacter pylori* in clinical specimens by molecular methods: a review. J Glob Antimicrob Resist 2016;4:35–41.

85. Allcock S, Young EH, Holmes M, et al. Antimicrobial resistance in human populations: challenges and opportunities. Glob Health Epidemiol Genom 2017;2:e4.

86. Rousham EK, Unicomb L, Islam MA. Human, animal and environmental contributors to antibiotic resistance in low-resource settings: integrating behavioural, epidemiological and One Health approaches. Proc Biol Sci 2018;285(1876) [pii:20180332].

87. Garg P, Sinha S, Chakraborty R, et al. Emergence of fluoroquinolone-resistant strains of *Vibrio cholerae* O1 biotype El Tor among hospitalized patients with cholera in Calcutta, India. Antimicrob Agents Chemother 2001;45(5):1605–6.

88. McLinden T, Sargeant JM, Thomas MK, et al. Component costs of foodborne illness: a scoping review. BMC Public Health 2014;14:509.

89. Buzby JC, Roberts T. The economics of enteric infections: human foodborne disease costs. Gastroenterology 2009;136(6):1851–62.

90. O'Neill J. Antimicrobial resistance: tackling a crisis for the health and wealth of nations. Review on Antimicrobial Resistance 2014. Available at: http://amr-review.org/Publications. Accessed April 2, 2019.

91. Scharff RL. Economic burden from health losses due to foodborne illness in the United States. J Food Prot 2012;75(1):123–31.

92. Bentsi-Enchill AD, Hombach J. Revised global typhoid vaccination policy. Clin Infect Dis 2019;68(Supplement_1):S31–3.

93. Yousafzai MT, Qamar FN, Shakoor S, et al. Ceftriaxone-resistant *Salmonella* Typhi outbreak in Hyderabad City of Sindh, Pakistan: high time for the introduction of typhoid conjugate vaccine. Clin Infect Dis 2019;68(Supplement_1):S16–21.

94. Baker S, The HC. Recent insights into *Shigella*. Curr Opin Infect Dis 2018;31(5): 449–54.

95. Tribble DR. Antibiotic therapy for acute watery diarrhea and dysentery. Mil Med 2017;182(S2):17–25.

96. Tang XJ, Yang Z, Chen XB, et al. Verification and large scale clinical evaluation of a national standard protocol for *Salmonella* spp./*Shigella* spp. screening

using real-time PCR combined with guided culture. J Microbiol Methods 2018; 145:14–9.

97. Baker KS, Campos J, Pichel M, et al. Whole genome sequencing of *Shigella sonnei* through PulseNet Latin America and Caribbean: advancing global surveillance of foodborne illnesses. Clin Microbiol Infect 2017;23(11):845–53.

98. Brown JD, Willcox SJ, Franklin N, et al. *Shigella* species epidemiology and antimicrobial susceptibility: the implications of emerging azithromycin resistance for guiding treatment, guidelines and breakpoints. J Antimicrob Chemother 2017; 72(11):3181–6.

99. Fallone CA, Chiba N, van Zanten SV, et al. The Toronto consensus for the treatment of *Helicobacter pylori* infection in adults. Gastroenterology 2016;151(1): 51–69.e14.

100. Mahachai V, Vilaichone RK, Pittayanon R, et al. *Helicobacter pylori* management in ASEAN: the Bangkok consensus report. J Gastroenterol Hepatol 2018;33(1): 37–56.

101. Zagari RM, Rabitti S, Eusebi LH, et al. Treatment of *Helicobacter pylori* infection: a clinical practice update. Eur J Clin Invest 2018;48(1). https://doi.org/10.1111/eci.12857.

102. Levy SB. Antibiotic resistance: an ecological imbalance. Ciba Found Symp 1997;207:1–9 [discussion 9–14].

103. Heymann DL, Jay J, Kock R. The One Health path to infectious disease prevention and resilience. Trans R Soc Trop Med Hyg 2017;111(6):233–4.

104. Kahn LH. Antimicrobial resistance: a One Health perspective. Trans R Soc Trop Med Hyg 2017;111(6):255–60.

105. Nadimpalli M, Delarocque-Astagneau E, Love DC, et al. Combating global antibiotic resistance: emerging one health concerns in lower-and middle-income countries. Clin Infect Dis 2018;66(6):963–9.

106. Mendelson M, Røttingen JA, Gopinathan U, et al. Maximising access to achieve appropriate human antimicrobial use in low-income and middle-income countries. Lancet 2016;387(10014):188–98.

107. Hoelzer K, Bielke L, Blake DP, et al. Vaccines as alternatives to antibiotics for food producing animals. Part 1: challenges and needs. Vet Res 2018;49(1):64.

108. Jansen KU, Knirsch C, Anderson AS. The role of vaccines in preventing bacterial antimicrobial resistance. Nat Med 2018;24(1):10–9.

109. Basu S, Paul DK, Ganguly S, et al. Efficacy of high-dose *Lactobacillus rhamnosus* GG in controlling acute watery diarrhea in Indian children: a randomized controlled trial. J Clin Gastroenterol 2009;43(3):208–13.

110. Mathipa MG, Thantsha MS. Probiotic engineering: towards development of robust probiotic strains with enhanced functional properties and for targeted control of enteric pathogens. Gut Pathog 2017;9:28.

111. Steffen R, Jiang ZD, Gracias Garcia ML, et al. Rifamycin SV-MMX® for treatment of travellers' diarrhea: equally effective as ciprofloxacin and not associated with the acquisition of multi-drug resistant bacteria. J Travel Med 2018;25(1). https://doi.org/10.1093/jtm/tay116.

Invasive Pneumococcal and Meningococcal Disease

Deirdre Fitzgerald, MBBS[a], Grant W. Waterer, MBBS, PhD[b],*

KEYWORDS

- Pneumococcal • Meningococcal • Invasive • Epidemiology • Treatment

KEY POINTS

- Pneumococcal disease decreased with effective vaccines but is on the rise again.
- Treatment of invasive pneumococcal disease includes the combination of a beta-lactam and a macrolide.
- Steroids should be used in pneumococcal meningitis, but not in pneumococcal pneumonia.
- There is increasing awareness of the cardiovascular complications of invasive pneumococcal disease.
- Meningococcal disease remains a significant problem and antibiotic resistance is increasing.

INVASIVE PNEUMOCOCCAL DISEASE

Epidemiology

Streptococcus pneumoniae is the most common bacterial cause of community-acquired pneumonia,[1] and can cause a variety of diseases ranging from invasive pneumococcal disease (IPD) to asymptomatic colonization of the nasopharynx. The broad spectrum of presentations relates both to the virulence of the bacteria and to host factors.

S pneumoniae virulence is highly dependent on its polysaccharide capsule, of which more than 90 serotypes have been identified. More invasive serotypes (eg, 1, 7, and 14) are more likely to cause infection when acquired and are much less likely to be found in the nose.[2] Less invasive serotypes (eg, 9N, 12F, 22F, and 23A) are more likely to persist and spread, reaching a greater number of vulnerable hosts who may develop disease despite the lower virulence of the pathogen.[3]

Neither Dr D. Fitzgerald nor Dr G.W. Waterer have any conflicts of interest to declare.
[a] Department of Respiratory Medicine, Sir Charles Gardiner Hospital, Verdun Street, Nedlands, Perth 6009, Australia; [b] University of Western Australia, Royal Perth Hospital, Wellington Street, Perth 6000, Australia
* Corresponding author.
E-mail address: grant.waterer@uwa.edu.au

Infect Dis Clin N Am 33 (2019) 1125–1141
https://doi.org/10.1016/j.idc.2019.08.007
id.theclinics.com

S pneumoniae was estimated to be responsible for 4 million episodes of disease in the United States in 2004, at a cost of $7.7 billion (USD) including direct medical care and loss of productivity and work.[4] Worldwide, pneumococcal disease accounts for 1.6 million deaths annually and was responsible for 5% of child mortality in 2008.[5] IPD is defined as the identification of pneumococci in a normally sterile specimen, for example, blood or cerebrospinal fluid (CSF). Although less common than pneumococcal pneumonia, due to the high specificity of the diagnosis, the incidence of IPD is commonly used as a surrogate for the burden of pneumococcal disease in a given population. Incidence rates of IPD vary considerably depending on the age group, comorbidities, frequency of immunocompromise, socioeconomic status, geographic location, and, importantly, vaccination status of the population studied.

The groups most affected by IPD, irrespective of geographic location, are children and older adults. Incidence in infants younger than 2 years ranged from 23.7 per 100,000 in Hong Kong to 54.2 per 100,000 in the United Kingdom and more than 677 per 100,000 in Mozambique, before widespread initiation of vaccination programs.[6–8] Feikin and colleagues[9] compared datasets from multiple continents, including Australia, North America, and Europe, and demonstrated rates ranging from 4.7 to 280.3 per 100,000 in children younger than 5 years. In the United States between 1993 and 2003, 95.3 per 100,000 children younger than 5 years developed IPD per annum, versus 40.6 per 100,000 adults.[10] Similar trends have been demonstrated worldwide, although a bimodal incidence is seen if adult incidence rates are subdivided into age groups of older than and younger than 65 years, with higher rates in the older cohort.[7] The epidemiology and distribution of pneumococcus have changed dramatically over the past 20 years with the development of the pneumococcal conjugate vaccines targeting specific, common, and invasive serotypes.

Transmission of pneumococcus is by respiratory droplet spread, with the nasopharynx of infants and young children acting as the organism's main reservoir. A cross-sectional study in the United States found nasopharyngeal carriage rates of 23% to 32%, with higher rates in younger children, those attending day care and those living with smokers.[11] Worldwide, rates from 4.5% to 90.0% have been reported, with higher rates of carriage in low-income and middle-income countries.[12,13]

Vaccines

Pneumococcal vaccination programs began in the 1970s with a 14-valent polysaccharide version, subsequently replaced by the 23-valent version (PPV-23) still in use today. Polysaccharide vaccines reduce rates of IPD in healthy adults but are not immunogenic in infants younger than 2 years, the cohort with the highest morbidity and mortality secondary to pneumococcus.[14] In addition, the effects of PPV-23 appear to wane over time[15] and it does not have any effect of nasal carriage. At present, PPV-23 is recommended for all adults at risk of pneumococcal disease and all who are older than 65 years.

A polysaccharide-protein conjugate vaccine was developed to overcome deficiencies in the PPV-23, especially in infants. The 7-valent vaccine, first introduced in the United States in 2000, covered serotypes that accounted for at least 70% of pediatric invasive strains in the United States at that time (4, 6B, 9V,14, 18C, 19F, and 23F).[16] The effects of PCV-7 in reducing vaccine-type (VT) IPD were almost immediately appreciated with substantial reductions in incidence of IPD (69% decrease in children <2 years old) within 12 months.[17] Decreases in hospitalizations for meningitis were observed.[18] A significant reduction in IPD incidence was also noted in adults, indicating evidence of herd immunity due to the eradication of nasal carriage in infants.[17] This effect was replicated in a number of studies worldwide, however, an increase in IPD due to non–vaccine type (NVT) pneumococcal serotypes was also noted, particularly serotype 19A and 7F.[9,10,19,20]

Two further PCVs have been developed to combat the emergence of NVT serotypes, PCV-10 (PCV-7 + serotypes 1, 5, 7F) and PCV-13 (PCV-10 + serotypes 6A, 7F, 19A). Both PCV-10 and PCV-13 have been associated with significant reductions in the incidence of IPD.[19–22] Unfortunately, pediatric and adult studies in many countries report stable or increasing IPD incidence in more recent years, predominantly due to NVT serotypes.[19,22,23] It also appears that the effect of PCV-13 in relation to serotype 3 has been minimal and there has been no change in the incidence of this serotype since the vaccine was introduced.[22] This may reflect lower immunogenicity for serotype 3. Finally, serotype 19A is believed to be one of the more common causes of pleural infection and its emergence post–PCV-7 as the most common NVT isolate is believed to at least partially account for the alarming increase in empyema rates during the early 2000s. The incidence of empyema has now reduced to pre–PCV-7 levels, attributed predominantly to PCV-13 inclusion of this virulent serotype.[24]

Given the substantial benefits seen with the conjugate vaccine, consideration has been given to replacing PPV-23 with PCV-13 in adults. A randomized controlled trial of PCV-13 versus placebo was undertaken in the Netherlands.[25] The CAPITA trial demonstrated 75% vaccine efficacy against vaccine-type IPD and 45.6% efficacy in pneumococcal pneumonia, without any difference in all-cause pneumonia rates. Herd immunity from the administration of PCV-7 and PCV-10, from 2006 and 2010 onward could also not be out-ruled as a contributor to the effect. Whether replacing PPV-23 with PCV-13 in adults as a cost-effective strategy remains a contentious area, with different countries taking different views on the value of additional individual protection on top of the herd immunity from pediatric programs.

Current developments in the field of pneumococcal vaccination predominantly focus on increasing vaccine valency. A 15-valent vaccine incorporating serotypes 22F and 33F has been developed. These serotypes are believed have invasive potential and account for significant proportions of NVT-IPD.[26] Immunoglobulin responses to PCV-15 in a pediatric population were numerically lower for all serotypes compared with PCV-13 and did not meet noninferiority criteria in 3 of the 13 shared serotypes, similar to trends seen in PCV-13 compared with PCV-10 and for PCV-10 compared with PCV-7.[27] This raises concern that increasingly higher valency vaccines will lose efficacy. Novel vaccine targets including common pneumococcal antigens such as pneumolysin toxin (dPly) and histidine-triad protein D (PhtD), as well as methods of increasing their immunogenicity, are currently under investigation.

Antibiotic Resistance

Since the first reported resistant isolate in 1967, the emergence of resistant strains of pneumococci has been a growing concern. Risk factors for acquisition of resistance include previous antibiotic use; recent respiratory tract infection; time spent in day care, nursing homes, or long-term care facilities; extremes of age; and nosocomial infection.[28] Incidence rates for penicillin nonsusceptibility worldwide vary considerably from continent to continent, with rates of only 3.1% in the United States[29] to 79.7% in Korea.[30] Although serotype 19A, a frequently resistant pneumococcus, is no longer ubiquitous following widespread use of PCV-13, other serotypes prone to resistance have become more common. For example, serotype 35B, previously only found in nasopharyngeal carriage samples, has been increasing in incidence post–PCV-13 and has high rates of penicillin nonsusceptiblity.[13,31]

In addition to penicillin, resistance to macrolides, lincosamides, tetracyclines, co-trimoxazole, and fluoroquinolones has also been documented and is of growing concern.[3,12,28] Resistance to macrolides as high as 85% has been recorded in Hong Kong,[12] whereas rates in Canada are 25%[23] and in the United Kingdom are as low as 7%.[19]

Host Factors

Many of the factors that predispose to IPD also predispose to increased severity and higher case fatality rates. Older patients account for a substantial proportion of IPD incidence (27.3%) but a significantly higher proportion of deaths (48%) with a fatality rate of 31.7% in the older than 75 years age group.[32] Any chronic disease, including chronic obstructive pulmonary disease, smoking, diabetes, chronic heart failure, liver disease, and chronic kidney disease, results in higher rates of IPD.[33] Cases of IPD are twice as likely to have asthma as controls.[34] Preterm infants have significantly higher risk of IPD than those born at term, highlighting the need for timely vaccination in this cohort.[35]

Exposure to cigarette smoke, either by actively smoking or passive inhalation, has a dose-response relationship with the incidence of IPD, although risk can return to normal if the exposure is removed.[36] Opioid use is also associated with increased risk of IPD.[37]

Immunosuppression, whether due to medications, human immunodeficiency virus (HIV), or asplenia, is an important risk factor for IPD. In a population of 36 million people with private health cover in the United States, 17% had a risk factor for IPD, of whom 36% were classified as immunosuppressed (defined by presence of cancer, organ transplant, asplenia, HIV, or chronic kidney disease).[33] The incidence rate ratio for IPD in these high-risk individuals varied depending on their underlying condition, but reached 21.7 times for chronic kidney disease, followed by progressively lower rates in HIV, asplenia, cancer, and organ transplantation compared with healthy individuals. Patients who develop pneumococcal infection on a background of immunosuppression are less likely to present with pneumonia and more likely to have bacteremia without focus and septic shock, as well as being almost 3 times as likely to die as their nonimmunosuppressed counterparts.[38] In a prospective study assessing pediatric patients with IPD, predominantly with meningitis, screening for immunosuppression identified an abnormality in 16%, and a primary immunodeficiency in 10%.[39] Patients who have acquired immunodeficiency due to immunosuppressive medications have a suppressed response to pneumococcal vaccines and are potentially at higher risk of invasive disease.[40]

HIV is an important risk factor for development of IPD with rates of up to 100 times that of noninfected individuals in early studies.[41] Although rates of IPD have decreased significantly since the advent of highly active antiretroviral therapy, conjugate pneumococcal vaccination remains highly recommended in this cohort.

Viral infection commonly occurs in conjunction with pneumococcal infection. Temporal correlations between incidence of viral infection, both influenza and respiratory syncytial virus, and IPD are reproducible year after year.[42] There are likely a number of mechanisms by which viral infections increased the risk of IPD, including that viral neuraminidase upregulates the platelet activating factor receptor (PAFR; a major pneumococcal binding site) on human epithelial cells.[43]

Sickle cell disease can commonly cause functional asplenia resulting in high risk of infection with encapsulated bacteria. Children with sickle cell disease have a higher incidence of IPD and a higher mortality in association with the disease.[44] Despite a 53% reduction in incidence post-PCV7, the outcomes remain persistently worse than children without sickle cell disease, suggesting that the current vaccination program is suboptimal in this group.

Clinical Presentation

The most common presentation of IPD remains bacteremic pneumonia, which accounts for 40% to 80% of cases in most studies.[3,10,15] Meningitis and bacteremia without focus make up most of the remainder. Other rarer presentations include empyema, peritonitis, endocarditis, and septic arthritis.

Diagnosis

The gold standard for diagnosis of IPD is culture from an ordinarily sterile site, for example, CSF, blood or pleura, or peritoneal or synovial fluid. Administration of antibiotics before sampling can decrease the sensitivity of CSF culture by almost 50%, and similar effects can be expected for blood cultures. Since computer tomography scanning has become readily available, a tendency to perform neuroimaging before lumbar puncture has developed, although this is recommended only in cases of raised intracranial pressure.[45] Delays in antibiotic administration are known to be detrimental,[46,47] so treatment should be prioritized if investigations cannot be carried out immediately.

The pneumococcal antigen test is a rapid immunochromatographic assay that detects the presence of the C polysaccharide antigen, common to all types of S pneumoniae, in urine.[48] In patients with bacteremia, the test has demonstrated high sensitivity in invasive disease.[48] Molecular methods with high sensitivity and specificity are now widely available and a standard of care in most centers for CSF and respiratory samples. As live organisms are not required for a positive result, polymerase chain reaction testing remains positive for several days after antibiotic initiation.[49]

Treatment

Early initiation of appropriate antimicrobial therapy is critical in IPD.[46] Current diagnostic tests do not provide rapid antibiotic sensitivity, so empiric therapy remains the standard and should be based on local antibiotic sensitivity patterns and an assessment of risk factors for antibiotic nonsusceptibility.[28] The best evidence around treatment of pneumococcal disease not surprisingly comes from pneumonia, where evidence points to the best empiric therapy being the combination of 2 antipneumococcal antibiotics, in particular a beta-lactam (most often a third-generation cephalosporin) and a macrolide. This recommendation is based largely on a large number of observational studies showing a substantial mortality advantage of the combination of a macrolide.[50] Prospective, randomized controlled data are limited to 2 studies of all-pathogen community-acquired pneumonia, one unable to show that beta-lactam therapy was not inferior to combination therapy,[51] and a second study[52] in which 40% of the apparent monotherapy arm actually received combination therapy with a macrolide and enrolled very few patients with severe IPD where the benefit of combination therapy has mostly been demonstrated. Fluroquinolones are reasonable alternatives when there is significant beta-lactam allergy. In the setting of pneumococcal meningitis, there is some support for adding rifampicin in combination with a cephalosporin if the strain is highly likely to be beta-lactam resistant.[53]

Duration of antibiotic therapy is controversial, but a meta-analysis of 5 randomized trials showed no improved outcomes for therapy over 7 days.[54] In meningitis, the recommended duration of antibiotic therapy is typically longer, that is, 10 days if the patient has a beta-lactam–susceptible infection and 14 days if the bacteria is beta-lactam resistant.[53]

The preadministration (preferably) or coadministration of corticosteroids with antibiotics is now considered standard of care in pneumococcal meningitis.[55] This follows data demonstrating improved survival and improved neurologic outcomes in patients with meningitis,[56] although this benefit may be limited to pneumococcal disease[57] and was not seen in low socioeconomic areas.[53]

A more recent controversy is the routine use of corticosteroids in pneumonia, in which pneumococci are the most common pathogen. Multiple meta-analyses have suggested a benefit of steroids in severely ill patients; however, these are based on small, flawed studies.[58] In particular, the study that is the major driver of benefit in the meta-analyses has large differences in renal function at baseline favoring the active group,[59] and the only other study with a positive mortality advantage[60] has been repeatedly identified as a significant outlier with results (principally 0% mortality in patients with community-acquired pneumonia requiring intensive care) that have not been remotely replicated in similar studies. The best designed study, in patients with severe disease and a C-reactive protein greater than 150 μg/mL,[61] did not demonstrate a survival advantage or difference in organ failure. A composite endpoint, driven by less radiological progression of disease at 72 hours, was favorable to steroids, but what this means in the absence of any important clinical endpoint is unclear. Equally several studies highlighting significant risks of steroids,[62] especially in patients with influenza, cause real concern over the risk-benefit profile of steroids. Until a patient group with a clear benefit has been established, corticosteroids should not be used unless there is another clear indication due to comorbid diseases or the criteria for refractory shock is present as per the current Surviving Sepsis Guidelines.[63]

Outcomes

The case fatality rate for IPD has remained relatively static at approximately 20% to 25% overall, possibly due to the increasing prevalence of comorbidities and immunosuppression.[10,15] Penicillin resistance does not appear to affect survival, but there may be worse outcomes in patients with cephalosporin resistance.[64] Certain serotypes have been associated with increased mortality (including 3, 6B, 9N, 11A, 16F, 19F, 19A) but the implicated serotypes commonly differ between studies.

Cardiac events, including acute myocardial infarction, angina, congestive cardiac failure, and arrhythmia, frequently occur in association with pneumonia and contribute to mortality.[65,66] A study of all-cause pneumonia identified cardiac events in 22% of patients[65] and a major cardiac event complicated the initial hospital admission in 20% of cases of pneumococcal pneumonia, associated with a fourfold increased risk of death.[66] Most of these occurred during the hospitalization; however, a significant minority occurred between 20 and 90 days after the admission, highlighting that acute physiologic factors are not the only driver of cardiovascular pathology.

Animal studies have shown that the pneumococcus directly invades the myocardium via the same receptors as are used to translocate to the CSF (PAFR and laminin receptor).[67] Pneumococci invade the myocardium but remain extracellular and cause minimal inflammation, facilitating ongoing bacterial growth, release of pneumolysin, and myocyte death. These changes result in conduction abnormalities and abnormal contractility. Bactericidal antibiotics cause bacterial lysis and the resultant inflammation results in scar formation and remodeling, which may contribute to the later-onset cardiac events that can occur over the following months to years. Unfortunately, we currently do not know the optimal strategy to prevent cardiac events acutely or subsequently, with only one small randomized controlled trial of 1 month of 300 mg of aspirin showing apparent benefit.[68] Further studies in this area are desperately needed.

In patients with meningitis, neurologic sequalae are all too common and appear to be even more frequent with pneumococcus. These include hearing loss, cranial nerve palsies, hemiparesis and quadriparesis, and aphasia, occurring in more than 25% of patients.[69] Cognitive impairment affects 32% of patients with meningitis, again with worse outcomes in those with pneumococcal infection.[70]

INVASIVE MENINGOCOCCAL DISEASE
Epidemiology

The human nasopharynx remains the only known reservoir of *Neisseria meningitidis* and spread is via respiratory droplet transmission. IMD most commonly affects infants younger than 1 year, with a second peak in adolescence.[71] There are currently 13 serogroups in circulation, determined by distinct capsular polysaccharides (A, B, C, W135, X, Y, D, H, I, K, L, Z, and 29E), although only the first 6 of these are typically pathogenic. The polysaccharide capsule is encoded by a single locus and horizontal exchange of serogroup-specific capsule biosynthesis genes can lead to serogroup switch between clonal complexes, most likely during co-colonization of the nasopharynx.[72]

The distribution of serogroups varies worldwide. Serogroup A, once a common cause of disease in the United States, essentially disappeared from the developed world in the 1950s for unexplained reasons. Since that time, Meningococcus A has remained common in developing countries, particularly in the so-called "Meningitis Belt" of sub-Saharan Africa.

Serogroup B is more commonly identified in developed countries and, before introduction of conjugate vaccines covering non-B serogroups, accounted for a third of meningococcal disease.[73] Serogroup B typically affects younger children and has lower mortality rates but can cause prolonged epidemics, such as one lasting more than 14 years in New Zealand, leading to development of a strain-specific vaccine.[74]

Serogroup C meningococcus accounted for a stable proportion of endemic disease in developed countries with few outbreaks until the 1990s. It is, however, a pathogenic subtype and is rarely found in carriage specimens.[75] A hyperinvasive clone (ST-11) previously associated with serogroup B emerged in Canada in 1986 with a serogroup C polysaccharide capsule and spread worldwide over the following decade.

The previously rare serogroup W135 is an emerging threat and, carrying the clonal complex ST-11, was the cause of a significant European outbreak following a pilgrimage to the Hajj.[76] W135 meningococcal disease has been found to be associated with higher case fatality rates and remains an increasing threat in parts of Africa.[77]

Serogroup Y meningococcus is most commonly seen in the United States, but has become the second commonest cause of IMD in Europe with significantly increased incidence over the past 20 years.[71,78] Meningococcus Y tends to affect older people and infants younger than 6 months, and is more commonly associated with pneumonia.[78] Serogroup X has been rarely identified to date, but outbreaks in Africa have occurred.[79]

Carriage rates in the general population range from 5% to 20%.[73] Carriage is highest in young adults, probably due to behavioral changes in that age group with increased socializing and close contact[73] and in association with crowding.[80] The relationship between carriage and infection is unclear. The distribution of isolates differs significantly between the carried population and those that cause disease in industrialized countries; rates of carriage are not associated with rates of disease and therefore cannot be used to forecast epidemics.[75] Contrary to these findings, serial sampling of the nasopharynx of a population in Ghana, performed over 8 years, demonstrated 3 sequential waves of colonizing isolates matching those obtained from disease specimens.[79] The 3 strains responsible for all cases during the study period accounted for 71% of the colonizing strains. It appears, therefore, that the association between carriage and invasive disease varies geographically.

Vaccines

Early polysaccharide vaccines targeted serogroup C outbreaks in the military but were poorly immunogenic in infants. Quadrivalent polysaccharide vaccines covering serogroups A, C, W, and Y were developed, but similarities between serogroup B capsular polysaccharide and human glycoproteins limited the development of meningococcus B vaccines.

The dramatic increase in serogroup C IMD in the United Kingdom in the 1990s prompted development of the monovalent meningococcal C conjugate vaccine.[81] After introduction into the vaccination schedule for infants in 1999, there was a significant decrease in meningococcal C disease with vaccine efficacy of 97% in teenagers and 92% in toddlers and evidence of a herd immunity effect.[82] Immunization schedules in the United Kingdom and other countries now reflect evidence of improved efficacy in older children, administering 1 dose of MenC vaccine at 1 year followed by a quadrivalent conjugate vaccine (Men ACWY) at 14 years.

Three conjugate quadrivalent (ACWY) vaccines with similar efficacy have been developed (Menactra, Menveo, and Nimenrix). The difficulties developing a vaccine for serogroup B meningococcus were overcome by development of a strain-specific conjugate vaccine with an alternative target, the outer membrane vesicle (OMV). Subsequently, the 4CMenB vaccine was developed, containing 4 immunogenic components (3 proteins and OMV). This vaccine has proven to be immunogenic in infants and appears to reduce carriage of other serogroups also.[83] The 4CMenB vaccine has now been incorporated in vaccine schedules in many European countries.

In the developed world, rates of meningococcal disease overall have declined substantially in the past 20 years. In the United States, annual incidence of 0.12 per 100,000 is now the norm.[84] European surveillance data from 2016 revealed a rate of 0.6 per 100,000.[84] Disease secondary to serogroup C, in particular, has declined to record lows worldwide.[85]

Large-scale epidemics occurring in Africa in the 1990s stimulated development of a conjugate serogroup A monovalent vaccine (MenAfriVac) and, with the leadership of the Meningitis Vaccine Project, vaccination began in 2010. As of 2015, 235.6 million people have been vaccinated, with dramatic reductions in disease and carriage rates in sub-Saharan Africa.[86]

Antibiotic Resistance

Alarming reports of increasing rates of resistance to penicillin in some countries have resulted in a recommendation that cephalosporins be used first-line in suspected meningococcal disease and treatment rationalized when sensitivity testing has been performed.[87] Strains with reduced susceptibility, but not resistance, to cephalosporins also have been identified.[88] Rifampicin resistance remains rare, but fluoroquinolone resistance is increasing, with levels as high as 70% measured in parts of China.[89] Gonococcal resistance is far more common and concerns of horizontal transfer of mutated genes coding for penicillin-binding protein from *Neisseria gonorrhoeae* to *Neisseria meningitidis* have been raised.[90]

Host Factors

Overcrowding and increases in close contact are recognized risk factors for increased transmission of meningococcus, first documented in military barracks[91] and subsequently in universities and schools.[92] Furthermore, increased household density is recognized to increase rates of transmission.[93] The increased likelihood of IMD development when a new strain is encountered is highlighted by the higher incidence among freshmen in university dorms versus dormitory students further on in their university career and among children within 1 month of relocation or going on vacation.[92,94]

Close contacts (family members, those cohabitating, and kissing partners) are at highest risk of transmission of an invasive strain.[95] Recent outbreaks of meningococcal C disease among men who have sex with men (MSM) have caused concern in the United States, Europe, and Asia. HIV, when reported, was present in just over half, conferring a 10-fold increased risk but not fully explaining the 4.4-fold increase in development of IMD in MSM versus controls.[96] There is some evidence of urogenital colonization by pathogenic strains rarely found in nasal carriage, suggestive of sexual transmission.[90]

The most commonly recognized immune compromise predisposing to IMD is complement deficiency, which can confer a 10,000-fold increased risk of infection.[97] Treatment with eculizumab, a monoclonal antibody that inhibits complement activation, is associated with similar effects. HIV infection is associated with up to an 11-fold greater incidence of IMD.[98] Asplenia is frequently reported to be a risk factor for IMD and, given the risk of overwhelming sepsis in response to other encapsulated bacteria, this seems logical; however, evidence is limited and most studies of asplenic patients have found extremely low rates of IMD.[99] Vaccination is recommended for all of these groups in most guidelines but there are reports of vaccine failure in patients treated with eculizumab.

Exposure to cigarette smoke has been demonstrated to increase nasopharyngeal carriage of meningococcus.[100] Case-control studies have found that passive exposure is also associated with IMD, particularly in children.[93,94] Presence of comorbidities including cancer, chronic obstructive pulmonary disease, and heart disease are significantly associated with IMD in older adults,[93] and viral upper respiratory tract infection frequently precedes presentation with IMD.[94] The upper respiratory tract of patients with IMD is more frequently colonized with respiratory pathogens than controls, including influenza and mycoplasma.[80]

Clinical Presentation

Meningococcal disease most commonly presents as meningitis, meningococcal septicemia, or both. The presenting features depend on the age of the patients, as meningitis occurs more frequently in young people whereas adults present more commonly with sepsis alone. Pneumonia, septic arthritis, and osteomyelitis also can occur, but are much less frequent.[71,76,78] The presenting features may relate to the causative strain, for example, pneumonia is more common in serogroup Y cases[78]; however, both are more common in older patients and so this may be a spurious association.

Given the high morbidity and mortality associated with meningitis, early identification of the condition is paramount. Unfortunately, specific signs and symptoms are rare, and the classic triad of fever, neck stiffness, and altered mental status is seen in only 44% of cases.[69] At least 2 of headache, fever, neck stiffness, and altered mental status occurred in 95% of all cases of meningitis, and physicians should maintain a high index of suspicion in patients with these symptoms.[69] Typical presenting features of meningitis are less common in adults with meningococcal meningitis than pneumococcal meningitis (27% vs 58%).[69] Furthermore, focal neurologic deficits, seizures, and comatose presentations are seen more frequently with pneumococcal disease.[69] A petechial rash in the context of meningitis is more specific for meningococcus but is not pathognomonic, as almost 10% with a rash will have an alternative causative bacteria.

Meningococcal sepsis in adults may initially present with a flulike illness but can rapidly progress to fulminant sepsis with disseminated intravascular coagulation, purpura fulminans (development of painful, well-demarcated, purple cutaneous bullae, potentially involving muscle and bone), and septic shock. Similar to adults, children with meningococcal disease often have a preceding respiratory tract infection and present initially with nonspecific symptoms, such as fever and irritability. Infants may be noted to have poor feeding whereas children older than 5 are more likely to report a headache. These symptoms typically begin approximately 15 to 22 hours before admission to hospital. More specific signs of sepsis, including change in skin color, leg pain, and peripheral vasoconstriction, occur approximately 6 to 7 hours after symptom onset, meningitis-specific symptoms occur at 12 to 15 hours, and progression to decreased consciousness and seizures occurs at 15 to 24 hours.[101] Headache and nuchal stiffness are less common in meningococcal meningitis versus other pathogens, particularly in infants. The typical petechial rash is present in 42% to 70% of children and, as in adults, is not specific for meningococcal disease.

Diagnosis

As with IPD, although culture remains a gold standard, molecular tests are increasingly becoming essential for rapid diagnosis. This is particularly true when antibiotics have been given before culture, as culture of meningococci suffer from the same limitations as pneumococci in this setting. No urine test is available for IMD, but unlike IPD, it can be diagnosed by finding meningococci on skin scrapings of patients with a petechial rash.

Treatment

Although meningococci are much less likely to be resistant to penicillin than pneumococci, emerging nonsusceptible strains have resulted in a recommendation for empiric therapy with a third-generation cephalosporin until susceptibilities are known. Options for the initial intravenous treatment of meningococcal meningitis are presented in **Table 1**, noting that many of the alternatives to third-generation cephalosporins require careful monitoring of serum levels.

Table 1
Options for initial intravenous treatment of meningococcal meningitis

	Total Daily Dose	
Antibiotic	**Children >3 mo**	**Adults**
Penicillin G	4×10^6 units every 4 h	4×10^6 units every 4 h
Ceftriaxone	50 mg/kg every 12 h	2 g every 12 h
Cefotaxime	50 mg/kg every 6 h	2 g every 4–6 h
Cefepime	50 mg/kg every 8 h	2 g every 8–12 h
Ampicillin	75 mg/kg every 6 h	2–3 g every 4 h
Vancomycin	15 mg/kg every 6 h	15–20 mg/kg every 8–12 h
Rifampicin	6.7 mg/kg every 8 h	600 mg every 24 h
Meropenem	40 mg/kg every 8 h	2 g every 8 h
Chloramphenicol	25 mg/kg every 6 h	1 g every 6 h
Moxifloxacin	10 mg/kg every 24 h	400 mg every 24 h

As with pneumococcal disease, the duration of antimicrobial therapy is a source of controversy. As with IPD, there are no data supporting long durations over shorter ones.[54] Unlike pneumococcal meningitis, preantibiotic administration of corticosteroids has not been shown to be beneficial, but when the pathogen is not known, administration is recommended in the setting of meningitis, as there is no evidence of harm in meningococcal disease.

A major difference from IPD is that in IMD chemoprophylaxis of close contacts is highly recommended because of the epidemic nature of the disease, with studies showing a reduction in reducing secondary infection by 89%.[102] Therefore, identification of potential contacts is critical once meningococcal infection has been identified. Chemoprophylaxis is typically with rifampicin or ciprofloxacin, with ceftriaxone recommended in pregnancy or when significant contraindications to the other options are present.

Outcomes

Despite advances in medical management, case fatality rates in meningococcal disease remain between 5% and 15%.[71,78,103] Higher mortality rates are seen in meningococcemia (vs meningitis), older patients, and specific serogroups (W135). Adverse physical outcomes have been described in up to a quarter of patients, including neurologic deficits (5%–11%) and skin scarring and amputation (3.0%–7.6%).[103] Cognitive function and psychiatric sequelae are also common in all age groups.

SUMMARY

Despite dramatic advances in the prevention of pneumococcal and meningococcal disease worldwide, case fatality rates remain static and vaccination programs will struggle to keep up with the bacterium's ability to adapt and spread. Preventing further resistance by improving antimicrobial stewardship is essential. Future developments are focused on the development of universal vaccines and improved diagnostic tools rather than novel anti-infectives.

REFERENCES

1. Jain S, Self WH, Wunderink RG, et al. Community-acquired pneumonia requiring hospitalization among U.S. adults. N Engl J Med 2015;373(5):415–27.
2. Brueggemann AB, Griffiths DT, Meats E, et al. Clonal relationships between invasive and carriage *Streptococcus pneumoniae* and serotype- and clone-specific differences in invasive disease potential. J Infect Dis 2003;187(9): 1424–32.
3. Fenoll A, Ardanuy C, Linares J, et al. Serotypes and genotypes of *S. pneumoniae* isolates from adult invasive disease in Spain: a 5-year prospective surveillance after pediatric PCV13 licensure. The ODIN study. Vaccine 2018; 36(52):7993–8000.
4. Huang SS, Johnson KM, Ray GT, et al. Healthcare utilization and cost of pneumococcal disease in the United States. Vaccine 2011;29(18):3398–412.
5. World Health Organisation. Immunization, vaccines and biologicals 2013. Available at: https://www.who.int/immunization/monitoring_surveillance/burden/estimates/Pneumo_hib/en/. Accessed March 5, 2019.
6. Ho PL, Chiu SS, Chow FK, et al. Pediatric hospitalization for pneumococcal diseases preventable by 7-valent pneumococcal conjugate vaccine in Hong Kong. Vaccine 2007;25(39–40):6837–41.

7. Miller E, Andrews NJ, Waight PA, et al. Herd immunity and serotype replacement 4 years after seven-valent pneumococcal conjugate vaccination in England and Wales: an observational cohort study. Lancet Infect Dis 2011;11(10):760–8.

8. Roca A, Sigauque B, Quinto L, et al. Invasive pneumococcal disease in children <5 years of age in rural Mozambique. Trop Med Int Health 2006;11(9):1422–31.

9. Feikin DR, Kagucia EW, Loo JD, et al. Serotype-specific changes in invasive pneumococcal disease after pneumococcal conjugate vaccine introduction: a pooled analysis of multiple surveillance sites. PLoS Med 2013;10(9):e1001517.

10. Lexau CA, Lynfield R, Danila R, et al. Changing epidemiology of invasive pneumococcal disease among older adults in the era of pediatric pneumococcal conjugate vaccine. JAMA 2005;294(16):2043–51.

11. Lee GM, Kleinman K, Pelton S, et al. Immunization, antibiotic use, and pneumococcal colonization over a 15-year period. Pediatrics 2017;140(5).

12. Ho PL, Lam KF, Chow FK, et al. Serotype distribution and antimicrobial resistance patterns of nasopharyngeal and invasive Streptococcus pneumoniae isolates in Hong Kong children. Vaccine 2004;22(25–26):3334–9.

13. Sandgren A, Sjostrom K, Olsson-Liljequist B, et al. Effect of clonal and serotype-specific properties on the invasive capacity of Streptococcus pneumoniae. J Infect Dis 2004;189(5):785–96.

14. Falkenhorst G, Remschmidt C, Harder T, et al. Effectiveness of the 23-valent Pneumococcal Polysaccharide Vaccine (PPV23) against pneumococcal disease in the elderly: systematic review and meta-analysis. PLoS One 2017; 12(1):e0169368.

15. Shapiro ED, Berg AT, Austrian R, et al. The protective efficacy of polyvalent pneumococcal polysaccharide vaccine. N Engl J Med 1991;325(21):1453–60.

16. Richter SS, Heilmann KP, Dohrn CL, et al. Pneumococcal serotypes before and after introduction of conjugate vaccines, United States, 1999-2011(1.). Emerg Infect Dis 2013;19(7):1074–83.

17. Whitney CG, Farley MM, Hadler J, et al. Decline in invasive pneumococcal disease after the introduction of protein-polysaccharide conjugate vaccine. N Engl J Med 2003;348(18):1737–46.

18. Hsu HE, Shutt KA, Moore MR, et al. Effect of pneumococcal conjugate vaccine on pneumococcal meningitis. N Engl J Med 2009;360(3):244–56.

19. Waight PA, Andrews NJ, Ladhani NJ, et al. Effect of the 13-valent pneumococcal conjugate vaccine on invasive pneumococcal disease in England and Wales 4 years after its introduction: an observational cohort study. Lancet Infect Dis 2015;15(6):629.

20. Weinberger R, von Kries R, van der Linden M, et al. Invasive pneumococcal disease in children under 16 years of age: incomplete rebound in incidence after the maximum effect of PCV13 in 2012/13 in Germany. Vaccine 2018;36(4): 572–7.

21. Andrews NJ, Waight PA, Burbidge P, et al. Serotype-specific effectiveness and correlates of protection for the 13-valent pneumococcal conjugate vaccine: a postlicensure indirect cohort study. Lancet Infect Dis 2014;14(9):839–46.

22. Ladhani SN, Collins S, Djennad A, et al. Rapid increase in non-vaccine serotypes causing invasive pneumococcal disease in England and Wales, 2000-17: a prospective national observational cohort study. Lancet Infect Dis 2018; 18(4):441–51.

23. Demczuk WHB, Martin I, Desai S, et al. Serotype distribution of invasive Streptococcus pneumoniae in adults 65 years of age and over after the introduction

of childhood 13-valent pneumococcal conjugate vaccination programs in Canada, 2010-2016. Vaccine 2018;36(31):4701–7.

24. Wiese AD, Griffin MR, Zhu Y, et al. Changes in empyema among U.S. children in the pneumococcal conjugate vaccine era. Vaccine 2016;34(50):6243–9.

25. Bonten MJ, Huijts SM, Bolkenbaas M, et al. Polysaccharide conjugate vaccine against pneumococcal pneumonia in adults. N Engl J Med 2015;372(12): 1114–25.

26. Moore MR, Link-Gelles R, Schaffner W, et al. Effect of use of 13-valent pneumococcal conjugate vaccine in children on invasive pneumococcal disease in children and adults in the USA: analysis of multisite, population-based surveillance. Lancet Infect Dis 2015;15(3):301–9.

27. Greenberg D, Hoover PA, Vesikari T, et al. Safety and immunogenicity of 15-valent pneumococcal conjugate vaccine (PCV15) in healthy infants. Vaccine 2018; 36(45):6883–91.

28. Ruhe JJ, Myers L, Mushatt D, et al. High-level penicillin-nonsusceptible *Streptococcus pneumoniae* bacteremia: identification of a low-risk subgroup. Clin Infect Dis 2004;38(4):508–14.

29. CDC. ABCs Report: *Streptococcus pneumoniae* 2017. 2017. Available at: https://www.cdc.gov/abcs/reports-findings/survreports/spneu17.html. Accessed March 5, 2019.

30. Song JH, Lee NY, Ichiyama S, et al. Spread of drug-resistant *Streptococcus pneumoniae* in Asian countries: Asian Network for Surveillance of Resistant Pathogens (ANSORP) Study. Clin Infect Dis 1999;28(6):1206–11.

31. French N, Gordon SB, Mwalukomo T, et al. A trial of a 7-valent pneumococcal conjugate vaccine in HIV-infected adults. N Engl J Med 2010;362(9):812–22.

32. Marrie TJ, Tyrrell GJ, Majumdar SR, et al. Effect of age on the manifestations and outcomes of invasive pneumococcal disease in adults. Am J Med 2018;131(1): 100 e1–e7.

33. Zhang D, Petigara T, Yang X. Clinical and economic burden of pneumococcal disease in US adults aged 19-64 years with chronic or immunocompromising diseases: an observational database study. BMC Infect Dis 2018;18(1):436.

34. Talbot TR, Hartert TV, Mitchel E, et al. Asthma as a risk factor for invasive pneumococcal disease. N Engl J Med 2005;352(20):2082–90.

35. Riise OR, Laake I, Vestrheim D, et al. Preterm children have higher risk than full-term children of invasive pneumococcal disease during the first 2 years of life. Pediatr Infect Dis J 2018;37(7):e195–200.

36. Nuorti JP, Butler JC, Farley MM, et al. Cigarette smoking and invasive pneumococcal disease. Active Bacterial Core Surveillance Team. N Engl J Med 2000; 342(10):681–9.

37. Wiese AD, Griffin MR, Schaffner W, et al. Opioid analgesic use and risk for invasive pneumococcal diseases: a nested case-control study. Ann Intern Med 2018;168(6):396–404.

38. Sangil A, Xercavins M, Rodriguez-Carballeira M, et al. Impact of vaccination on invasive pneumococcal disease in adults with focus on the immunosuppressed. J Infect 2015;71(4):422–7.

39. Gaschignard J, Levy C, Chrabieh M, et al. Invasive pneumococcal disease in children can reveal a primary immunodeficiency. Clin Infect Dis 2014;59(2): 244–51.

40. van Aalst M, Langedijk AC, Spijker R, et al. The effect of immunosuppressive agents on immunogenicity of pneumococcal vaccination: a systematic review and meta-analysis. Vaccine 2018;36(39):5832–45.

41. Janoff EN, Breiman RF, Daley CL, et al. Pneumococcal disease during HIV infection. Epidemiologic, clinical, and immunologic perspectives. Ann Intern Med 1992;117(4):314–24.

42. Weinberger DM, Harboe ZB, Viboud C, et al. Pneumococcal disease seasonality: incidence, severity and the role of influenza activity. Eur Respir J 2014;43(3): 833–41.

43. McCullers JA, Bartmess KC. Role of neuraminidase in lethal synergism between influenza virus and Streptococcus pneumoniae. J Infect Dis 2003;187(6): 1000–9.

44. Payne DB, Sun A, Butler JC, et al. PspA family typing and PCR-based DNA fingerprinting with BOX A1R primer of pneumococci from the blood of patients in the USA with and without sickle cell disease. Epidemiol Infect 2005;133(1): 173–8.

45. Tunkel AR, Hartman BJ, Kaplan SL, et al. Practice guidelines for the management of bacterial meningitis. Clin Infect Dis 2004;39(9):1267–84.

46. Auburtin M, Wolff M, Charpentier J, et al. Detrimental role of delayed antibiotic administration and penicillin-nonsusceptible strains in adult intensive care unit patients with pneumococcal meningitis: the PNEUMOREA prospective multicenter study. Crit Care Med 2006;34(11):2758–65.

47. Bodilsen J, Dalager-Pedersen M, Schonheyder HC, et al. Time to antibiotic therapy and outcome in bacterial meningitis: a Danish population-based cohort study. BMC Infect Dis 2016;16:392.

48. Smith MD, Sheppard CL, Hogan A, et al. Diagnosis of *Streptococcus pneumoniae* infections in adults with bacteremia and community-acquired pneumonia: clinical comparison of pneumococcal PCR and urinary antigen detection. J Clin Microbiol 2009;47(4):1046–9.

49. Bryant PA, Li HY, Zaia A, et al. Prospective study of a real-time PCR that is highly sensitive, specific, and clinically useful for diagnosis of meningococcal disease in children. J Clin Microbiol 2004;42(7):2919–25.

50. Wunderink RG, Waterer G. Advances in the causes and management of community acquired pneumonia in adults. BMJ 2017;358:j2471.

51. Garin N, Genne D, Carballo S, et al. beta-Lactam monotherapy vs beta-lactam-macrolide combination treatment in moderately severe community-acquired pneumonia: a randomized noninferiority trial. JAMA Intern Med 2014;174(12): 1894–901.

52. Postma DF, van Werkhoven CH, van Elden LJ, et al. Antibiotic treatment strategies for community-acquired pneumonia in adults. N Engl J Med 2015;372(14): 1312–23.

53. McGill F, Heyderman RS, Michael BD, et al. The UK joint specialist societies guideline on the diagnosis and management of acute meningitis and meningococcal sepsis in immunocompetent adults. J Infect 2016;72(4):405–38.

54. Karageorgopoulos DE, Valkimadi PE, Kapaskelis A, et al. Short versus long duration of antibiotic therapy for bacterial meningitis: a meta-analysis of randomised controlled trials in children. Arch Dis Child 2009;94(8):607–14.

55. Brouwer MC, Heckenberg SG, de Gans J, et al. Nationwide implementation of adjunctive dexamethasone therapy for pneumococcal meningitis. Neurology 2010;75(17):1533–9.

56. de Gans J, van de Beek D, European Dexamethasone in Adulthood Bacterial Meningitis Study Investigators. Dexamethasone in adults with bacterial meningitis. N Engl J Med 2002;347(20):1549–56.

57. Brouwer MC, McIntyre P, Prasad K, et al. Corticosteroids for acute bacterial meningitis. Cochrane Database Syst Rev 2015;(9):CD004405.
58. Waterer G, Bennett L. Improving outcomes from community-acquired pneumonia. Curr Opin Pulm Med 2015;21(3):219–25.
59. Nafae R, Ragab M, Amany F, et al. Adjuvant role of corticosteroids in the treatment of community-acquired pneumonia. Egypt J Chest Dis Tuberc 2013;62: 439–45.
60. Confalonieri M, Urbino R, Potena A, et al. Hydrocortisone infusion for severe community-acquired pneumonia: a preliminary randomized study. Am J Respir Crit Care Med 2005;171(3):242–8.
61. Torres A, Sibila O, Ferrer M, et al. Effect of corticosteroids on treatment failure among hospitalized patients with severe community-acquired pneumonia and high inflammatory response: a randomized clinical trial. JAMA 2015;313(7): 677–86.
62. Waljee AK, Rogers MA, Lin P, et al. Short term use of oral corticosteroids and related harms among adults in the United States: population based cohort study. BMJ 2017;357:j1415.
63. Rhodes A, Evans LE, Alhazzani W, et al. Surviving sepsis campaign: international guidelines for management of sepsis and septic shock: 2016. Intensive Care Med 2017;43(3):304–77.
64. Hanada S, Iwata S, Kishi K, et al. Host factors and biomarkers associated with poor outcomes in adults with invasive pneumococcal disease. PLoS One 2016; 11(1):e0147877.
65. Perry TW, Pugh MJ, Waterer GW, et al. Incidence of cardiovascular events after hospital admission for pneumonia. Am J Med 2011;124(3):244–51.
66. Musher DM, Rueda AM, Kaka AS, et al. The association between pneumococcal pneumonia and acute cardiac events. Clin Infect Dis 2007;45(2):158–65.
67. Brown AO, Mann B, Gao G, et al. *Streptococcus pneumoniae* translocates into the myocardium and forms unique microlesions that disrupt cardiac function. PLoS Pathog 2014;10(9):e1004383.
68. Oz F, Gul S, Kaya MG, et al. Does aspirin use prevent acute coronary syndrome in patients with pneumonia: multicenter prospective randomized trial. Coron Artery Dis 2013;24(3):231–7.
69. van de Beek D, de Gans J, Spanjaard L, et al. Clinical features and prognostic factors in adults with bacterial meningitis. N Engl J Med 2004;351(18):1849–59.
70. Hoogman M, van de Beek D, Weisfelt M, et al. Cognitive outcome in adults after bacterial meningitis. J Neurol Neurosurg Psychiatry 2007;78(10):1092–6.
71. Cohn AC, MacNeil JR, Harrison LH, et al. Changes in *Neisseria meningitidis* disease epidemiology in the United States, 1998-2007: implications for prevention of meningococcal disease. Clin Infect Dis 2010;50(2):184–91.
72. Swartley JS, Marfin AA, Edupuganti S, et al. Capsule switching of *Neisseria meningitidis*. Proc Natl Acad Sci U S A 1997;94(1):271–6.
73. Caugant DA, Hoiby EA, Magnus P, et al. Asymptomatic carriage of *Neisseria meningitidis* in a randomly sampled population. J Clin Microbiol 1994;32(2): 323–30.
74. Oster P, Lennon D, O'Hallahan J, et al. MeNZB: a safe and highly immunogenic tailor-made vaccine against the New Zealand *Neisseria meningitidis* serogroup B disease epidemic strain. Vaccine 2005;23(17–18):2191–6.
75. Yazdankhah SP, Kriz P, Tzanakaki G, et al. Distribution of serogroups and genotypes among disease-associated and carried isolates of *Neisseria meningitidis*

from the Czech Republic, Greece, and Norway. J Clin Microbiol 2004;42(11): 5146–53.

76. Aguilera JF, Perrocheau A, Meffre C, et al. Outbreak of serogroup W135 meningococcal disease after the Hajj pilgrimage, Europe, 2000. Emerg Infect Dis 2002;8(8):761–7.

77. Mustapha MM, Marsh JW, Krauland MG, et al. Genomic epidemiology of hypervirulent serogroup W, ST-11 *Neisseria meningitidis*. EBioMedicine 2015;2(10): 1447–55.

78. Rosenstein NE, Perkins BA, Stephens DS, et al. The changing epidemiology of meningococcal disease in the United States, 1992-1996. J Infect Dis 1999; 180(6):1894–901.

79. Leimkugel J, Hodgson A, Forgor AA, et al. Clonal waves of *Neisseria* colonisation and disease in the African meningitis belt: eight- year longitudinal study in northern Ghana. PLoS Med 2007;4(3):e101.

80. Moore PS, Hierholzer J, DeWitt W, et al. Respiratory viruses and mycoplasma as cofactors for epidemic group A meningococcal meningitis. JAMA 1990;264(10): 1271–5.

81. Snape MD, Pollard AJ. Meningococcal polysaccharide-protein conjugate vaccines. Lancet Infect Dis 2005;5(1):21–30.

82. Ramsay ME, Andrews N, Kaczmarski EB, et al. Efficacy of meningococcal serogroup C conjugate vaccine in teenagers and toddlers in England. Lancet 2001;357(9251):195–6.

83. Gossger N, Snape MD, Yu LM, et al. Immunogenicity and tolerability of recombinant serogroup B meningococcal vaccine administered with or without routine infant vaccinations according to different immunization schedules: a randomized controlled trial. JAMA 2012;307(6):573–82.

84. Lagrou K, Peetermans WE, Jorissen M, et al. Subinhibitory concentrations of erythromycin reduce pneumococcal adherence to respiratory epithelial cells in vitro. J Antimicrob Chemother 2000;46(5):717–23.

85. Bijlsma MW, Bekker V, Brouwer MC, et al. Epidemiology of invasive meningococcal disease in the Netherlands, 1960-2012: an analysis of national surveillance data. Lancet Infect Dis 2014;14(9):805–12.

86. Daugla DM, Gami JP, Gamougam K, et al. Effect of a serogroup A meningococcal conjugate vaccine (PsA-TT) on serogroup A meningococcal meningitis and carriage in Chad: a community study [corrected]. Lancet 2014;383(9911):40–7.

87. Latorre C, Gene A, Juncosa T, et al. *Neisseria meningitidis*: evolution of penicillin resistance and phenotype in a children's hospital in Barcelona, Spain. Acta Paediatr 2000;89(6):661–5.

88. Deghmane AE, Hong E, Taha MK. Emergence of meningococci with reduced susceptibility to third-generation cephalosporins. J Antimicrob Chemother 2017;72(1):95–8.

89. Chen M, Guo Q, Wang Y, et al. Shifts in the antibiotic susceptibility, serogroups, and clonal complexes of *Neisseria meningitidis* in Shanghai, China: a time trend analysis of the Pre-Quinolone and Quinolone Eras. PLoS Med 2015;12(6): e1001838 [discussion: e].

90. Harrison OB, Cole K, Peters J, et al. Genomic analysis of urogenital and rectal *Neisseria meningitidis* isolates reveals encapsulated hyperinvasive meningococci and coincident multidrug-resistant gonococci. Sex Transm Infect 2017; 93(6):445–51.

91. Glover JA. Observations on the meningococcus carrier-rate in relation to density of population in sleeping quarters. J Hyg (Lond) 1918;17(4):367–79.

92. Bruce MG, Rosenstein NE, Capparella JM, et al. Risk factors for meningococcal disease in college students. JAMA 2001;286(6):688–93.
93. Fischer M, Hedberg K, Cardosi P, et al. Tobacco smoke as a risk factor for meningococcal disease. Pediatr Infect Dis J 1997;16(10):979–83.
94. Hadjichristodoulou C, Mpalaouras G, Vasilopoulou V, et al. A case-control study on the risk factors for meningococcal disease among children in Greece. PLoS One 2016;11(6):e0158524.
95. Kristiansen BE, Tveten Y, Jenkins A. Which contacts of patients with meningococcal disease carry the pathogenic strain of *Neisseria meningitidis*? A population based study. BMJ 1998;317(7159):621–5.
96. Folaranmi TA, Kretz CB, Kamiya H, et al. Increased risk for meningococcal disease among men who have sex with men in the United States, 2012-2015. Clin Infect Dis 2017;65(5):756–63.
97. Densen P. Complement deficiencies and meningococcal disease. Clin Exp Immunol 1991;86(Suppl 1):57–62.
98. Cohen C, Singh E, Wu HM, et al. Increased incidence of meningococcal disease in HIV-infected individuals associated with higher case-fatality ratios in South Africa. AIDS 2010;24(9):1351–60.
99. Arnott A, Jones P, Franklin LJ, et al. A registry for patients with asplenia/hyposplenism reduces the risk of infections with encapsulated organisms. Clin Infect Dis 2018;67(4):557–61.
100. Stuart JM, Cartwright KA, Robinson PM, et al. Effect of smoking on meningococcal carriage. Lancet 1989;2(8665):723–5.
101. Thompson MJ, Ninis N, Perera R, et al. Clinical recognition of meningococcal disease in children and adolescents. Lancet 2006;367(9508):397–403.
102. Purcell B, Samuelsson S, Hahne SJ, et al. Effectiveness of antibiotics in preventing meningococcal disease after a case: systematic review. BMJ 2004;328(7452):1339.
103. Cabellos C, Pelegrin I, Benavent E, et al. Invasive meningococcal disease: what we should know, before it comes back. Open Forum Infect Dis 2019;6(3):ofz059.

Opportunistic Infections in Transplant Patients

Rebecca Kumar, MD[a], Michael G. Ison, MD, MS[a,b],*

KEYWORDS

- Transplantation • Organ transplant • Infection • Cytomegalovirus • BK virus
- Polyoma virus • Nocardia • Toxoplasmosis

KEY POINTS

- Although opportunities infections can occur at any time, most occur between 1 and 12 months post-transplant.
- Monitoring of CMV immunity may be useful to guide duration of primary and secondary prophylaxis for CMV post-transplant.
- Routine screening for BK viremia is effective in reducing the incidence of BK virus nephropathy when linked with reduction of immunosuppression for viral loads $\geq$ 10,000 copies/mL.
- The new inactivated, adjuvanted zoster vaccine has been proven safe and immunogenic post-kidney transplant and should be considedred for all at risk transplant recipients.
- TMP-SMX remains the prophylactic agent of choice to prevent both Pneumocystis and Toxoplasmosis post-transplant.

INTRODUCTION

Since the first transplant was performed in 1954, transplants have become increasingly common with excellent patient and graft outcomes in large part owing to advances in surgical technique, immunosuppression, and antimicrobial prophylaxis. In 2017 alone, 34,770 solid organ transplants (SOT) were performed in the United States.[1] For patients who have undergone SOT, infection remains a common complication owing to the regimens required to prevent rejection. Opportunistic infections,

Disclosures: R. Kumar is supported through T32 AI095207 (NIH). M.G. Ison reports being a paid member of the DSMB for GlaxoSmithKlein and Shionogi; personal consulting fees from Celltrione, Genentech/Roche, Janssen, Seqirus, Shionogi, Viracor Eurofins, and VirBio; payments to Northwestern University by AiCuris, Chimerix, Emergent BioScience, Genentech/Roche, Gilead, Janssen, and Shire for research; and for having served as an nonpaid consultant for GlaxoSmithKlein, Romark, and Vertex.
^a Division of Infectious Diseases, Northwestern University Feinberg School of Medicine, Chicago, IL, USA; ^b Division of Organ Transplantation, Northwestern University Feinberg School of Medicine, Chicago, IL, USA
* Corresponding author. Division of Infectious Diseases, Northwestern University Feinberg School of Medicine, 645 North Michigan Avenue Suite 900, Chicago, IL 60611.
E-mail address: mgison@northwestern.edu

Infect Dis Clin N Am 33 (2019) 1143–1157
https://doi.org/10.1016/j.idc.2019.05.008
0891-5520/19/© 2019 Elsevier Inc. All rights reserved.

which are infections that are generally of lower virulence within a healthy host but cause more severe and frequent disease in immunosuppressed individuals, typically occur in the period 1 month to 1 year after transplantation.[2] This article focuses on opportunistic infections in the SOT recipient.

Risk for infection is influenced by a multitude of factors, including the epidemiologic exposures, the "net state of immunosuppression," use of infection prophylaxis and monitoring, and time of infection relative to the time of transplant.[2,3] Epidemiologic exposures can be obvious exposures (ie, recent vacation to coccidioidomycosis regions) or more obscure and remote (ie, military service in the jungles of Vietnam in the 1960s). An estimation of the net state of immunosuppression provides a way of risk stratifying for the development of opportunistic infections.[2] No single assay or score that adequately defines the net state of immunosuppression has been developed or validated. As a result, the clinician must assess all contributors to immunosuppression, including current and past immunosuppression, the presence of intentional and unintentional cytopenias, metabolic conditions (ie, malnutrition, diabetes, uremia), replicating viruses that produce immune evasion proteins as part of their replication (ie, cytomegalovirus [CMV], Epstein-Barr virus, and human immunodeficiency virus), and defects in mucocutaneous barriers. It is not only important to understand the duration and temporal sequence of immunosuppression, but also to understand the relative impact of the specific immunosuppression level (ie, higher or lower than expected exposure). Most transplant recipients receive antimicrobial prophylaxis against and/or laboratory monitoring for the presence of specific infections. These approaches generally decrease the incidence and delays the onset of the relevant opportunistic infections. As such, the use of such prevention strategies may alter the timing of relevant infections. For example, CMV may develop 1 to 3 months after transplantation without prophylaxis but will occur later (1–2 months after stopping prophylaxis) in patients who are given valganciclovir.

Perhaps the most important factor in predicting the risk of opportunistic infection is the time of presentation of illness relative to the transplant procedure. Classically, infections occur in 3 time periods.[2,3] In the first period, during the first month after transplantation, almost all of the infections are due to typical postoperative nosocomial infections; rarely, patients will develop recipient origin infections or donor-derived infections. During the period of peak immunosuppression, typically month 1 to 12 after transplantation, the majority of infections are classic opportunistic infections, including CMV, aspergillus, Nocardia, and toxoplasmosis. Use of prophylaxis will result in a later onset of opportunistic infections development.[4] Late infections, those occurring more than 1 year after transplantation, are typically community-acquired infections although opportunistic infections may rarely occur. These infections may be more prolonged and result in more complications than in otherwise healthy patients.

VIRAL OPPORTUNISTIC INFECTIONS
Cytomegalovirus

Despite advances in antiviral therapy for the prevention and treatment of CMV, this herpes virus remains one of the most common opportunistic infections complicating the course of organ transplant recipients. CMV is a highly prevalent infection with 60% to 80% of adults patients generally being latently infected. Most patients become infected in their teens and most initial infections are minimally symptomatic. Once infected, CMV remains latent in numerous cell types, including—but not limited to—macrophage, fibroblast, and endothelial cells.[5] A wide range of triggers may result in reactivation, which can occur in immunocompetent and immunocompromised patients, although it is far more common in transplant recipients.

Perhaps the most important factor in defining the risk of developing CMV after transplantation is the donor and recipient CMV serostatus. The greatest risk is associated with transplanting organs from CMV infected donors into uninfected recipients (CMV D+/R–). Seropositive recipients have an intermediate risk, with a slightly higher risk in seropositive donors relative to seronegative donors. The risk of developing CMV disease is lowest among seronegative donor and recipient pairs (D–/R–). Disease may still occur rarely in D–/R– patients, especially if they have received large numbers of blood products or are exposed to infected close contacts, such as children.[5,6]

An emerging way to further risk stratify the risk of developing CMV disease is through the assessment of CMV-specific immunity. Although a number of approaches have been studied, including interferon-gamma release assays (T-Spot.CMV [Oxford Immunotec, Marlborough, MA, USA] and QuantiFERON-CMV [Qiagen, Germantown, MD, USA]), immunohistochemical staining, major histocompatibility complex multimer staining, and the detection of polyfunctional CMV-specific responses, no one assay has been found superior to another. Data from a range of studies suggest that the detection of CMV-specific immunity is associated with a lower risk of infection when detected before transplantation, after transplantation, or after treatment for CMV. As a result, studies are ongoing to determine if routine use of these assays can guide decisions about the need for prophylaxis, viral load surveillance, or the need for secondary prophylaxis.[6] Two recent studies demonstrated the feasibility of such approaches.[7,8]

There are 3 commonly used strategies for prevention of CMV after transplantation: universal prophylaxis, preemptive therapy, and a combination of both known as surveillance after prophylaxis.[6] Universal prophylaxis involves giving patients who are at risk a fixed duration of antiviral therapy.[6] Preemptive therapy involves monitoring CMV levels in the blood at regular intervals, typically weekly, to detect early viral replication. If a threshold value is reached, antiviral treatment is started to prevent progression to disease.[6] Studies to determine the optimal treatment threshold are only beginning to be defined and depend on the transplant type, the risk of disease, and the induction and maintenance therapy used in the patient; as such, each center should define the optimal threshold appropriate for their populations.[6] Although current guidelines suggest that either approach is acceptable, there are differences between the 2 approaches. Prophylaxis is associated with rare instances of early CMV infection, is generally easy to implement, provides prophylaxis against herpes simplex virus and varicella zoster virus (VZV), and is associated with lower rates of graft rejection and organ loss while being associated with the rare development of resistance and higher direct costs of the medication, higher rates of late-onset CMV, and the side effects of therapy, including cytopenias. Preemptive therapy is associated with lower rates of late-onset CMV, less drug toxicity, high rates of rejection and graft loss, greater complexity ensuring compliance with testing, and the lack of prophylaxis against herpes simplex virus and VZV without adding additional therapies. Additionally, preemptive therapy is associated with the rare development of resistance as well.[6] Individual centers need to define the optimal approach based on priorities and resources available locally. Surveillance after prophylaxis is a hybrid of the 2 approaches, involving active surveillance with serum viral loads at specific time intervals after prophylaxis has been discontinued.[6] Although this approach is growing in popularity, the transition to preemptive monitoring typically starts when frequency of laboratory testing decreases and studies of such hybrid approaches have not clearly demonstrated significant clinical usefulness.[9–11]

Historically, high-dose valacyclovir and oral ganciclovir have been used for the prevention of CMV; most centers use oral valganciclovir. For patients who cannot take oral therapy, IV ganciclovir can be used. Valganciclovir is approved for prevention of CMV as 900 mg/d with recommendations for adjustment of dosing based on renal function. Nonetheless, cytopenias may be frequent and some centers have attempted to use a lower dose (450 mg once daily for patients with normal renal function). The use of lower dose valganciclovir has been demonstrated to be associated with an increased risk of breakthrough infection and the development of ganciclovir resistance.[12] The initial study comparing 3 months of oral ganciclovir with valganciclovir demonstrated that valganciclovir was associated with a lower risk of developing CMV while on therapy (2.9% vs 10.4% for oral ganciclovir). More than one-half of patients in both groups eventually developed CMV.[13] Further, valganciclovir was associated with a higher rate of tissue-invasive CMV disease in liver transplant recipients. To address the high rate of late-onset CMV, a study compared 100 days with 200 days of valganciclovir prophylaxis in high-risk (D+/R+) kidney transplant recipients. Two hundred days of valganciclovir prophylaxis was associated with a lower incidence of CMV (16.1% vs 36.8%) but a higher incidence of leukopenia (19% vs 4%).[14] Given the high incidence of CMV and the risk of developing CMV pneumonitis, extended prophylaxis has been demonstrated to be beneficial among lung transplant recipients. Twelve months or more of therapy for lung recipients is associated with lower rates of CMV disease (4 vs 32%) and infection (10% vs 64%) when compared with 3 months of prophylaxis.[15] Often extended therapy is limited by cytopenias and therapy may have to be discontinued early. As a result of these data, most experts recommend 3 months of prophylaxis for intermediate-risk transplant recipients (R+), 6 months of prophylaxis for high risk populations (D+/R–, patients who receive potent lymphocyte depletions, and recipients of intestinal transplants) and 12 or more months of prophylaxis for lung transplant recipients.[5,6] Although letermovir, a novel terminase inhibitor, is approved for prophylaxis in hematopoietic stem cell transplant recipients, studies of the efficacy in kidney transplant recipients are ongoing (NCT03443869) and this agent currently will generally not be used in SOT recipients until efficacy data are available.[16]

Clinical disease can present with asymptomatic viremia, CMV syndrome (fever, fatigue, myalgias, cytopenias, and viremia) and tissue-invasive disease. Beyond the indirect effects of ongoing viral replication, CMV can also cause other indirect effects, including activation of other herpes viruses, triggering graft dysfunction and rejection, and enhancement of the risk of developing opportunistic infections.[5,6] Detection begins with clinical suspicion. All patients with fever, neutropenia, and symptoms consistent with end-organ disease should prompt testing for CMV. Although viral culture and CMV antigenemia assays can be used, quantitative polymerase chain reaction is considered the gold standard for screening for CMV and monitoring response to therapy. Nonetheless, polymerase chain reaction has its limitations. Up to 15% of patients with CMV colitis may not have detectable CMV in blood samples and viral titers may not directly correlate with the extent of disease. Additionally, quantitative viral load results vary greatly by the sample tested (ie, whole blood vs serum), the specific assay, and whether the results are calibrated to an external standard. Before the availability of an external standard, interlaboratory results varied by up to 3 logs.[17] Standardization has decreased this variability and testing with the same standardized platform across laboratories reduces the interlaboratory variability to within 0.5 logs.[18] As such, serial monitoring is most reliable when using the same assay system, optimally in the same laboratory. Last, pathology may be critical for the diagnosis of end-organ disease. When biopsies are performed, the use of immunohistochemical staining increases sensitivity in detecting infection over standard hematoxylin and eosin staining.

For patients who develop CMV, antiviral therapy with ganciclovir, valganciclovir, cidofovir, and foscarnet can be used for the treatment of CMV. Most patients are treated with intravenous (IV) ganciclovir or oral valganciclovir. A randomized trial documented that oral valganciclovir can be used to treat most patients with CMV viremia, although IV ganciclovir is generally preferred for patients with severe CMV disease, CMV pneumonitis, and CMV colitis.[5,6] Treatment is typically continued until at least 1, and often 2, viral loads are below the limit of detection. Many centers then follow with a period of secondary prophylaxis, although emerging data question the routine use of such prophylaxis.[6] Resistance should be considered with clinical or virologic failure after 2 weeks of effective therapy. Resistance is generally documented with the use of genotypic resistance testing. The results of therapy and the urgency of patient illness can guide therapy. Standard therapies used include high-dose ganciclovir, foscarnet, and cidofovir. A number of experimental therapies and approaches are available using CMV Ig, adaptive infusion of CMV-specific T cells, leflunomide, artesunate, maribavir (NCT02931539) or letermovir (NCT03728426).[5,6]

BK Polyomavirus

BK polyomavirus remains latent in uroepithelium cells after initial infection, which typically occurs in early childhood. Although asymptomatic shedding can occur in immunocompetent patients, it is more common among transplant recipients. Clinical disease can include hemorrhagic cystitis and BK virus nephropathy.[19] Although BK virus nephropathy can occur very rarely in nonrenal transplant patients, it causes BK virus nephropathy in up to 15% of kidney transplant recipients in the absence of routine screening.[19] Fortunately, replication typically can be detected initially in the urine in 20% to 40% of patients after renal transplantation. In patients with persistent replication, 10% to 20% will develop viremia 2 to 4 months after initial detection of viruia. Those with persistent viremia may go on to develop BK virus nephropathy 1 to 3 months after the initial detection of viremia.[20] Risk factors for the development of BK virus nephropathy come from donor organ characteristics (ie, deceased donor, female gender, high BK polyomavirus antibody titers, HLA mismatches), recipient characteristics (ie, age, low or absent BK virus-specific antibody titers, male gender), and transplant-specific factors (ie, stent use and immunosuppression used for induction and maintenance).[19] Further, recent data suggest that donor viuria may be associated with an increased risk of developing.[21]

Because viuria and viremia predate the development of BK virus nephropathy in most patients, routine screening of renal transplant recipients coupled with modulation of immunosuppression has been shown to be cost effective and to decrease the risk of the development of BK virus nephropathy. Current guidelines recommend monthly screening for viremia until month 9 then screening every 3 months until 2 years with prolonged screening in pediatric transplant patients. Patients with persistent viremia of greater than 1000 copies/mL for 3 weeks or an increase to greater than 10,000 copies/mL should prompt a reduction of immunosuppression and more frequent monitoring. No prospective study has demonstrated the optimal approach to reduction of immunosuppression and current guidelines suggest a 50% decrease of 1 agent first, with further decreases in immunosuppression if viremia persists or progresses.[19] Patients with persistent viremia greater than 10,000 copies/mL are presumed to have BK virus nephropathy. Although biopsies can be performed, the infection can be patchy and negative biopsies do not exclude disease. At least 2 passes should be collected and the biopsies should be stained by polyoma-specific immunohistochemical stains. Likewise, the presence of lymphocytic infiltration may represent response to infection and not rejection. Other findings, such as C4D deposits, endarteritis, fibrinoid vascular necrosis, and glomerulitis, should be documented before diagnosing concurrent rejection.[19] Because of the possibility of concurrent rejection, patients with presumed BK virus nephropathy who have changes from baseline creatinine should undergo biopsy.

Patients with presumed or biopsy-proven BK virus nephropathy are generally managed with a decrease in immunosuppression. If this measure fails to improve viremia or there is progressive renal dysfunction, adjunctive agents, including cidofovir, leflunomide, or IgIV, may be given.[19] No studies have consistently shown 1 agent to be superior to another, and improvement is typically delayed after onset of therapy. Patients receiving treatment for BK virus nephropathy should have regular blood counts, BK viral loads, and renal function assessed every other week; patients given leflunomide should have liver function tests monitored at the same interval, and patients receiving low-dose cidofovir should also be screened for CMV because exposure to low-dose cidofovir may cause resistance. Historically, fluoroquinolones were considered options for treatment, but multiple randomized studies failed to document clinical efficacy.[22–24]

JC Polyomavirus

JC virus seroprevalence increases with age, but it is estimated about 50% to 90% of adults have exposure to the virus.[25] JC polyomavirus causes 2 types of disease in transplant patients: JC polyomavirus-associated nephropathy and progressive multifocal leukoencephalopathy. JC polyomavirus-associated nephropathy accounts for up to 10% of polyomavirus BK nephropathy in renal transplant patients and should be considered when there is biopsy-proven polyomavirus BK nephropathy, but negative BK viral loads in the blood and urine. Testing blood for JC virus will confirm the diagnosis and serve as a marker to monitor response to disease. The management of JC polyomavirus-associated nephropathy is identical to that for BK virus nephropathy.

Thankfully, progressive multifocal leukoencephalopathy is a rare complication in SOT recipients with an incidence of about 0.1%.[26] The development of progressive multifocal leukoencephalopathy typically occurs 1 year or later after transplantation.[2] It is made by a combination of clinical syndrome, demyelination on imaging, and JV in the cerebrospinal fluid (CSF).[2] The onset is typically subacute and neurologic deficits include altered mental status, motor deficits (hemiparesis or monoparesis), limb ataxia, gait ataxia, and visual symptoms such as hemianopia and diplopia. Seizures can occur, typically in just less than one-half of patients. Imaging demonstrates patchy or confluent white matter changes typically in the corpus callosum, brainstem, pyramidal tracts, and cerebellum. Detection of JC virus on CSF helps to confirm the diagnosis, but is only 72% to 92% sensitive. Patients without detectable JC virus may require brain biopsy to confirm diagnosis.[27] Progressive disease occurs in most patients, leading to death in most. Decreasing immunosuppression and consideration of experimental therapies, including brincidofovir, cytarabine, cidofovir, topotecan, mirtazapine, mefloquine, or adoptive T-cell therapy are possible treatment strategies.

Varicella Zoster Virus

Most adults listed for organ transplantation (98%–96%) are immune to VZV through either past primary infection or vaccination.[28] Because the Oka varicella vaccine is a live vaccine, all solid organ candidates should be screened before transplantation, regardless of vaccine history or prior infection. If found to be negative they should receive varicella vaccine at least 14 days before transplantation or starting immuno-suppressive therapy to prevent primary infection.[29]

The development of herpes zoster (HZ) is a challenging complication in transplant recipients. HZ typically occurs after 6 months after transplantation with most cases developing late. The incidence of HZ is approximately 8% to 11% after transplantation, significantly higher than immunocompetent patients.[30,31] Further, postherpetic neuralgia can be very debilitating.[2,30] Localized dermatomal HZ can generally be treated with oral valacyclovir or famciclovir; oral acyclovir is generally not recommended because of inadequate blood levels. Patients with progressive disease, multidermatomal disease, or disease involving the trigeminal ganglion or the geniculate ganglion should be treated with IV acyclovir. The addition of steroids is generally not done for transplant patients. Although the live-attenuated zoster vaccine (Zostavax) is not recommended in transplant recipients, the new inactivated adjuvanted zoster vaccine (Shingrix) can be given safely to transplant recipients.[32] A recently completed randomized study demonstrated significant boosting of humoral and cell-mediated immune responses in kidney transplant recipients. Although these patients will be studied over time to assess the impact of clinical disease, centers are beginning to recommend vaccination 6 to 12 months after transplantation.

Patients who have evidence of primary varicella should be admitted and treated with IV acyclovir because of the risk of severe and progressive disease. Most recommend adding IV immunoglobulin or varicella zoster immune globulin. Patients who are nonimmune to VZV should receive a varicella zoster immune globulin or IV immunoglobulin within 10 days of exposure. Adjunctive oral valacyclovir can be considered in patients presenting beyond 10 days after exposure or as an adjunct to immunoglobulin therapy. Most recommend using antivirals for 3 to 4 weeks.[30]

BACTERIAL OPPORTUNISTIC INFECTIONS
Nocardia

Nocardia infections typically affect somewhere between 0.7% and 3.5% of SOT recipients.[33] The most frequent site of infection is the lungs although disseminated disease, particularly central nervous system (CNS) involvement, is not uncommon. Nocardia infections occur in the setting of T-cell suppression, with infection occur most commonly in patients with transplant, human immunodeficiency virus infection (CD4 count of <100), and corticosteroid use.[33] Infection usually occurs within the initial 1- to 12-month period after transplantation.[2,33] As with any opportunistic infection, increases in immunosuppression increase the risk of infection.[33]

Although it is thought that trimethoprim-sulfamethoxazole (TMP-SMX) helps to prevent Nocardia, emerging data suggest that breakthrough infections do occur and breakthrough bacteria may retain susceptibility to TMP-SMX.[34,35] As such, the use of TMP-SMX prophylaxis should not remove nocardia from the differential diagnosis in patients presenting with nodular pneumonias, cutaneous lesions, or brain lesions. In addition, involvement of the eyes, kidney, bone, joints, and pericardium have been described.[33] Biopsy is often needed to diagnose the infection. Although full susceptibility testing should be sought, contemporary diagnostic strategies, such as sequencing, may give early species-level identification, which can help with the selection of empiric regimens. Typically, initial therapy includes combination therapies, including high-dose TMP-SMX and a second agent, including aminoglycosides, carbapenems, third-generation cephalosporins, minocycline, fluoroquinolones, or linezolid. Patients with severe disease or disease involving the CNS typically are started on intravenous therapy with TMP-SMX or a carbapenem plus amikacin. In such patients, when they have clinically improved and after at least 6 weeks of IV therapy, step down to susceptibility-directed oral therapy can be recommended. Generally, treatment is continued for at least 1 year.[33]

Listeria

Listeria is generally transmitted by food and is typically associated with deli meats; cases involving dairy-based ice cream have also been reported recently.[36] Typical infection involves fever and diarrhea; however, invasive listeriosis tends to occur most frequently in the elderly, immunosuppressed, and pregnant women. In the transplant population, infection frequently presents as meningitis or meningoencephalitis. When listeria is suspected, ampicillin or penicillin should be part of the empiric regimen with TMP-SMX as an alternative for penicillin allergic patients. Patients with proven listeria and CNS disease often will have aminoglycosides added for synergy. Although there are few data, TMP/SMX prophylaxis likely decreases the risk of developing of listeriosis.[37]

Tuberculosis

Tuberculosis (TB) occurs about 20 to 74 times more frequently in the transplant population when compared with the general population.[38,39] TB can develop as a result of reactivation of latent TB present in the recipient, transmission from the donor, or de novo acquisition, especially when traveling to endemic regions after transplantation.[38–42] Routine risk factors for TB are risk factors in transplant recipients, including residing, working, or volunteering in a homeless shelter, hospital, or correctional facility; close contact with someone with TB; or prolonged travel or residence in an endemic region. The best approach to decrease the risk of posttransplant TB is to screen candidates using either tuberculin skin testing or one of the interferon-gamma release assays. Although guidelines suggest screening patients with epidemiologic risk for latent TB or those who have radiologic evidence of asymptomatic TB, many centers routinely screen all candidates. Tuberculin skin testing requires returning to the transplant center for reading and can have false-positive results from other mycobacteria or prior BCG vaccination. Interferon-gamma release assays have the advantage of being a laboratory test that can be easily drawn and requires no additional follow-up with the patient. The assay has a positive control tube to help screen for anergy and uses peptides that minimize false-positive results owing to other mycobacteria and prior BCG vaccination. Repeat screening while on the waitlist is generally not needed absent new exposures. Those who have a positive TB screening test or who have a known TB exposure, irrespective of testing results, are generally treated for latent TB. Although a number of regimens are available, isoniazid 300 mg plus vitamin B_6 daily for 9 months is often used because it avoids agents with significant drug interactions with immunosuppression and therefore may be continued after transplantation if the transplant occurs before therapy is completed.[39] Despite the concern for the risk of adverse effects, even pre-liver transplant patients generally can tolerate this regimen, although close monitoring of liver function testing is needed.[43] Alternatively, patients can use 4 months of rifampin 600 mg daily or weekly directly observed isoniazid-rifapentine for 12 weeks; these approaches require the patient remaining on clinical hold until after therapy is completed because of drug interaction issues that limit their use after transplantation.[39,44]

Clinicians should have a high index of suspicion for TB in patients with relevant exposures and new pulmonary findings, particularly cavitary disease. Additionally fever of unknown origin and sepsis can be the presenting symptoms in patients, particularly with donor-derived TB.[40] The evaluation should include induced sputum and bronchoalveolar lavage (BAL) for patients with pulmonary disease and cultures of blood, local tissue and relevant fluids (ie, CSF) should be performed. In patients with proven or suspected TB, the initial treatment is similar to other nontransplant patients. Often rifabutin is used instead of rifampin to minimize drug interactions. Generally, 6 months of therapy is adequate for transplant patients with rapid response to treatment. Optimized regimens can be selected by based on resistance data from cultured isolates.[41]

FUNGAL OPPORTUNISTIC INFECTIONS
Pneumocystis jirovecii

Pneumocystis jirovecii causes pneumocystis pneumonia in immunosuppressed hosts. Before the use of prophylaxis, disease typically occurs 1 to 6 months after transplantation and affected around 10% of patients.[2,45] With the routine use of prophylaxis, pneumocystis pneumonia typically occurs late, months to years after prophylaxis has been discontinued.[46,47] Infection is a result of environmental exposure. Clinically patients present typically with a subacute onset of shortness of breath, cough, and fever. Patients often note worsening dyspnea with exertion. Frequently patients will seek the care of local doctors who will diagnose bronchitis or pneumonia and often will present antibiotics directed at community-acquired agents. When the patient does not improve, they will refer the patient to the transplant center, where the diagnosis is eventually made. Bilateral infiltrates may be present on chest radiographs, although computed tomography scans have a greater sensitivity at detecting changes.

The use of prophylaxis can prevent the development of infection. TMP-SMX is first line for prophylaxis, but if a patient is unable to tolerate this regimen, atovaquone or dapsone may be used. As noted, TMP-SMX can serve as prophylaxis for toxoplasmosis but it is unclear if alternative agents are as beneficial. Thus, if a patient is unable to tolerate TMP-SMX owing to nonhypersensitivity reactions, they should be rechallenged once the initial adverse reaction has resolved.[48] If TMP-SMX is absolutely contraindicated, then second-line agents that are appropriate include atovaquone and dapsone.

Endemic Mycosis

Endemic mycoses are fungal infections that are more prevalent in specific regions such as the Ohio and Mississippi River Valleys in the case of blastomycosis and histoplasmosis and the desert Southwest in the case of coccidioidomycosis.[49] Because cell-mediated immunity is critical for the control of these fungal infections, they are more common among transplant recipients and presentations may begin with indolent symptoms before disease progresses. The risk of disease is greatest in those with exposure, so careful assessment of both donor and recipient environmental exposure is important to discern.

Blastomycosis is caused by *Blastomyces dermatitidis*, which is most commonly present in the Ohio and Mississippi Rivers Valleys, upper Midwest, and US states and Canadian provinces that border the Great Lakes and the St. Lawrence Seaway. It is a relatively uncommon infection that most often presents later after transplantation. Most cases occur in the first 2 years after transplantation. There have been no documented cases of donor-derived blastomycosis infections.[50] Transmission is typically through the inhalation of fungal spores or direct cutaneous inoculation. Infection typically occurs within the lungs, and extrapulmonary symptoms (involvement of the genitourinary, central nervous, cutaneous, etc) occurs in 25% to 40% of these patients.[51] A definitive diagnosis is generally made through culture, although the detection of the polysaccharide cell well antigen in urine, serum, BAL fluid, or CSF is another possible route to diagnosis. Sensitivity of the antigen is 62% to 83% and cross-reaction can occur with other endemic mycoses. The preferred therapy for patients with proven or suspected infections depends on the severity and location of infections. Patients with mild, localized disease can be treated with itraconazole; other newer azoles, such as voriconazole, posaconazole, and isavuconazole, have been used in rare reports. For moderate to severe disease, disseminated disease, or disease involving the CNS, initial therapy with a lipid formulation of amphotericin followed by step down therapy with an azole is recommended; for CNS disease, step down therapy is typically voriconazole or fluconazole. Therapy is typically continued for about 12 months.[49]

Coccidioidomycosis, caused by *Coccidioides immitis* and *C posadasii*, is endemic to the southwestern United States, areas of Mexico adjacent to the US border, and parts of Central and South America. In endemic regions, the incidence can be as high as 1.4% to 6.9%, with most cases developing within the first year after transplantation.[49] Donor-derived infection is well-documented and typically presents early after transplantation with severe infections and mortality approaching 30%.[52] Inhalation is the primary mode of transmission, with pulmonary infections representing the most common site of infection; less than 1% have extrapulmonary infections. Culture is the gold standard for diagnosis, although polymerase chain reaction and antigen detection may speed diagnosis of the infection. Unlike other endemic infections, serology plays an important role in risk stratifying patients and identifying infections. Given the variability of the sensitivity of available enzyme immunoassays, immunodiffusion-based assays, and complement-fixing anticoccidioidal antibodies, sensitivity increases with the combination of assays for testing patients with potential disease.[49] Further, serologic testing of donors and recipients may identify patients at risk of donor-derived or reactivation disease; for screening, enzyme immunoassay is the preferred modality. Treatment with fluconazole remains the first choice for initial therapy for stable patients with acute or chronic pulmonary disease; amphotericin followed by fluconazole is recommended for patients with severe acute pulmonary or disseminated disease. High-dose fluconazole is recommended for meningeal disease.[49] The initial therapy for 6 to 12 months is generally followed by lifelong secondary prophylaxis. Patients living in endemic regions or with donors who are seropositive for coccidiomycosis should receive at least 6 to 12 months of fluconazole-based prophylaxis; some centers in endemic regions use targeted prophylaxis at those who have preexisting or new seropositivity.[53]

Histoplasmosis is caused by *Histoplasma capsulatum*, which is endemic to the river regions of the United States, Mexico, and Central and South America as well as other regions globally. Infections remain relatively infrequent (<1%) even in endemic regions and is typically a late complication. Most infections are from primary inhalation after transplantation, although rare donor-derived disease has been described.[49,54] The most common presentation in transplant recipients is a subacute infection that progresses to severe disseminated infections over 2 to 4 weeks.[49] Hepatosplenomegaly, pancytopenia, liver enzyme elevations, and mucocutaneous findings are common among patients with disseminated histoplasmosis. Diagnosis frequently relies on cultures from BAL or tissue biopsy, although growth may take weeks to occur. Urine, blood, BAL fluid, and CSF antigen detection allows for more rapid diagnosis and has a sensitivity of 70% to 92%. Molecular diagnostic and $(1–3)-\beta-D$-glucan assays can also be used.[49] Patients with mild to moderate disease can be treated with itraconazole; other newer azoles, such as voriconazole, posaconazole, and isavuconazole, have been used in rare reports. Patients with severe disease should be treated with a lipid formulation of amphotericin followed by step down therapy with an azole. Therapy is recommended for at least 1 year.[49] Immune reconstitution syndrome has been described in patients with disseminated histoplasmosis who have reduction of immunosuppression, which is still recommended to speed recovery from the illness. Patients who have active histoplasmosis within 2 years of transplantation or develop disease after transplantation may benefit from secondary itraconazole prophylaxis, although the optimal duration of secondary prophylaxis has not been defined.[55]

Cryptococcus

Cryptococcus neoformans and C gattii account for approximately 8% of invasive fungal infections in organ recipients, with an estimated incidence of 0.2% to 5.0%.[56] Cryptococcal infections typically occur 1 year or more after transplantation.[2] Most cases of cryptococcosis occurs as a result of reactivation, although primary inhalation can also cause disease. Donor-derived cryptococcosis has been described, especially from donors who are immunosuppressed, although some donors without clear risk factors have also resulted in transmission.[57] Presentation is often insidious with fevers, respiratory symptoms, headaches, and meningeal symptoms typically present. Most cases represent disseminated disease with CNS involvement. Diagnosis is generally established through the detection of serum or CSF cryptococcal antigen detection and cultures. Initial therapy with a lipid formulation of amphotericin B and 5-flucytosine is preferred with transition to fluconazole-based therapy after clinical and microbiologic response.[56] Secondary prophylaxis is typically continued for at least 1 year after the completion of therapy. Importantly, repeat lumbar puncture or placement of lumbar drains may be required to control elevated CSF pressure. Last, although a decrease in immunosuppression is a cornerstone for the management of cryptococcal disease in transplant recipients, immune reconstitution syndrome may occur and require enhanced immunosuppression to manage.[58]

Toxoplasmosis

Toxoplasmosis is caused by the parasite Toxoplasma gondii. Infection can lead to asymptomatic persistence of the protozoa in the cystic form, which can then reactive in the setting of immune suppression.[59] Infection typically occurs as a result of reactivation or as a donor-derived infection and is therefore more common among recipients of heart transplants; the highest risk is in seropositive donors into seronegative recipients.[59] De novo acquisition of infections from exposure to rare or undercooked meats in addition to feces of infected cats. The seroprevalence is low (11%) in the United States.

The use of TMP-SMX prophylaxis can decrease the risk of active disease after transplantation from 50% to 75% to 2%.[60] Although most recommend at least 1 year of prophylaxis in D+/R– transplants, the optimal duration of prophylaxis has not been well-studied. In sulfa-allergic patients, atovaquone is preferred, although there are limited data on the efficacy of this approach. Clinical disease includes fever, hepatosplenomegaly, lymphadenopathy, visual changes, and focal neurologic findings; arrhythmias and congestive heart failure can be present when toxoplasmosis myocarditis is present. Diagnosis typically relies on biopsy, although the availability of molecular diagnostics has improved the sensitivity of diagnosing toxoplasmosis. Treatment includes induction with pyrimethamine, sulfadiazine, and leucovorin for a minimum of 6 weeks followed by lifelong TMP-SMX suppression.[59]

SUMMARY

As surgical techniques and immunosuppression have advanced, the outcomes of transplants have improved over the past several decades. A key limiting factor for transplant recipients is the persistent threat of opportunistic infections. Thankfully, new approaches to prophylaxis and treatment have reduced the frequency and improved the outcomes of common posttransplant opportunistic infections.

REFERENCES

1. Organ procurement and transplantation network. Available at: https://optn.transplant.hrsa.gov/. Accessed October 22, 2018.
2. Fishman JA. Infection in organ transplantation. Am J Transplant 2017;17(4): 856–79.
3. Fishman JA, Rubin RH. Infection in organ-transplant recipients. N Engl J Med 1998;338(24):1741–51.
4. Helfrich M, Dorschner P, Thomas K, et al. A retrospective study to describe the epidemiology and outcomes of opportunistic infections after abdominal organ transplantation. Transpl Infect Dis 2017;19(3).
5. Razonable RR, Humar A. Cytomegalovirus in solid organ transplant recipients - guidelines of the American Society of Transplantation infectious disease community of practice. Clin Transplant 2019;e13512.
6. Kotton CN, Kumar D, Caliendo AM, et al. The third international consensus guidelines on the management of cytomegalovirus in solid-organ transplantation. Transplantation 2018;102(6):900–31.
7. Kumar D, Mian M, Singer L, et al. An interventional study using cell-mediated immunity to personalize therapy for cytomegalovirus infection after transplantation. Am J Transplant 2017;17(9):2468–73.
8. Westall GP, Cristiano Y, Levvey BJ, et al. A randomized study of quantiferon-CMV-directed versus fixed duration valganciclovir prophylaxis to reduce late CMV following lung transplantation. Transplantation 2019;103(5):1005–13.
9. Boillat Blanco N, Pascual M, Venetz JP, et al. Impact of a preemptive strategy after 3 months of valganciclovir cytomegalovirus prophylaxis in kidney transplant recipients. Transplantation 2011;91(2):251–5.
10. Lisboa LF, Preiksaitis JK, Humar A, et al. Clinical utility of molecular surveillance for cytomegalovirus after antiviral prophylaxis in high-risk solid organ transplant recipients. Transplantation 2011;92(9):1063–8.
11. van der Beek MT, Berger SP, Vossen AC, et al. Preemptive versus sequential prophylactic-preemptive treatment regimens for cytomegalovirus in renal transplantation: comparison of treatment failure and antiviral resistance. Transplantation 2010;89(3):320–6.
12. Stevens DR, Sawinski D, Blumberg E, et al. Increased risk of breakthrough infection among cytomegalovirus donor-positive/recipient-negative kidney transplant recipients receiving lower-dose valganciclovir prophylaxis. Transpl Infect Dis 2015;17(2):163–73.
13. Paya C, Humar A, Dominguez E, et al. Efficacy and safety of valganciclovir vs. Oral ganciclovir for prevention of cytomegalovirus disease in solid organ transplant recipients. Am J Transplant 2004;4(4):611–20.
14. Humar A, Lebranchu Y, Vincenti F, et al. The efficacy and safety of 200 days valganciclovir cytomegalovirus prophylaxis in high-risk kidney transplant recipients. Am J Transplant 2010;10(5):1228–37.

15. Palmer SM, Limaye AP, Banks M, et al. Extended valganciclovir prophylaxis to prevent cytomegalovirus after lung transplantation: a randomized, controlled trial. Ann Intern Med 2010;152(12):761–9.

16. Marty FM, Ljungman P, Chemaly RF, et al. Letermovir prophylaxis for cytomegalovirus in hematopoietic-cell transplantation. N Engl J Med 2017;377(25): 2433–44.

17. Pang XL, Fox JD, Fenton JM, et al. Interlaboratory comparison of cytomegalovirus viral load assays. Am J Transplant 2009;9(2):258–68.

18. Hirsch HH, Lautenschlager I, Pinsky BA, et al. An international multicenter performance analysis of cytomegalovirus load tests. Clin Infect Dis 2013;56(3):367–73.

19. Hirsch HH, Randhawa PS, AST Infectious Diseases Community of Practice. Bk polyomavirus in solid organ transplantation - guidelines from the American Society of Transplantation infectious diseases community of practice. Clin Transplant 2019;e13528.

20. Hirsch HH, Knowles W, Dickenmann M, et al. Prospective study of polyomavirus type bk replication and nephropathy in renal-transplant recipients. N Engl J Med 2002;347(7):488–96.

21. Grellier J, Hirsch HH, Mengelle C, et al. Impact of donor bk polyomavirus replication on recipient infections in living donor transplantation. Transpl Infect Dis 2018; 20(4):e12917.

22. Knoll GA, Humar A, Fergusson D, et al. Levofloxacin for bk virus prophylaxis following kidney transplantation: a randomized clinical trial. JAMA 2014; 312(20):2106–14.

23. Lee BT, Gabardi S, Grafals M, et al. Efficacy of levofloxacin in the treatment of bk viremia: a multicenter, double-blinded, randomized, placebo-controlled trial. Clin J Am Soc Nephrol 2014;9(3):583–9.

24. Patel SJ, Knight RJ, Kuten SA, et al. Ciprofloxacin for bk viremia prophylaxis in kidney transplant recipients: results of a prospective, double-blind, randomized, placebo-controlled trial. Am J Transplant 2019;19(6):1831–7.

25. Brew BJ, Davies NW, Cinque P, et al. Progressive multifocal leukoencephalopathy and other forms of JC virus disease. Nat Rev Neurol 2010;6(12):667–79.

26. Mateen FJ, Muralidharan R, Carone M, et al. Progressive multifocal leukoencephalopathy in transplant recipients. Ann Neurol 2011;70(2):305–22.

27. Cinque P, Scarpellini P, Vago L, et al. Diagnosis of central nervous system complications in HIV-infected patients: cerebrospinal fluid analysis by the polymerase chain reaction. AIDS 1997;11(1):1–17.

28. Zuckerman RA, Limaye AP. Varicella zoster virus (VZV) and herpes simplex virus (HSV) in solid organ transplant patients. Am J Transplant 2013;13(Suppl 3):55–66 [quiz 66].

29. Harpaz R, Ortega-Sanchez IR, Seward JF, Advisory Committee on Immunization Practices (ACIP) Centers for Disease Control and Prevention (CDC). Prevention of herpes zoster: recommendations of the advisory committee on immunization practices (ACIP). MMWR Recomm Rep 2008;57(RR-5):1–30 [quiz CE2-4].

30. Pergam SA, Limaye AP, AST Infectious Diseases Community of Practice. Varicella zoster virus in solid organ transplantation. Am J Transplant 2013;13(Suppl 4): 138–46.

31. Martin-Gandul C, Stampf S, Hequet D, et al. Preventive strategies against cytomegalovirus and incidence of alpha-herpesvirus infections in solid organ transplant recipients: a nationwide cohort study. Am J Transplant 2017;17(7):1813–22.

32. Vink P, Ramon Torrell JM, Sanchez Fructuoso A, et al. Immunogenicity and safety of the adjuvanted recombinant zoster vaccine in chronically immunosuppressed

adults following renal transplant: a phase III, randomized clinical trial. Clin Infect Dis 2019 [pii:ciz177].

33. Restrepo A, Clark NM, Infectious Diseases Community of Practice of the American Society of Transplantation. Nocardia infections in solid organ transplantation: guidelines from the infectious diseases community of practice of the American Society of Transplantation. Clin Transplant 2019;e13509.

34. Hemmersbach-Miller M, Stout JE, Woodworth MH, et al. Nocardia infections in the transplanted host. Transpl Infect Dis 2018;20(4):e12902.

35. Majeed A, Beatty N, Iftikhar A, et al. A 20-year experience with nocardiosis in solid organ transplant (sot) recipients in the southwestern united states: a single-center study. Transpl Infect Dis 2018;20(4):e12904.

36. Mazengia E, Kawakami V, Rietberg K, et al. Hospital-acquired listeriosis linked to a persistently contaminated milkshake machine. Epidemiol Infect 2017;145(5): 857–63.

37. van Veen KE, Brouwer MC, van der Ende A, et al. Bacterial meningitis in solid organ transplant recipients: a population-based prospective study. Transpl Infect Dis 2016;18(5):674–80.

38. Bumbacea D, Arend SM, Eyuboglu F, et al. The risk of tuberculosis in transplant candidates and recipients: a TBnet consensus statement. Eur Respir J 2012; 40(4):990–1013.

39. Subramanian AK, Theodoropoulos NM, Infectious Diseases Community of Practice of the American Society of T. Mycobacterium tuberculosis infections in solid organ transplantation: guidelines from the infectious diseases community of practice of the American Society of Transplantation. Clin Transplant 2019;e13513.

40. Morris MI, Daly JS, Blumberg E, et al. Diagnosis and management of tuberculosis in transplant donors: a donor-derived infections consensus conference report. Am J Transplant 2012;12(9):2288–300.

41. Santoro-Lopes G, Subramanian AK, Molina I, et al. Tuberculosis recommendations for solid organ transplant recipients and donors. Transplantation 2018; 102(2S Suppl 2):S60–5.

42. Kay A, Barry PM, Annambhotla P, et al. Solid organ transplant-transmitted tuberculosis linked to a community outbreak - California, 2015. MMWR Morb Mortal Wkly Rep 2017;66(30):801–5.

43. Theodoropoulos N, Lanternier F, Rassiwala J, et al. Use of the quantiferon-tb gold interferon-gamma release assay for screening transplant candidates: a single-center retrospective study. Transpl Infect Dis 2012;14(1):1–8.

44. Nwana N, Marks SM, Lan E, et al. Treatment of latent mycobacterium tuberculosis infection with 12 once weekly directly-observed doses of isoniazid and rifapentine among persons experiencing homelessness. PLoS One 2019;14(3): e0213524.

45. Faure E, Lionet A, Kipnis E, et al. Risk factors for pneumocystis pneumonia after the first 6 months following renal transplantation. Transpl Infect Dis 2017;19(5).

46. Neofytos D, Hirzel C, Boely E, et al. Pneumocystis jirovecii pneumonia in solid organ transplant recipients: a descriptive analysis for the swiss transplant cohort. Transpl Infect Dis 2018;20(6):e12984.

47. Martin SI, Fishman JA, AST Infectious Diseases Community of Practice. Pneumocystis pneumonia in solid organ transplantation. Am J Transplant 2013;13(Suppl 4):272–9.

48. McLaughlin MM, Galal A, Richardson CL, et al. Switch to atovaquone and subsequent re-challenge with trimethoprim-sulfamethoxazole for pneumocystis prophylaxis in a kidney transplant population. Transpl Infect Dis 2017;19(6).

49. Miller R, Assi M, AST Infectious Diseases Community of Practice. Endemic fungal infections in solid organ transplant recipients - guidelines from the American Society of Transplantation Infectious Diseases community of practice. Clin Transplant 2019;e13553.

50. Challener D, Abu Saleh O. Disseminated blastomycosis in a transplant patient. Transpl Infect Dis 2018;20(2):e12870.

51. Miller R, Assi M, AST Infectious Diseases Community of Practice. Endemic fungal infections in solid organ transplantation. Am J Transplant 2013;13(Suppl 4): 250–61.

52. Kusne S, Taranto S, Covington S, et al. Coccidioidomycosis transmission through organ transplantation: a report of the OPTN ad hoc disease transmission advisory committee. Am J Transplant 2016;16(12):3562–7.

53. Blair JE, Ampel NM, Hoover SE. Coccidioidomycosis in selected immunosuppressed hosts. Med Mycol 2019;57(Supplement_1):S56–63.

54. Singh N, Huprikar S, Burdette SD, et al. Donor-derived fungal infections in organ transplant recipients: guidelines of the American Society of Transplantation, infectious diseases community of practice. Am J Transplant 2012;12(9):2414–28.

55. Abdala E, Miller R, Pasqualotto AC, et al. Endemic fungal infection recommendations for solid-organ transplant recipients and donors. Transplantation 2018; 102(2S Suppl 2):S52–9.

56. Baddley JW, Forrest GN, AST Infectious Diseases Community of Practice. Cryptococcosis in solid organ transplantation- guidelines from the American Society of Transplantation Infectious Diseases community of practice. Clin Transplant 2019;e13543.

57. Camargo JF, Simkins J, Schain DC, et al. A cluster of donor-derived cryptococcus neoformans infection affecting lung, liver, and kidney transplant recipients: case report and review of literature. Transpl Infect Dis 2018;20(2):e12836.

58. Singh N, Lortholary O, Alexander BD, et al. An immune reconstitution syndrome-like illness associated with cryptococcus neoformans infection in organ transplant recipients. Clin Infect Dis 2005;40(12):1756–61.

59. La Hoz RM, Morris MI, Infectious Diseases Community of Practice of the American Society of Transplantation. Tissue and blood protozoa including toxoplasmosis, Chagas disease, leishmaniasis, babesia, acanthamoeba, balamuthia, & naegleria in solid organ transplant recipients - guidelines from the infectious diseases community of practice of the American Society of Transplantation. Clin Transplant 2019;e13546.

60. Baden LR, Katz JT, Franck L, et al. Successful toxoplasmosis prophylaxis after orthotopic cardiac transplantation with trimethoprim-sulfamethoxazole. Transplantation 2003;75(3):339–43.

UNITED STATES POSTAL SERVICE®

Statement of Ownership, Management, and Circulation
(All Periodicals Publications Except Requester Publications)

1. Publication Title	2. Publication Number	3. Filing Date
INFECTIOUS DISEASE CLINICS OF NORTH AMERICA	001 – 556	9/18/2019

4. Issue Frequency	5. Number of Issues Published Annually	6. Annual Subscription Price
MAR, JUN, SEP, DEC	4	$330.00

7. Complete Mailing Address of Known Office of Publication *(Not printer) (Street, city, county, state, and ZIP+4®)*

ELSEVIER INC.
230 Park Avenue, Suite 800
New York, NY 10169

Contact Person
STEPHEN R. BUSHING

Telephone *(Include area code)*
215-239-3688

8. Complete Mailing Address of Headquarters or General Business Office of Publisher *(Not printer)*

ELSEVIER INC.
230 Park Avenue, Suite 800
New York, NY 10169

9. Full Names and Complete Mailing Addresses of Publisher, Editor, and Managing Editor *(Do not leave blank)*

Publisher *(Name and complete mailing address)*

TAYLOR BALL, ELSEVIER INC.
1600 JOHN F KENNEDY BLVD. SUITE 1800
PHILADELPHIA, PA 19103-2899

Editor *(Name and complete mailing address)*

KERRY HOLLAND, ELSEVIER INC.
1600 JOHN F KENNEDY BLVD. SUITE 1800
PHILADELPHIA, PA 19103-2899

Managing Editor *(Name and complete mailing address)*

PATRICK MANLEY, ELSEVIER INC.
1600 JOHN F KENNEDY BLVD. SUITE 1800
PHILADELPHIA, PA 19103-2899

10. Owner *(Do not leave blank. If the publication is owned by a corporation, give the name and address of the corporation immediately followed by the names and addresses of all stockholders owning or holding 1 percent or more of the total amount of stock. If not owned by a corporation, give the names and addresses of the individual owners. If owned by a partnership or other unincorporated firm, give its name and address as well as those of each individual owner. If the publication is published by a nonprofit organization, give its name and address.)*

Full Name	Complete Mailing Address
WHOLLY OWNED SUBSIDIARY OF REED/ELSEVIER, US HOLDINGS	1600 JOHN F KENNEDY BLVD. SUITE 1800 PHILADELPHIA, PA 19103-2899

11. Known Bondholders, Mortgagees, and Other Security Holders Owning or Holding 1 Percent or More of Total Amount of Bonds, Mortgages, or Other Securities. If none, check box ▶ ☐ None

Full Name	Complete Mailing Address
N/A	

12. Tax Status *(For completion by nonprofit organizations authorized to mail at nonprofit rates) (Check one)*
The purpose, function, and nonprofit status of this organization and the exempt status for federal income tax purposes:
☒ Has Not Changed During Preceding 12 Months
☐ Has Changed During Preceding 12 Months *(Publisher must submit explanation of change with this statement)*

PS Form **3526**, July 2014 *(Page 1 of 4 (see instructions page 4))* PSN: 7530-01-000-9931 **PRIVACY NOTICE:** See our privacy policy on www.usps.com

---

13. Publication Title	14. Issue Date for Circulation Data Below
INFECTIOUS DISEASE CLINICS OF NORTH AMERICA	JUNE 2019

15. Extent and Nature of Circulation		Average No. Copies Each Issue During Preceding 12 Months	No. Copies of Single Issue Published Nearest to Filing Date
a. Total Number of Copies *(Net press run)*		235	238
b. Paid Circulation *(By Mail and Outside the Mail)*	(1) Mailed Outside-County Paid Subscriptions Stated on PS Form 3541 *(Include paid distribution above nominal rate, advertiser's proof copies, and exchange copies)*	135	158
	(2) Mailed In-County Paid Subscriptions Stated on PS Form 3541 *(Include paid distribution above nominal rate, advertiser's proof copies, and exchange copies)*	0	0
	(3) Paid Distribution Outside the Mails Including Sales Through Dealers and Carriers, Street Vendors, Counter Sales, and Other Paid Distribution Outside USPS®	44	51
	(4) Paid Distribution by Other Classes of Mail Through the USPS *(e.g., First-Class Mail®)*	0	0
c. Total Paid Distribution *(Sum of 15b (1), (2), (3), and (4))*	▶	179	209
d. Free or Nominal Rate Distribution *(By Mail and Outside the Mail)*	(1) Free or Nominal Rate Outside-County Copies included on PS Form 3541	44	15
	(2) Free or Nominal Rate In-County Copies included on PS Form 3541	0	0
	(3) Free or Nominal Rate Copies Mailed at Other Classes Through the USPS *(e.g., First-Class Mail)*	0	0
	(4) Free or Nominal Rate Distribution Outside the Mail *(Carriers or other means)*	44	15
e. Total Free or Nominal Rate Distribution *(Sum of 15d (1), (2), (3) and (4))*	▶	44	15
f. Total Distribution *(Sum of 15c and 15e)*	▶	223	224
g. Copies not Distributed *(See Instructions to Publishers #4 (page #3))*	▶	12	14
h. Total *(Sum of 15f and g)*	▶	235	238
i. Percent Paid *(15c divided by 15f times 100)*	▶	80.27%	93.3%

* If you are claiming electronic copies, go to line 16 on page 3. If you are not claiming electronic copies, skip to line 17 on page 3.

16. Electronic Copy Circulation		Average No. Copies Each Issue During Preceding 12 Months	No. Copies of Single Issue Published Nearest to Filing Date
a. Paid Electronic Copies	▶		
b. Total Paid Print Copies (Line 15c) + Paid Electronic Copies (Line 16a)	▶		
c. Total Print Distribution (Line 15f) + Paid Electronic Copies (Line 16a)	▶		
d. Percent Paid (Both Print & Electronic Copies) (16b divided by 16c × 100)	▶		

☒ I certify that 50% of all my distributed copies (electronic and print) are paid above a nominal price.

17. Publication of Statement of Ownership

☒ If the publication is a general publication, publication of this statement is required. Will be printed ☐ Publication not required.
in the **DECEMBER 2019** issue of this publication.

18. Signature and Title of Editor, Publisher, Business Manager, or Owner	Date
STEPHEN R. BUSHING - INVENTORY DISTRIBUTION CONTROL MANAGER *Stephen R. Bushing*	9/18/2019

I certify that all information furnished on this form is true and complete. I understand that anyone who furnishes false or misleading information on this form or who omits material or information requested on the form may be subject to criminal sanctions (including fines and imprisonment) and/or civil sanctions (including civil penalties).

PS Form **3526**, July 2014 *(Page 3 of 4)* **PRIVACY NOTICE:** See our privacy policy on www.usps.com

Printed and bound by CPI Group (UK) Ltd, Croydon, CR0 4YY

08/05/2025

01864747-0004